D0876879

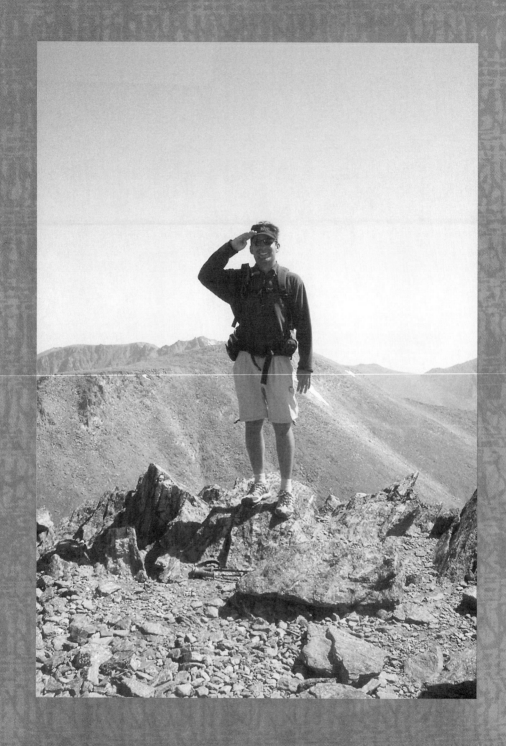

Best Summit Hikes
in Colorado

An opinionated guide to 50+
ascents of classic and little-known
peaks from 8,144 to 14,433 feet

James Dziezynski

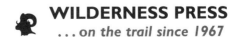

WILDERNESS PRESS
...on the trail since 1967

BERKELEY, CA

Best Summit Hikes in Colorado: An Opinionated Guide to 50+ Ascents of Classic and Little-Known Peaks from 8,144 to 14,433 Feet

1st EDITION August 2007
  3rd printing 2010

Front and back cover photos copyright © 2007 by James Dziezynski
Interior photos, except where noted, by James Dziezynski
Maps: James Dziezynski
Cover and book design: Lisa Pletka
Book editors: Glenda Lockhart and Eva Dienel

ISBN 978-0-89997-408-8

Manufactured in Canada

Published by: **Wilderness Press**
              1345 8th Street
              Berkeley, CA 94710
              (800) 443-7227; FAX (510) 558-1696
              info@wildernesspress.com
              www.wildernesspress.com

Visit our website for a complete listing of our books and for ordering information.
Distributed by Publishers Group West

Cover photos: *(front)* Top left: The trail to Uncompahgre Peak. Middle row (left to right):
                  Looking down from the summit of Mount Eolus; the start of the ridge to
                  Belleview Mountain at West Maroon Pass. Bottom row (left to right):
                  Approaching the summit of Red Cloud in the beautiful San Juans; sunset
                  at the Mount Sopris Trailhead.
                  (back) Ice Lakes Basin

Frontispiece: Mount Chapin's summit in Rocky Mountain National Park

SAFETY NOTICE: Although Wilderness Press and the author have made every attempt to
ensure that the information in this book is accurate at press time, they are not responsible
for any loss, damage, injury, or inconvenience that may occur to anyone while using this
book. You are responsible for your own safety and health while in the wilderness. The fact
that a trail is described in this book does not mean that it will be safe for you. Be aware that
trail conditions can change from day to day. Always check local conditions and know your
own limitations.

Acknowledgments

Extra special thanks go to the following people; without them this book would not exist: Jody Pratt, for her endless support and pure love of mountains; Nancy Coulter-Parker, for opening countless doors that allowed me to write about the outdoors; my parents, David and Lynne Dziezynski; Sheila Powell, for all her encouragement; and Kevin "The King" Bresler.

Special thanks: Paul Lenhart; Amy and Michael Karls; Nancy, Ronald, and Matt Pratt; John and Karyn Dziezynski and family; Tom and Kim Dziezynski and family; John, Megan, and Hazel Ragozzine; Christina Sheedy; Roslyn Bullas, Laura Keresty, and Eva Dienel at Wilderness Press; Paul and Mandy Bartok; David Besnette; Ryan Sheeler; Tom Goldpaugh; Ivette Romero; and Donald Anderson.

Also: James and Jeanette Baggett; Jennie and Arthur Dziezynski; Terry and Al Soucy; Kim and Brian Fitzgerald; Frankie and Alberta Baggett; Melissa and Ernie Siladji; Edith and Bill Sochon; Debbie Shupenis and family; Lorraine and Joe Lucian; Paul Retrum; Mike and Fred at Blank Gulch; Steve at Mount Huron; Marc Dziezynski; David T. Dziezynski; Celine and Jimmy Dziezynski; Kris Dziezynski; Bob Dziezynski; Joann Dziezynski; Janis and Adlai Shihab and family; the Powell family; Vicki Epley; Mike and Bev Kelley; Doug Schnitzspahn; Gina DeMillo; Karen Stedman; Pat Whittle; Sean Dougherty; Scott Neville; Lucas Tucker; Brian and Megan Hill; "CyricZ"; Althena Luna; Judith Saunders; Rose DeAngelis; Angelique Baffi; Maral Arslanian; "Aetherspoon"; Mark Zappone; Greg Miller; Jill Pananos; Chris Thompson; Amy Kukla; Christina Ward; "Chili" Dave; Andy Marker; Karina Manoim; Melissa Grossarth; Bruplex; Jon Copp; William Blair; Thóra Briem; Mike McCarthy; Mark Pfeil; Ben Fishelman; Melinda Kenneally; Cyrus Tata; Marie Willson; Eric B. Peterson; Sue Killoran; Big Dave Etzold; Rob Koosa; Lisa Aurigemma; Jon Copp; Ken and Judy Renner; Candice Blodgett; Marcus Woolf; Isaac Woods Stokes; Dina Stanziano; Michelle Theall and Karina Evertsen at *Women's Adventure;* John Linnell for State Songs (the soundtrack to this book!); Andy Blair and Laura Schmonses at NOLS; and my extra patient cat Xanadu!

For their support: Mindy Myers at Merrell, Michelle Wilkinson at National Geographic Maps, and the folks at Thales/Magellan GPS and Suunto. Finally, thanks to the immortal Albert Russell Ellingwood, my personal hero when it comes to climbing in Colorado.

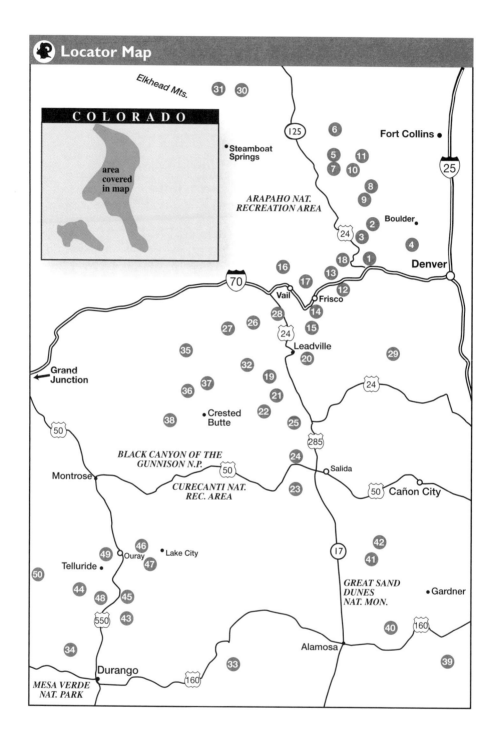

List of Peaks and Elevations

1 **James Peak** 13,294 ft.

2 **Navajo Peak** 13,409 ft.

3 **Jasper Peak** 12,923 ft.

4 **Guardians of the Flatirons: S. Boulder Peak** 8,549 ft + more

5 **Lead Mountain** 12,537 ft.

6 **Clark Peak** 12,951 ft.

7 **Mount Richthofen** 12,940 ft.

8 **Longs Peak** 14,255 ft.

9 **Mount Alice** 13,310 ft.

10 **Mount Ida** 12,880 ft. + more

11 **Mount Chapin** 12,454 ft. + more

12 **Mount Sniktau** 13,234 ft. + more

13 **The Citadel** 13,213 ft.

14 **Peak 1 – Tenmile Peak Traverse** 12,933 ft. + more

15 **Pacific Peak** 13,950 ft.

16 **Mount Powell** 13,534 ft.

17 **Deming Mountain** 12,902 ft.

18 **Vasquez Peak** 12,947 ft. + more

19 **Mount Elbert** 14,433 ft.

20 **Mount Sherman** 14,036 ft. + more

21 **Mount Hope** 13,933 ft.

22 **Huron Peak** 14,003 ft.

23 **Mount Ouray** 13,971 ft.

24 **Mount Shavano** 14,229 ft. + more

25 **Mount Yale** 14,196 ft.

26 **Fools Peak** 12,947 ft.

27 **Mount Thomas** 11,977 ft.

28 **Mount of the Holy Cross** 14,005 ft.

29 **Bison Peak** 12,431 ft.

30 **Mount Zirkel** 12,180 ft.

31 **Hahns Peak** 10,839 ft.

32 **Geissler Mountain** 13,301 ft. + more

33 **Summit Peak** 13,300 ft. + more

34 **Hesperus Mountain** 13,232 ft.

35 **Mount Sopris** 12,953 ft. + more

36 **Treasury Mountain** 13,462 ft.

37 **Belleview Mountain** 13,233 ft.

38 **East Beckwith Mountain** 12,432 ft. + more

39 **West Spanish Peak** 13,626 ft.

40 **Blanca Peak** 14,345 ft.

41 **Mount Adams** 13,931 ft.

42 **Eureka Mountain** 13,507 ft. + more

43 **Chicago Basin Trio: Windom Peak** 14,082 ft. + more

44 **Cross Mountain – Lizard Head Traverse** 12,935 ft. + more

45 **Storm King Peak** 13,752 ft.

46 **Uncompahgre Peak** 14,314 ft.

47 **Redcloud Peak** 14,034 ft + more

48 **Golden Horn** 13,769 ft.

49 **Mount Sneffels** 14,150 ft.

50 **Lone Cone** 12,613 ft.

Contents

The Hikes

Preface

Depending on whom you talk to, there are 52, 54, or 56 peaks that top 14,000 feet. Perhaps it is because of these show-stealing summits that I began to wonder how the peaks would measure up if we didn't consider elevation—indeed, if we threw out the tape measure and looked at other respectable mountain qualities like scrambling potential and dynamic routes. The more I scrutinized the "rules" that determined what was a 14er, the more I became convinced that a good summit is true no matter what the elevation. Four peaks in particular—Pacific Peak, Mount Hope, Mount Adams, and Mount Ouray—are incredible hikes, but without that tag of "14er," these four are often overlooked, despite being premier climbs. Heaven help the poor, humble peak less than 13,000 feet!

With that in mind, I began to write notes on what are truly the best Colorado summits in a number-blind world. After years of hiking and encouraging friends to check out the best peaks (known and unknown) in Colorado, I decided to write them down—thus the book you're holding in your hands. Most books group peaks either regionally or by elevation, but neither system ensures you'll get a collection of superb climbs. I decided that my book would be different.

The criteria for my selections were simple: great hikes that captured the different moods and motifs of Colorado's diverse mountains. As fun as it is to scratch off another 14er on the list, there's no denying the amazing allure of Bison Peak at 12,451 feet. Likewise, I was

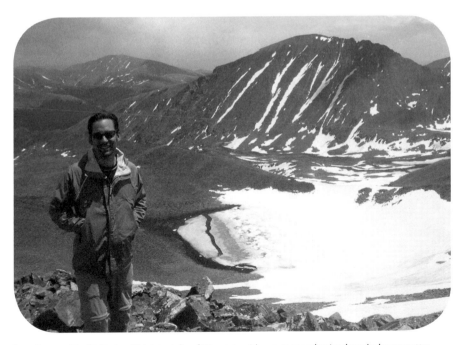

From the top of Pacific Peak, which is just shy of 14er status, it's easy to see why size doesn't always matter when it comes to deciding the best summits in Colorado.

not going to omit a great hike just because it is *over* 14,000 feet. A combination of natural beauty, intriguing human history, and adventurous paths make up the hikes in this book.

In the summer of 2006, I hiked every standard route in this book and many of the optional routes. I also climbed several peaks that just didn't make the cut; I couldn't in good faith call them the "best." Obviously, this is a subjective collection, but I'm confident that all of the peaks included in these pages represent the grand flavor of Colorado mountains: rugged beauty, hard-earned vistas, a glimpse into the secret society of plants and animals that call these peaks home, clean air, historical significance, and a chance to elevate our spirits both literally and physically.

Beyond the scope of this book there are still many more mountains to explore. In fact, I have purposely left out such wonderful peaks as Arrow and Vestal in the Grenadier Range. Both could have made the cut, but it's nice to have a few secrets in the world, don't you agree?

My hope is that you will get as much enjoyment and inspiration out of these peaks as I have. I hope they evoke beautiful emotions and help you forge lasting memories with friends. I hope they challenge you and bring you to new places, open new viewpoints, and occasionally give you a thrilling appreciation for the power of nature. Most of all, I hope you get out into the mountains and revel in the knowledge that you are back in the flow of elevated life, without the slightest doubt that what you're doing is the essence of truly living.

James Dziezynski
June 2007
Boulder, Colorado

Introduction

On a sunny Colorado afternoon long ago, a seemingly insignificant shellfish drifting in an ancient ocean peacefully passes from the world of the living. Rays of sunlight streaking through briny water illuminate the small creature as it gently settles into the muddy ooze of a silent, cretaceous sea floor. Chalky powder in the turbulent air above the waves blows out over the sea and coats the water with a slimy film. Eventually, the powder sinks to the bottom, effectively preserving our shellfish friend in the folds of history.

However, this is not the end of his story.

For ages thereafter, huge dinosaurs roam the continents, fly through the skies, and swim in the oceans, until their reign ends at the behest of some mysterious and unknown whim of fate. The great ocean that covers ancient Colorado then slowly recedes, creating lush rainforests. Violent volcanic eruptions initiate the creation of new mountains and wipe out old-world flora. Ultimately, these lava flows raise the mighty Sawatch Range to the sky. Across Colorado, enormous plates of land are driven upward, and the ocean ebbs.

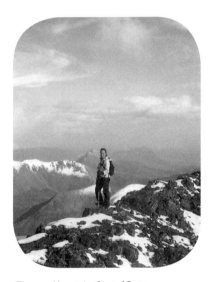

Treasury Mountain, Crested Butte

Fast-forward through the eons, and we find mammals making their way onto the scene. With their new hotshot brains, they begin to figure out a few of the more elementary secrets of the natural world. A select group of these critters gets rather smart; they slowly master the rudiments of survival and begin to probe into the world beyond hunting and gathering. Thanks to the major evolutionary coup of opposable thumbs and the ability to walk on two legs (thus freeing those thumbs up to do what they please), humans come onto the scene—roughly 65 million years after our little aquatic traveler settled in that prehistoric, fossilizing mud.

Eventually, one of these humans, a fellow called Plinius the Elder, gives our archaic shellfish a name: *Ammonis cornua*, translated: "Horns of Ammon." Ammon was an Egyptian deity who fancied a ram-horn headdress, which became his distinguishing feature. The name for the shellfish stuck and was later uploaded into the English lexicon as ammonite.

More time passed. Civilizations rose and fell. Poor Ammon was all but forgotten, despite his stylish headgear. Eventually, curious explorers from Spain found their way to those rocky mountains, dubbed the land "Colorado" (disregarding any naming rights of the folks who originally lived there), and sought refuge in the hills that touched the sky.

Perhaps the explorers believed that in those mountains they could harness something spiritual; after all, the gods of old were said to have perched upon the airy reaches of Mount Olympus. Maybe the "home of the gods" was all a metaphor; or maybe there really was something divine waiting on the tops of mountains. Still today, those lofty heights captivate us with a primal allure, appealing to our cravings to sense the world on high.

Those who dare reply to this invitation are ushered into a world of raw beauty, with each mountain a fickle host, as capable of unspeakable malice as of unimaginable beauty. For some of us, experiencing the mountains is an essential part of being alive, nearly equal to our need for fresh air, cool water, and warm sun.

Imagine a traveler sets off to climb a rarely visited ridge on a mountain once undersea. His mind teems with things important to him in his time. He is outfitted with apparel that would have been deemed miraculous a century before and that will likely be considered antiquated decades later. As he leaves the beaten path, his steps fall on rock that has seen the core of the earth, the bottom of the ocean, and now touches the parade of clouds floating through a blue September sky. Lowering his head to inhale the thin atmosphere, his eye catches a white anomaly in the otherwise tan and gray ground. He removes a glove to brush aside the dirt, and discovers what appears to be a drastically misplaced seashell. Picking up the primitive nautilus in his warm-blooded hand, he inspects his fortuitous find.

For the first time in 70 million years (give or take a day), our little ammonite friend again feels the warmth of the sun's rays. Troubles slip from the man's mind as he beholds history in his palm. He is connected with the past and with the spirit of the mountain. Thoughts are unfettered from language and time; his soul feels a primitive delight that cannot be put into words. This ephemeral moment eases something inside him; he feels at peace on the mountain. Resting the shell gently down in the dirt, he continues higher, his heart unburdened of many troubles.

The Colorado Rocky Mountains

Overview

Wind, water, fire, ice, and earth are the artists responsible for shaping Colorado's mountains. These elemental influences have made the landscape regions distinct both in character and contour. While all major mountains in Colorado are considered part of the broad North American Rocky Mountain Range (which runs from New Mexico to British Columbia), subranges within the chain have undergone varying degrees of elemental influence. As a result, these geological deviations give each mountain region a unique flavor.

For example, the glacially carved Sawatch Range is known for its gentle slopes and great elevations, greeting hikers like a kindly old grandfather. Crumbling marine shale gives mountains in the Maroon Bells-Snowmass Wilderness the essence of a great manor house in disrepair; it's a place where seemingly solid rocks embedded in the earth can pop out like rotten teeth. Pods of pristine peaks can be found in the sporadic outcrops and dramatic profiles of the Sangre De Cristo Range. Incredible sculptures of imposing granite define the remote Grenadier Range, daring you to enter their impressive kingdom.

There are many more subranges in Colorado, not to mention sub-subranges, such as the Spanish Peaks in the Sangre De Cristo Range of the Rocky Mountains. Geology is the primary factor in defining ranges, though categorization can be influenced by other whims. One example is the group of high Sawatch Mountains known as the Collegiate Peaks. These well-known mountains bear the names of prestigious eastern US universities, a far cry from the mellifluous names that had been bestowed upon them by native people. They differ little from surrounding Sawatch mountains, though it is interesting to note that they were initially grouped (before being named) according to mining boundaries.

However they are grouped on the map, as you spend more time in the mountains you will begin to unveil the "personalities" of individual peaks. Until one actually sets foot on the slopes, the objective data and raw facts serve merely to foster our curiosity. Experiencing the mountain with your own senses reveals the spirit of the peak. Each journey to the high country transforms that two-dimensional mark on the map into a vivid memory. And whether the mention of a mountain brings to mind warm memories, or recollections of chilling close calls, every step of the way will have been an adventure. Such are the adventures hikers yearn to live.

Geology and Biology: A Very Brief History

The definitive characteristic of the Rocky Mountains can be found right under your boots. Eons of change have put the "rock" into the Rocky Mountains. How these mountains were built is an intriguing tale. Fossils abound in compressed chronicles of stone, each representative of a past ecosystem. Dynamic transformations over the years have yielded a wealth of information and, conversely, have contributed to new scientific mysteries.

To summarize all the geological mayhem, Colorado's rock has been shaped by three primary forces: plate tectonics, volcanic eruptions, and glacial polishing. Starting at the bottom of the pile are the Precambrian foundations of igneous and metamorphic rock, formed some 600 million years ago when most of planet Earth was a volatile, volcanic work in progress. Very little is known about this period. To put it in perspective, scientists believe the most advanced form of life at the time was a multicelled piece of slimy bacteria. (Similar life-forms can be found today in the back of my refrigerator.)

Then, 300 million years ago, the land began to rise up as continental plates collided. This created enormous sand dunes and other soft formations that served as a holding place for the mountains to come. Much of the trademark flagstone adorning the buildings at the University of Colorado in Boulder was formed in this era. Around 250 million years ago, the gnawing power of erosion had whittled down this sandstone, making space for great lakes of silty water and nearly uninhabitable swamps. Rising temperatures made life demanding for primitive creatures. If that wasn't bad enough, an event known as the "Great Extermination," in which life was eradicated on a global scale, made survival for our prehistoric friends an incredible act of endurance. This period of unexplained catastrophe ushered out the old, slimy age, and introduced a new explosion of diverse life across the globe.

Between 250 and 100 million years ago, Colorado's climate transformed flat, muddy swamps into great tropical forests. Incredibly dense and lush, these forests were ideal homesteads for a variety of dinosaurs. The really big boys called Colorado home, including the biologically enigmatic sauropods such as Diplodocus, Apatosaurus, and Brontosaurus. These huge creatures had shockingly tiny brains, an anomaly that was offset by the fact that all they had to do was eat and grow bigger. Giant ferns grew in the verdant swamps, unchecked by dry weather or pollution. It was a great time for all. But, like all good things, it had to end.

Persistent erosion and changing temperatures began to have a profound effect on the landscape between 100 and 65 million years ago. Swampy basins lost their thickets of vegetation, resulting in marshy lakes that continued to expand onto flat tracts of land. All the hard work that plate tectonics had done to build up the land was nearly for naught. By the end of this era, most of Colorado was hundreds of feet underwater. This inland salty sea was host to incredible creatures, from gargantuan sea life to enormous flying reptiles. Seashells of ammonites and other critters from this period can be found today in several regions, notably the Elk and Gore ranges.

From about 60 to 38 million years ago, the mountains began to rebound. An uplift of plates elevated mountains to modest heights: 3,000 to 4,000 feet higher than the seas below. Water rose with the land, pooling in isolated lakes or disappearing completely. Fearsome predators such as the jawsome Tyrannosaurus Rex roamed the land. As a whole, the animals and plants of this era show a gradual downsizing trend. The great giants found food sources vanishing or else became snacks for smaller, more aggressive species. The times, they were a-changin', setting the stage for the huge alterations in the land. Scientists speculate that the famous "doom asteroid" struck Earth in this time period. (The asteroid theory is based on high levels of iridium found in rock/plant samples, suspected to be a direct result of a huge meteor slamming into Earth in the Yucatan Peninsula near the modern-day city of Cancun in Mexico.) This collision affected life-forms of all sizes and triggered volcanic flows throughout the region. The impact was felt on a global level, yet it was only the first act in a show that would take place over the next few million years. The greatest changes were just around the corner…

Colorado's defining era was about to begin. Roughly 37 million years ago, massive continental plates were thrust into motion. This movement slid the North American Plate westward over the steadfast Pacific Plate, unleashing torrents of volcanic lava and ash. Incredible pressure pushed the land higher and higher, transforming those unassuming 3,000-foot hills into crowns atop enormous peaks. For millions of years, the land was altered as heavy rains washed away volcanic ash. Geologists are a bit puzzled that the mountains formed in the region that is present-day Colorado. Normally, tectonic-based ranges rise a mere 20 to 600 miles from the oceanic coast. These mountains rose up thousands of miles inland, possibly indicating a distinctive geologic event, which has never been repeated.

Dinosaurs too big (or perhaps too dull in the skull) for the new land to support disappeared. Smaller, smarter, and faster was the order of the day. The last titans gave way to more adaptable creatures. Mammoths, camels, bison, lions, and other warm-blooded creatures flourished, replacing the reptiles who had ruled this domain for millions of years. This golden era introduced the reign of the giant mammals, a tenure that was to be very short lived. Of all the creatures in this ancient mammalian menagerie, only a select few would survive into the modern day.

About one million years ago, things began to calm down, and the Colorado we know today began to take shape. Rock that had lain for millions of years under seas was now sky high. The Colorado Plateau rose up from huge faults and rifts. Plate motions made mountains out of molehills; the Sangre De Cristo and Wet Mountains ranges in the east are direct results of this powerful subduction. Volcanic eruptions added to the artistry. One example: the striking, crumbling precipice of Lizards Head Peak just outside of Telluride is the durable throat of a long extinct volcano.

A mere 16,000 years ago, an ice age passed over the land. This was the last hurrah for the monster mammals, including the tusky mammoth. Only the hearty bison survived the advancing and receding glaciers, just to be hunted to near-extinction by white men in the 1800s. Glacial rivers smoothed and polished the land, carving deep cirques in the sides of mountains. In modern times, these glaciers are making their last stand as Colorado's mountains prepare for the next great geological event.

Poets would have us believe that mountains are static and permanent features, everlasting monuments that contrast with mankind's brief stint on earth. The less romantic truth is that mountains are constantly changing. Discrete modifications in height occur every few years, though it takes precision instruments to sense most changes. Events like the explosive eruption of Washington's Mount St. Helens in 1980 are business as usual for mountain ranges but have a long-lasting impact on humans when they occur in our lifetime. Mountains are no less subject than we are to the forces of nature, though they offer resilience that projects permanence.

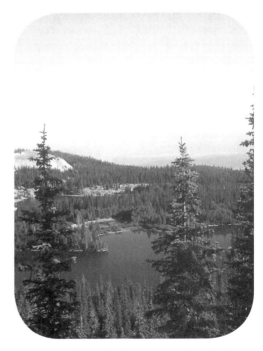

Colorado's dynamic landscape as viewed from the lower slopes of Mount Sopris

Laramide Orogeny

The Rocky Mountains owe their airy existence to a geological event known as the Laramide Orogeny. The word orogeny comes from the Greek language and means "mountain-building." In context, orogenies specifically describe mountains that have risen as a result of plate tectonics. To simplify what is an incredibly complex process, think of Earth's continents as floating plates akin to shards of broken ice on a pond. The "pond" that our continents float upon is called the lithosphere. When these shards collide, whole continents are shaped by the plates driving into one another until one finally yields and slides beneath the dominant shard—a process known as subduction. As the "defeated" plate drifts under the "victorious" plate, the land of the upper plate is pushed higher and higher, and the raw forms of mountains appear. After centuries of refinement at the behest of the elements, the mountains begin to take on the dramatic shapes we identify with our greatest peaks. The collision that formed Colorado's mountains is known as the Laramide Orogeny.

The Laramide Orogeny (named for the Laramie Mountains in eastern Wyoming) began roughly 80 million years ago, though the start of such a slow-acting phenomenon is difficult to pinpoint. The process continued for nearly 40 million years. As the North American continental plate slid westward, it eventually converged with the oceanic Pacific Plate, also know as the Farallon Plate. The North American Plate was the dominant of the two, and began to glide over the Pacific Plate, pushing it down.

Slowly, the Pacific Plate slid between the North American Plate and Earth's mantle—the last solid layer before the planet's molten core. Because of the relatively snug fit of these plates and the shallow angle of subduction, there was little volcanic activity. As the plates converged in fits and starts, the land grew increasingly higher from Alaska to Mexico.

Prototypes of the Rocky Mountains formed at this time. As the plates settled, cracks in the layers (called geologic faults) released high-pressure volcanic magma. These delayed eruptions occurred several million years after the start of the Laramide Orogeny. Major flows in the Sawatch and San Juan ranges contributed to the formation of mountains. Eventually, the plates locked into place and the magma was sealed below the earth, surfacing from time to time to heat a hot spring or to vent through fumaroles. The land stabilized over the centuries, making the Rocky Mountains a fixture on the continent, where they will continue to stand tall for generations to come.

Human History in the Colorado Rockies

After the Ice Age (roughly 11,000 years ago), the first human inhabitants took up residency in the Rockies. These primitive people endured harsh winters in pursuit of the great mammals that roamed in the valleys. Mammoths were coveted for the amount of meat they would yield and for their sturdy bones and ivory tusks, which could be shaped into tools. People migrated with the animals, leaving few permanent settlements in their wake.

Many of the tribes that formed over the years are familiar names: Apache, Arapahoe, Cheyenne, Crow, Shoshoni, Sioux, and Ute, to list a few. These people flourished as they mastered yearly patterns of migration. Autumn and winter were spent on the warmer, lower plains, while spring and summer were ideal times to hunt and forage in the mountains.

Undoubtedly lost in these annals of time are the first true ascents of the major mountains in Colorado. While most of these feats have gone undocumented, it is naïve to assume that the native people were any more exempt from the lure of the mountains than we are today. Alas, history is written from the perspective of the conqueror and not the conquered, and the mystery of who first set foot atop these peaks will remain unknown.

Amongst the first meddling Europeans to explore the Rockies was Francisco Vásquez de Coronado, the fabled ambassador of Spain who was, unfortunately, very good at his job. His journeys to the southern Rocky Mountains (mostly in New Mexico) in 1540 introduced native people to the ways of the white man. While there were a few beneficial results for the indigenous peoples from these encounters, such as the introduction of the horse and metalworking, the downside was a near eradication of the natives' culture, habitat, and spirituality.

The Spanish influence on the southern Rockies is evident today, with many peaks in the San Juan Mountains (itself an obviously Spanish moniker) named after Spanish explorers and missionaries. A select few mountains have reverted back to their native names in modern times.

A slow stream of Western European men began to infiltrate the Colorado region, mostly in search of fur and timber, and an uneasy alliance between the natives and newcomers was reached. In the late 1700s, as the nation of America came into being, people grew more curious in what lay in the uncharted lands to the west. The Scottish Canadian explorer Sir Alexander Mackenzie crossed the Rockies in 1793, on his way to the first transcontinental navigation of North America. He would later go on to discover the Arctic Ocean. The turbulent river that runs from Great Slave Lake, north to the Arctic, is named in his honor. Following in his footsteps, bold miners and fur traders set up the first European settlements in Colorado.

Shortly after Mackenzie's exploration, the fabled Lewis and Clark Expedition (1804–1806) set about making detailed descriptions of the land along the Missouri and Columbia rivers, which entailed crossing the Rocky Mountains. They encountered many of the native peoples on their journey, many of whom were peaceful, or at worst, ambivalent to the band of American

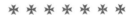

Lewis and Clark opened the door for many explorers: Kit Carson, Jim Bridger, Zebulon Pike, John Fremont, Jedediah Smith, and John Colter. These mountain men became larger than life for their exploits in the Wild West.

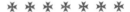

explorers. Lewis and Clark opened the door for many famous explorers, whose names are on our maps today: Kit Carson, Jim Bridger, Zebulon Pike, John Fremont, Jedediah Smith, and John Colter. These mountain men became larger than life for their exploits in the Wild West.

Miners doggedly combed the land for precious minerals in the Rocky Mountains region and finally hit gold in Colorado in1859. Gold deposits in the mineral-rich South Platte River region were the catalyst that led to an explosion in mining. "Pikes Peak or Bust" was the order of the day, as dreamy miners dug into the rocky earth in search of great wealth. William Green Russell, a native Georgian, was the first to establish a successful gold mine, just outside of the present-day city of Englewood. By the 1860s, Central City and Idaho Springs were major hubs of mining commerce, with cities on the plains such as Boulder, Golden, and Denver playing supporting roles.

Now that the land had tangible value, greed became a motivating factor in the extermination and relocation of the native people. Overpowered by the guns of the white man, the native tribes were hastily removed from the landscape as more and more settlers claimed legal ownership of the earth. Friction culminated in the disgraceful slaughter of peaceful Cheyenne and Arapahoe Indians in Kiowa County, a horrible event later known as the Sand Creek Massacre. On November 29, 1864 a cowardly group of Colorado militiamen mercilessly slaughtered an encampment of mostly elderly men, women, and children, killing over 200. This point marked the beginning of the end for the people who had called Colorado home for centuries.

As the gold mines in the high country began to sputter out, mining got a shot in the arm with the great silver discoveries outside of Leadville in 1879. More and more settlers stayed in Colorado after the lodes ran dry, moving to major cities and leaving ghost towns in their wake. The population grew as Colorado's agreeable climate, natural resources, and intrinsic beauty became widely known. Out-of-work miners turned to agriculture in the high country, and hundreds of ranches sprang up.

Colorado achieved statehood on August 1, 1876, becoming the 38th state of the United States. Since then, it has grown to become a major recreational and tourist destination. Mining experienced a modern boom during both world wars. Molybdenum, an element crucial in strengthening the armor plating on tanks and warships, became a major resource. The Climax Molybdenum Mine, on Fremont Pass outside of Leadville, continues to carry out operations to this day.

In modern times, skiing and other outdoors recreation have given new life to the high country. With our newfangled horseless carriages and high-tech Gore-Tex jackets, the backcountry has never been more accessible. The value of Colorado's wilderness in an era of development and industry is priceless; we must ensure future generations will enjoy the mountains as we do today by honoring and respecting the land.

Wildlife

High-elevation critters are a hearty bunch! Despite the harsh conditions experienced at altitude, animals of many sizes flourish, all the way up to 14,000 feet. Survival depends on clever adaptations to the environment. These creatures employ a great bag of tricks to endure year after year. Hibernation, torpor, seasonal fur camouflage, ingenious den designs, and unique physiological adaptations are amongst the strategies that are proven winners in the alpine kingdom.

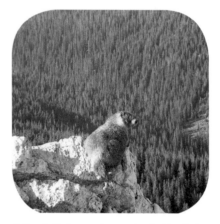

Yellow-bellied marmots are not as timid as their name implies.

Hikers and backpackers entering the backcountry need to respect local wildlife. Once on their turf, we need to play by their rules. They experience the world through a different set of sense organs, oftentimes superior to our own eyes, ears, and noses. And since neither man nor animal is looking for trouble, reducing the chances of a bad encounter is essential for both.

By now you should know, never feed the wildlife, no matter how cute or hungry they look. Feeding animals can make them reliant on hikers as a food source. At high-traffic areas such as Rocky Mountain National Park, the pudgy jaybirds and ground squirrels begging at popular trailheads prove many people disregard this rule. Wildlife must remain wild. An animal that retains the skills that have kept its kind alive for hundreds of years must not lose that proficiency by developing a craving for Cheetos.

Do not approach wild animals and never do anything that would frighten them. Animal behavior is unpredictable, and it is always best to give even the "friendly" animals their space. Slow-moving and less aggressive animals should not be stressed out by visitors trying to handle them. Take photographs from a safe distance.

To put it simply, be respectful, and acquiesce to them if you must. Life is hard enough in the high country; the last thing the animals that live there need is meddling humans to goof things up.

Mammal Roll Call

Furry friends are plentiful in the mountains. Largest of all are the impressive moose that live in pockets throughout marshy areas of the Rocky Mountains, notably in the Gore Range peaks outside of Vail. Moose are not native to Colorado. They were introduced in 1978 as a small group and have flourished, comprising about 600 animals today. With male bull moose averaging 1,100 pounds, they are not to be trifled with. Even the daintiest female moose can weigh 800 pounds when full grown. Moose are the largest members of the deer family (Cervidae), and their name comes from an Algonquin word meaning "twig-eater." These muscular mammals are relatively rare in Colorado, so consider yourself lucky if you spot one. (Note that bison, which can weigh up to 2,000 pounds, are not considered wild animals in Colorado. The only native populations that exist are on ranches, where they are raised for meat or hides.)

More commonly found are the moose's cousins, the elk. Elk originally roamed the plains east of the Rockies, but they have since adapted to conditions in lower high-altitude regions. Don't be surprised if you happen to see them higher on the mountain, as they will wander to the very tops of peaks when summer weather is agreeable. Elk are by nature herd animals, though young bucks are known to be a bit more adventurous and may leave the comfort of the group for short periods of time. Like moose, they are generally peaceful but can get aggressive during the rut (mating season). The famous bugle of elk during the mating season is a haunting call, a distinct tone that must be heard to be appreciated.

Deer round up the major members of the ungulate order (ungulates are the hoofed mammals). Mule deer make up the largest subfamily in the mountains. Although their role in life is primarily serving as prey for larger carnivores, mule deer are scrappy and rugged. While still herd animals, they often band in much smaller groups than elk, sometimes in families of only 4 to 6 members. I've encountered mule deer above 14,000 feet and even on the summits of some fairly rugged peaks (such as Mount Zirkel). Keep your eyes open, and you may spot them, too.

Black bears are perhaps the most feared of the mountain mammals and amongst the most misunderstood. Most are shy and will avoid confrontations with humans. Because they are omnivores, black bears are perfectly content to munch on berries and vegetation, hunting for meat only when they have to. Remember, however, they are still equipped with the finest in carnivore technology and are excellent swimmers and climbers. Unless you are Carl Lewis, you cannot outrun a black bear. Smaller black bears are often mistaken for large dogs, while larger black bears can easily be mistaken for bison. Some males can grow to weigh over 800 pounds and reach 6 feet tall, from ground to shoulder. With a healthy, glossy coat and a face that shows a relaxed dominance, it is easy to get captivated in the presence of such an incredible beast. Note that bear's fur changes with the seasons, fluctuating from near black to light brown. For information on bear encounters, read the section "What to Do if You Encounter a Black Bear," on page 15.

Grizzly bears (a.k.a. brown bear) are considered to be extinct in this area, but just to be safe, the Colorado Department of Natural Resources considers the grizz an endangered species. The last known grizzly was killed by hunters in the San Juan Mountains in 1979. There have been no confirmed sightings since, though reports come in every year of their existence. Wyoming does have confirmed grizzly populations however, and it is not far-fetched to think some of this group may wander into Colorado. Rumors persist of a small population in the Sawatch Range around Mount Elbert. While it may be easy for an inexperienced wildlife observer to confuse a grizzly and a black bear, they are quite different in both appearance and demeanor. Grizzly bears are brownish-yellow and are more muscular than black bears. Their enormous heads and muscular humps over the shoulders make them formidable and majestic animals. Grizzlies are more aggressive than black bears and are much more unpredictable. The good news in Colorado is that if there are any grizzlies in the state, they do well to stay out of sight.

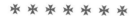

Large felines are nature's perfect predators; fast, stealthy, smart, and equipped to win any battle. You may have never seen a mountain lion, but I guarantee they've seen you! Nonetheless, most lions have no need to attack humans.

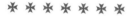

Mountain lions (a.k.a. cougar, puma, or panther) are the elusive kings of the mountain and the least predictable. Because they live as individuals, as opposed to in packs, their behavior can differ from cat to cat. Large felines are nature's perfect predators; fast, stealthy, smart, and equipped to win any battle. You may have never seen a mountain lion, but I guarantee they've seen you! Most lions have no need to attack humans and seem smart enough to avoid the trouble (not to mention expending the effort to attack a 200-pound human when that energy can be better used to take down a 400-pound elk). However, mountain lions have an instinct to pursue fast-moving creatures and several attacks on humans have occurred when people were running or biking. If presented with the opportunity of an easy kill, a hungry lion will stalk smaller people or children. Such tactics are generally thought to be acts of desperation by emaciated or older lions and are very rare, with the average being one attack per year over the past 120 years. The fact that lions have ample opportunity to attack oblivious hikers and normally choose not to indicates we are not their favorite targets. With their high intelligence and reliance on stealth, it may benefit both the mountain lion and the hiker that they stay in the shadows. For more information, read the section "What to Do if You Encounter a Mountain Lion," on page 14.

The lesser carnivores you may see include bobcats, badgers, coyotes, weasels, martens, red fox, and if you're extra lucky, the recently reintroduced lynx. There may be traces of of gray wolves in northern Colorado. Lynx were believed to be extinct in Colorado by 1973, but a successful reintroduction of 200 cats was initiated in 1999 in the San Juan Mountains. As of March 2006, this population seems to be doing well. Wolverines were extirpated in Colorado by the early 1900s, but rare sightings have been reported in the mountains.

Weasels often surprise people by hanging out on the summits of peaks. While they tend to inhabit lower-elevation regions, they may venture high to prey on unsuspecting rodents sheltered in high talus fields. Badgers are low-slung animals that resemble superskunks. I spotted one outside the town of Mancos, an impressive fellow sporting a fashionable gray and white coat. Coyotes are masters of adaptation and can live anywhere, from the slums of Los Angeles to the alpine boreal forests of Alaska. It is a special treat to hear the lonesome howl of the coyote echoing in the night—and to hear that howl answered by his fellows far away.

Mountain goats and Rocky Mountain bighorn sheep are often confused. Bighorn sheep are masters of the mountain, moving about steep cliffs with fearless ease. These nondomesticated cousins of farm sheep should not be called "rams," a term that denotes an uncastrated male sheep. Bighorn sheep are noted for their curled horns, which are used primarily in contests of strength between males during the mating season. By butting their heads with incredible force, they use the "Mike Tyson system" of wooing female mates—brute force. Bighorn sheep are the official state animal of Colorado and the mascot of Colorado State University.

Mountain goats are often snowy white (and keeping those coats clean is no easy task while cavorting on dirty mountaintops). Their name is a bit of a misnomer, as they are more closely related to antelopes than goats. Much like bighorn sheep, they are master rock climbers. On more than one occasion, I've seen lines of goats walk effortlessly across rock faces I would rate at least class 4 rock climbing (see section on class ratings on page 51). Adult mountain goats weighing 200 pounds can scale 60-degree slopes with ease. With their tufted beards and wise, expressive eyes, they are another species that can be gentle as a lamb or brazen as a bull. Be warned: an angry mountain goat can inflict some serious damage on an unassuming hiker, especially if said hiker is on a narrow ledge. Give them their space, and they will almost always peacefully pass on by.

Yellow-bellied marmots are amongst the most common critters in the mountains. These beaver-like rodents are charming and cute, but they do have a sinister side. Many have completely lost their fear of humans, boldly rummaging through backpacks or approaching hikers to beg for food. Many a tent has been gnawed through and many a food bag ripped asunder by marmots. Nighttime assaults on tents can be especially annoying, as the persistent pests not only threaten your food, they can rob you of precious sleep. Marmots are also quite curious about parked automobiles, and more than one has been known to chew clean through rubber hoses, lured by the sweet scent of brake fluid or antifreeze (both of which are obviously toxic). Marmots can be pesky at times, but the mountains wouldn't be the same without them.

Pikas are small, grayish, mouse-like animals with large ears. They can be seen popping in and out of rocky talus fields, industriously gathering straw and flowers for their dens. No doubt you have heard their trademark "rubber ducky" squeak at one time or another. Their soft gray fur is indicative of their relation to rabbits; they are of the same family. Amazingly, pikas do not hibernate in the winter. Instead, they rely on densely insulated burrows and large reserves of stored food to get them through the cold months. This incredible system makes them one of the elite animals that can actually endure winters above 14,000 feet. Biologists fear pikas may be headed toward extinction as development and pollution encroach on their environment.

Beavers are always hard at work in high-elevation ponds. Beavers that live in higher elevations develop thick and luxuriant coats, a trait that made them appealing to early fur trappers. Salt-loving porcupines are the second largest rodents in Colorado, behind beavers. River otters were believed extinct in Colorado by 1970, but efforts to reintroduce new populations have been successful, notably along the Dolores, South Platte, and Colorado rivers. These playful members of the weasel family are a delight to watch as they frolic on river banks, tumbling and swimming just for the fun of it. The unmistakable stench of the skunk indicates they too are out in the mountains. Mink and muskrat round out the smaller water-loving mammals. Like beavers and river otters, they are semiaquatic animals who live on the banks of rivers, ponds, and lakes.

Finally, how can we forget about the little guys? Uinta chipmunks are curious and bold, and too often their cuteness is rewarded with an ill-advised handout of pretzels or peanuts. They need to retain their foraging skills to get them through the winter, so please make a point of not sharing, even if they are agreeable to taking food from your hand. Golden-mantled ground squirrels are often mistaken for chipmunks, since they share the same habitats, color schemes, and personalities. An easy way to tell the two apart: chipmunks have stripes on their furry faces and squirrels do not. A variety of rabbits exist in Colorado. The mountain cottontail is the most common; as a result, these bunnies serve as a food source for coyotes, mountains lions, and other predators. Snowshoe hares are speedy animals whose coats change color with the seasons. The smallest of the mammals include field mice, pocket gophers, and shrews.

On the Wing: Major Birds of the Rocky Mountains

Bird-watching has gone mainstream in the past few years, proving that it's not only nerdy foreigners in giant Coke-bottle glasses who peep at the life in the sky (which is not to imply that I have ever subscribed to the stereotype that bird-watchers are necessarily nerdy, foreign, or visually impaired!). Birds in the Rocky Mountains are plentiful and come in a delightful array of colors. There are far too many to cover in this brief overview, but I'll note some of the most prevalent birds you'll encounter in the mountains. (Bird lovers should check out www.birding.com/wheretobird/Colorado.asp online or pick up a copy of *Birds of Colorado* by Stan Tekiela, published by Adventure Publications).

No other bird conveys majesty on the wing quite like the bald eagle. Bald eagles were nearly extinct in the lower US by the early 20th century, but they have made a great comeback, thanks to conservation efforts. (The only bald eagle born outside of North America was hatched in a zoo in Germany in May of 2006.) Today, a healthy population flourishes in Colorado. Females may have a wing span of 7 feet and are larger than their male counterparts. An interesting bit of eagle trivia: Native Americans are rumored to have set up eagle traps on the summit of Longs Peak, giving strength to the argument that John W. Powell wasn't the first person to stand atop that fabled 14er. Golden eagles are slightly smaller than bald eagles and have brownish-beige colorings. Incredibly agile in flight, these birds of prey mate for life and are one of the few threats to rodents living above 13,000 feet.

Peregrine falcons prefer cold mountain regions, migrating north to the Arctic, and south to the Rockies and other northern American mountain regions. Since they are seasonal visitors, your best chance to see peregrine falcons is during spring and early summer. They are unrivaled as the fastest animals on earth, capable of unleashing a freefall, diving attack that regularly exceeds 200 miles per hour! In this incredible display, called a stoop, the falcon folds its wings, extends the razor-sharp talons on its feet, and plummets at mind-bending speeds toward an unsuspecting bird below. The aim is to damage or completely sheer off a wing (a direct impact would injure both birds). When the disabled prey hits the ground, the falcon descends to finish off the job. If you are fortunate enough to witness a peregrine falcon stoop, the awesome image will remain in your mind for years to come.

Red-tailed hawks are smaller simulacrums of the golden hawk. Whenever you hear the telltale screech of a bird in movies or on TV, chances are you are hearing the distinct cry of the red-tailed hawk.

Ravens and crows can be found throughout Colorado. Both are large black birds with fancy ebony beaks. The two are difficult to differentiate. One major difference can be seen in their flying postures: crows tend to flap, flap, flap their wings, while ravens will flap a little and then soar through the air, similar to the way hawks fly.

Gray jays are friendly avian beggers with stylish gray and black markings. Jays relentlessly haunt campsites and picnic tables, looking for scraps of food. Mountain bluebirds are a striking electric blue color, painted the same hue as the clear mountain sky. As you make your way along mountain trails, several varieties of swallow may gleefully zip by you with an audible *thwipp*. Appropriately named redwinged blackbirds are distinguished by the bright red "arm band" on the shoulders of their black wings. Robins, owls, ducks, cranes, herons, and woodpeckers are also common in the mountains.

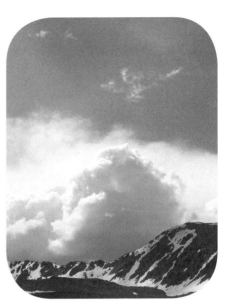

Storms roll into the Pacific Peak basin.

Ground-patrolling birds are abundant. White-tailed ptarmigans are extremely likable, peaceful fellows. They amble about on the tundra, only mildly concerned when hikers approach. "Mumbling" ptarmigans often have broods of adorable chicks in tow. Ptarmigans are masters of camouflage, with brownish, speckled, ground-imitating feathers in the summer and pure snow-white plumage in the winter. On one occasion, I came across pockets of nearly invisible white ptarmigans huddled against the cold in a January subzero whiteout. Their hearty, stoic, stick-it-out approach to winter earns my respect. The more fidgety pheasant is equally good at camouflage but has a bad habit of abandoning its guise when hikers come too near. The loud and frantic flapping of startled pheasants has been scaring the living daylights out of hikers since time immemorial. There are other grouse species in Colorado, none of them as bizarre as the rarely seen Gunnison sage-grouse. Looking like a ruffled member of avian aristocracy, the male of this species has a distinctive white ring of feathers on its neck that it inflates with air sacs during mating rituals—what lady-grouse could resist such a display?

Last, but not least, are the iridescent hummingbirds that hover about in search of nectar. Usually blue-green or yellowish in color, hummingbirds are often mistaken for large bugs upon first sight. Despite their small size, they are curious creatures, prone to investigating bright-colored clothing and backpacks.

Something Fishy

Fish in the pure, cold mountain streams are the object of anglers' affections (and often the objects of their meals as well). The only trout truly native to Colorado's higher mountain lakes is the sleek cutthroat trout; other members of the trout family have been introduced. These include the speckled rainbow trout, brown trout, and brook trout. The mountain whitefish is another native species; it prefers to live in lower-elevation rivers. Introduced and stocked species include the landlocked Kokanee salmon and lake trout.

Fishing is a big industry in Colorado, and those hoping to participate need to acquire a license from the Colorado Department of Wildlife (http://wildlife.state.co.us/Fishing/; 303-297-1192). Many high-altitude lakes are stocked by aerial drops in the spring, making for fine fishing throughout the summer and autumn months.

Animal Encounters

What to Do if You Encounter a Mountain Lion

Mountain lion encounters are rare, since the big cat is an elusive animal. In areas where human development infringes on habitat and territory (such as Boulder and Colorado Springs) the chance of seeing lions increases. Hikers are seldom bothered by mountain lions; attacks on humans usually happen as a result of the chase-and-kill reflex triggered by a runner, biker, or jogger.

Unlike bears and other predators, mountain lion behavior is highly unpredictable. Lions may quietly stalk unsuspecting passers-by until they have exited the cat's territory without incident. Other times, lions will burst out of the woods for no apparent reason other than to attack. If you come across a mountain lion, do not run! Mountain lions (who can run close to 45 miles per hour) can easily chase down a human (who, on average, can run about 20 miles per hour). If you come upon a lion, look at it without directly gazing into its eyes (focus on the feet). Slowly back away; if the animal is focused on you, talk firmly but calmly.

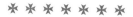

If you come across a mountain lion, do not run! Mountain lions (who can run close to 45 miles per hour) can easily chase down a human (who, on average, can run about 20 miles per hour).

More extreme measures need to be taken if the lion has an active interest in you. When a lion perks up and begins stalking you, you must act. Do everything you can to make yourself look bigger, including opening your coat or waving around your hiking poles and arms. Groups of hikers should huddle together and make noise, throwing rocks or sticks at the lion. Try to pick up potential weapons without crouching down. Do not turn your back on a mountain lion. Children and smaller people, usually women, should get behind larger companions. If the confrontation has gotten to this stage, aggressive scare tactics should repel mountain lions (who aren't used to having their prey fight back).

In the worst-case scenario—an attack— fight back with all you have. Punch, kick, swing, bite, scratch, and aim for the eyes or nose. Try to stay on your feet and get back up if you get knocked over. Mountain lions attacks usually come in one or two powerful waves; these cats are not endurance fighters. This is not universally true, however, as emaciated lions may fight to the last. Never play dead with mountain lions. This apocryphal defense only applies to some grizzly bears. A mountain lion will seize the opportunity of passive prey by administering a deadly bite to the neck. Climbing trees is another bad idea. Mountain lions are proficient climbers, and you'll only end up out on a limb. If you successfully fend off the animal, leave the area immediately. You'll probably be roughed up if you've survived an attack. Keep your guard up; patient mountain lions are capable of regrouping and finishing off wounded prey. Report any attacks to the local sheriff or wildlife bureau.

What to Do if You Encounter a Black Bear

Feared, hated, and reviled for centuries, black bears have earned an unfair reputation as bloodthirsty killers. They are nowhere near as aggressive as grizzly bears, yet they carry the burden of being associated with their ferocious cousins. Many are shy and will run away at the first sight of humans. Most conflicts occur in areas where human and bear habitats overlap (even then, bears are more prone to raid a garbage can than attack a person). Most black bear attacks are defensive in nature, with the attacker usually defending a kill or protecting cubs.

Black bear attacks are rare, but they do happen, most often when a hiker surprises a bear or comes too near a den with cubs. If you encounter a black bear, give it space. If the bear does not go away, you need to leave the area—even if it means missing out on a coveted summit. Black bears aren't looking to pick a fight. If you see them stand up on their hind legs, it is not always an aggressive action; they are simply trying to get a better view of things. If a bear becomes uncomfortable, it will begin growling, slapping the ground, or clamping its jaws as a warning. This is your cue to leave. Back away slowly and do not turn your back on the bear; as with mountain lions, look at the animal but not directly into its eyes.

One thing to note is that most of the audible and visible displays of a black bear are defense mechanisms designed to scare you off. Even the "bluff charge" where a bear runs at you while growling is more often than not a (terrifying) warning, telling you to get lost. In most circumstances, there is no reason to intimidate the bear. Quietly leaving the area is the best decision for both of you.

While their habits are somewhat predictable, that does not mean black bears will never assault humans. When they decide to attack, they will not bother with the defensive behavior noted above. An aggressive bear may casually walk over on all fours without barking or growling, giving the illusion of a harmless saunter. A seemingly calm bear coming toward you is a threat. At this point, you must take measures to fend it off, including making yourself look larger. Yell out loud and throw rocks, sticks, and whatever else is around at the bear. Do not run, but slowly back away. Bears are excellent runners, swimmers, and tree-climbers. Again, research has shown most black bear attacks are defensive in nature, usually by a sow protecting her cubs. Measured swats or light bites that do not break the skin are extremely effective in frightening off intrusive hikers.

In the rare case of an all-out attack, fight back. As with mountain lions, do not play dead. Most black bears only you want out of their territory, and playing dead leaves you in the danger zone, with a greater chance of being killed. Bear spray may give you peace of mind, but its effectiveness in real life is marginal, at best. A determined bear will continue to attack through the pain, and you may end up blinding yourself in the confusion.

The key to bear safety is to avoid confrontations that may turn ugly. Be smart and respect bears of all sizes.

Tips and Common Sense When Dealing with Wildlife

- Always give animals ample space and respect. Elk, deer, and other "gentle" wildlife can attack if frightened or threatened.
- Never attempt to feed any wildlife, period.

- When scaring away smaller animals, like marmots, aim carefully when throwing sticks or stones. Your goal is to scare them, not injure them.
- A loud whistle is a good first-line defense against animals that get too close.
- Be especially cautious when in close company of mountain goats and bighorn sheep. These encounters often happen on high ledges or ridges, where a well-timed head-butt could create a nasty fall.
- Report any animal attacks to park rangers or to the Colorado Division of Wildlife.
- Stay alert during dusk and dawn, as these are prime hunting conditions for predators.
- When hiking in remote areas, make as much ambient noise as you can, such as conversations, singing, whistling, etc. In situations like these, that friend who is an endless chatterbox becomes a valuable commodity. You want to make yourself known, so as not to scare any animals in the area. Bear bells are encouraged.

Additional Tips for Those Who Hike Alone

- Use a bear bell or other noisemaking device. I have two when I go out solo, and I secure one to each of my hiking poles. The natural motion of the poles makes them loudly ring out.
- Avoid using an MP3 player, iPod, or Walkman, especially in treeline.
- Leave a detailed plan of where you'll be hiking with a friend or family member. Include your route, trailhead, what gear you'll be wearing, and what time you expect to be home. Include emergency phone numbers to contact for the person keeping an eye on you.
- Remember to keep your first-aid kit stocked; it goes without saying that you should bring one on every hike.
- Stay calm during one-on-one encounters with wild animals. Even if you're terrified, maintaining a confident demeanor and dominant posture will help in confrontations with predators.

Trees, Plants, Fungi, and Flowers

Alpine Flowers

Alpine flowers are amongst the most rugged and beautiful in the world. Wildflowers bloom in every hue, often together in a single meadow. Seeing natural bouquets in remote mountain meadows is a treat even for the most macho of hikers. Of the hundreds of purple, red, blue, yellow, pink, and orange flowers, there are a few that stand out. My personal favorite is the whimsical elephant's head, a pink specimen that grows in watery areas between 8,000 and 11,000 feet. Flowers on the stalk resemble a totem pole of miniature pachyderms, each with a gleefully raised trunk. Mountain columbine, the state flower of Colorado, comes in a variety of shades. Columbine alternates colored stripes (usually light blue, purple, or red) with white petals that spread out like a parasol. Monk's hood is a popular purple perennial that is a relative of the buttercup. Indian paintbrush is a red or white flower that looks like a tussled thistle. In years of heavy rainfall, the "paintbrush" part of the plant may bloom fiery red. Other flowers of note include lupine, cinquefoil, Parry's primrose, wild roses, buttercup, spring beauty, larkspur, white phlox, king's crown, and marsh marigolds. A good book to consider if you'd like to learn more about alpine flowers is the budget-friendly *Colorado Flowers and Trees* by James Kavanagh, published by Waterford Press.

One of the best surprises to be found in Colorado's backcountry is wild berry. Raspberries, blueberries, mountain strawberries, huckleberries, and blackberries are amongst the treats growing wild. Shrubs that produce such berries usually bloom in late summer, mostly in areas close to a steady water supply. Wild strawberries are a unique and succulent surprise, just edging out wild raspberries as my personal favorite.

Fungus Among Us

Wild mushrooms are another mountain delicacy. Unless you are well-versed in mycology, however, never attempt to eat unknown fungus. Many mushrooms are poisonous and can make you very sick. For those who know what they are looking for, keep in mind that many wilderness areas require a permit to gather mushrooms. Permits are usually free and serve as a way for biologists to monitor the growth of certain mushrooms; call the Park Service ahead of time to find out more.

Areas with high precipitation, such as the central San Juans, host a variety of quirky mushrooms that make colorful decorations along the trail. The poisonous fly agaric is like a mushroom you'd find in a fairytale, with its bright red dome speckled with white faux barnacles. Shaggy stems are yellow mushrooms that look like they were molded from fluffed custard. Giant boletuses resemble huge ground sponges in color and texture. Those in the know will keep an eye out for tasty morel mushrooms, prized culinary delicacies that proliferate in the wake of forest fires. (Connoisseurs will actually follow wildfires around the country, in hopes of scavenging a harvest of morels).

If you are interesting in learning more about Colorado's mushrooms, check out the Colorado Mycological Society's web page, at www.cmsweb.org. This comprehensive website is the place for information on the different types of fungus and mushrooms growing in Colorado's mountains.

Notable Shrubs

Hikers have a love/hate relationship with the various mountain willows found in the high country. These are amongst the toughest plants on Earth and are the only widespread vegetation found in the high arctic regions. On the plus side, many willows color the landscape in autumn with tranquil reds and yellows. Occasionally they work well as emergency handholds, and dense thickets can provide shelter when fast-moving thunderstorms appear out of the blue. Their sturdy roots also help keep soil from being washed off steep slopes. On the negative side, many willows grow over 6 feet tall and present a veritable obstacle course for bushwhackers. Besides being extremely difficult to navigate through in thick patches, the

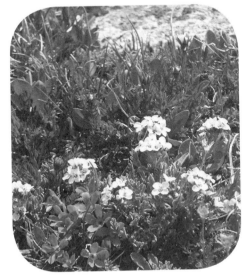

Alpine flowers are tough and beautiful.

branches are scratchy, and their dense roots can disguise swampy holes just waiting to swallow your boots. Trying to navigate a willow patch in winter can make the most mild-mannered hiker explode in expletives, especially after post-holing for an hour to hike half a mile.

As you ascend higher, you will encounter the group of thick, low-lying shrubs collectively known as the krumholtz, a German word meaning "twisted wood." The presence of these shrubs denotes the termination of treeline, which can happen anywhere between 10,400 and 12,200 feet in Colorado. Shrubs forming the krumholtz are incredibly tough; they had better be if they hope to withstand the fury of the elements on a daily basis. Versions of subalpine fir, Englemann spruce, and limber pine are reconfigured in dwarfed proportions to better adapt to their harsh environment. They grow in dense outcrops, usually protected by rocks. Year after year, they endure weeks of subzero temperatures, hurricane-force winds, torrential downpours, and a very brief growing season. Although they may appear lifeless, many of the shrubs you'll encounter in the krumholtz are hundreds of years old. Be respectful of such wizened elders when you trek in alpine regions.

Topping out the list of high-altitude plants are the tiny alpine avens, a vital food source for resident pikas. Growing in small, dense patches, avens are surrounded by brawny, bright green stalks that resemble little ferns. Yellow or white flowers bloom in the summer and early autumn. Avens have developed amazing alpine adaptations: long taproots grow deep into the scarce alpine soil to suck up fleeting moisture, thick "hairs" protect stems and leaves from wind damage, and red pigmentation is used to filter out powerful ultraviolet rays and to efficiently convert sunlight into heat.

Major Trees

Conifers (trees whose seeds are encased in woody cones) dominate the mountainsides where conditions are favorable to growth. Englemann spruce, Douglas fir, subalpine fir, and lodgepole pine grow in areas that are cool and have adequate water supplies. Drier regions (usually the sunnier south-facing hills and valleys) are more suited to ponderosa pines. Blue spruce and western hemlock are other common trees growing between 8,000 and 12,000 feet.

Aspen trees are symbolic of Colorado's forests. They are deciduous (Latin for "temporary") trees, meaning they shed their leaves to conserve energy when cold weather arrives. Colorado's aspen trees are known as quaking or trembling aspen because of the way sunlight plays off their rounded leaves and because of the "shimmery" sound they make when the wind blows. Aspens are members of the willow family. Each stand of trees is actually one living unit, with every tree sharing a common network of roots. Trees that spawn from this network (known as clones, because they share identical genetic markers) live between 80 and 140 years before dying off and letting new trees generate from the root system. These roots go deep enough into the ground to resist the devastating effects of fire and avalanches; this is why you will see aspen stands rebound in areas affected by these phenomena, while other trees take years or decades to repopulate. Modern biologists have proposed the oldest living thing on earth may be an enormous aspen stand in Utah known as "Pando" (see sidebar, page 19). The powdery film on the bark of Aspen trees serves as a natural sunscreen; in a pinch, it can also work as a very basic sun block for human skin.

Lower elevations find other deciduous trees: poplar, cottonwood, and balsam trees are common near rivers and lakes. Because of their fibrous make-up, these trees split poorly, rot easily, and are ill-suited for burning. If you are hunting for campfire wood, stick with the sappy (but burnable) evergreen trees or dried aspen logs.

All Hail Pando, King Of All Living Things!

Pando is a fitting name for a great king, wouldn't you agree? Pando (Latin for "I spread") refers to an enormous quaking aspen colony located near Fish Lake in the Wasatch Range in southern Utah. Formed from a single seed, the "Trembling Giant" encompasses over 107 acres and is estimated to be at least 80,000 years old. The trees that make up Pando are genetic clones that share a common, archaic network of roots. Trees that sprout from this matrix live approximately 140 years and are replaced by fresh saplings on a regular basis. Pando supported roughly 47,000 trees as of 2006!

Pando is considered to be a single organism; think of the individual trees that grow from the shared roots as being like hairs on a human head. They live, grow, and die with the genesis of new trees come from a single living source. While it is impossible to weigh such a massive growth, biologists say Pando makes a great case for the heaviest living thing on earth (in direct competition with the fabled redwood trees in California). Ideal climate conditions have helped the colony live for so long. Some biologists think Pando may be closer to a million years old. To put it into human terms: modern man (*Homo sapiens*) came onto the scene about 40,000 years ago and migrated to the Americas about 10,000 years ago.

Pando's survival strategies have endured fire, ice, wind, and heat. Assuming water levels in Utah do not drastically change, Pando's reign could carry on for thousands more years. Long live the King!

Safety in the Mountains

Altitude: This Is Your Brain on Thin Air; Any Questions?

Note: The following overview is not a substitute for attaining a deeper knowledge of altitude-related symptoms. Wilderness first-aid courses are great opportunities to learn more and are advised for those spending a great deal of time at altitude. Suggested reading: *Altitude Illness: Prevention and Treatment* by Stephen Bezruchka, M.D., and *Going Higher* by Charles Houston, M.D., both published by The Mountaineers Books.

We humans have grown rather fond of oxygen. The air we breathe enables our intricate respiratory systems to relay oxygen to the vital organs of our bodies. At altitude, decreased oxygen levels cause the body to alter how it utilizes the invaluable gas. The series of adaptations that occur at high elevations are known as acclimatization. Simply put, acclimatizing allows your body to properly function when the concentration of oxygen in the air is reduced.

First off, it's important to know what happens to the air at altitude. "Thin air" is a layman's term used to describe the paucity of oxygen at higher elevations, due to lower atmospheric pressure. At sea level, oxygen levels are "compressed" by the weight of the atmosphere; therefore, at sea level, oxygen molecules are abundant. As you ascend higher, the weight of the atmosphere lessens, meaning the particles of air have more space to move around. As a result, less dense air will contain smaller concentrations of oxygen. Air circulating the summit of Colorado's highest peaks, 14,000 feet above sea level, will contain roughly one third of the oxygen found in the air at sea level.

People used to living at sea level begin to feel the effects of altitude around 5,000 feet. Journeys to higher elevations can provoke severe changes; life-threatening ailments associated with altitude have occurred as low as 8,000 feet. Knowing what is happening to your body is key to functioning well at altitude. A little understanding will aid in making each trip to altitude an enjoyable one. The most important thing to remember: ascending slowly and avoiding overexertion are vital in adapting to altitude. And if you begin to feel bad—real bad—descent is the smartest decision and the easiest way to feel better.

How Our Bodies Adapt to Altitude

Our body has three major involuntary systems that change to cope with altitude, though how proficiently it does so is different for each individual. Rate of respiration, heart rate, and increased red blood cell production all work to bring oxygen levels to adequate levels when a person is confronted with decreased oxygen. Most obvious to the hiker is an increased rate of respiration. By breathing faster (even at rest), we are able to coax more oxygen out of the air. When respiration takes priority, simple tasks such as drinking from a water bottle or holding a conversation can leave one winded. Above 13,000 feet, it is normal to rest and catch your breath every few steps.

One's heart rate increases to efficiently pump each oxygen-reduced packet of blood through the body. Anyone who has felt the curious heart-pounding result from simple tasks at altitude knows it doesn't take much to trigger the familiar throbbing sensation in the chest. Opening the wrapper of a candy bar or fighting with the stubborn cap on summit register tubes can leave one wheezing!

Red blood cell production is a much slower process than respiration and heart rate, taking approximately a month to fully adapt at a given altitude. For those spending weeks or months at altitude, this is the final step to being fully comfortable at high elevations. The more red blood cells present in the body, the more carriers there are for oxygen. Blood initially gets thicker at elevation due to dehydration. The blood remains thick as the body acclimates to the increased presence of red blood cells.

Other bodily functions are affected by these primary changes in body rhythms. Diuresis is inevitable; as the body speeds up, it needs to expel more extraneous fluid. Peeing a lot is not necessarily a bad thing. Urine color is a good indicator of hydration. Clear urine is a sign of proper hydration, while thicker yellow or foul-smelling urine is an indication the body needs more water/fluids. It can be annoying if you're trying to get a good night's sleep, but not peeing a lot at altitude can be a sign your body is not making the proper adjustments. (Don't be alarmed, just pay attention if this happens.)

Digestion can also be affected by altitude, as there is often not enough oxygenated blood in the digestive tract to break down fatty foods. As a result, appetites may diminish (though psychological factors may play a part in this too). Sour or acidic stomachs are common at altitude; regular antacids are helpful in making your tummy feel better. Increased flatulence is a comical (if you're a guy) side effect, though more discreet individuals (usually women) can find this a bit embarrassing. Hey, you're up in the mountains, let it rip! Farting can relieve pressure and actually make you feel better, so don't hold it in!

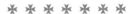

High-altitude edema or peripheral edema is a temporary swelling of the face, eyes, fingers, and ankles. Using hiking poles can help reduce the possibility of peripheral edema in the hands.

Along with digestion, you may need to "go number two" more than you would at home. This is normal; as things speed up in your body, so will your metabolism. Having to poop more is natural. Cheeky NOLS (National Outdoors Leadership School) instructors have dubbed the telltale light brown piles of unacclimated hikers "NOLS gold." Lighter-colored feces are a result of nutrients passing through the body too quickly to be fully absorbed. A yucky side effect is the appeal of such nutrient rich piles to animals—that is why it is important to properly dispose of human waste. Make a hole at least 8 inches deep for human waste and cover it up; pack out any non-biodegradable materials.

High-altitude edema or peripheral edema is a temporary swelling of the face, eyes, fingers, and ankles. This condition is more prevalent in women, though it will affect most people going up to 14,000 feet to some degree. A less scientific term for this condition is "sausage fingers." By itself, it is not a threat, but an early indicator of other possible symptoms, notably AMS (acute mountain sickness). Again, there's no reason to be alarmed, but pay attention. Using hiking poles (which keep the fingers active in the act of gripping) can help reduce the possibility of peripheral edema in the hands. Prolonged peripheral edema can split the skin on the thumb and fingertips, sometimes below the finger nail. This can be a painful condition that makes some simple chores (like priming a pump-pressure stove) difficult.

How Long Does It Take to Acclimate? How Long Do the Effects Last?

Full acclimatization takes about one month for most people, though most feel strong at high altitude (over 5,000 feet) after three to four days. The rate of ascent is an important factor: acclimating from sea level to 8,000 feet is easier than adapting from 8,000 feet to 16,000 feet. If properly ascending, hikers in Colorado generally feel "normal" after

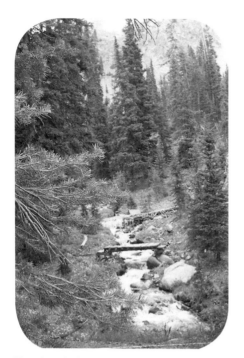

"Camp low, climb high" is a good motto when acclimating.

two to three days above 10,000 feet. After approximately six to 10 days, your body will have completed most major high-altitude-related adjustments; it takes roughly seven to 14 days to lose the major benefits of acclimatization.

Illnesses and Symptoms of Altitude Sickness

Just about everyone who ventures up to altitude gets a sampling of accute mountain sickness (AMS) at one time or another. In mild cases (which are most common), the condition is bearable, though a little uncomfortable. Slight headaches, nausea, loss of appetite, malaise (a vague lack of energy or ability to think clearly), and sleeplessness are common and can often be dealt with by using over-the-counter pain relievers. For fast relief (that has worked for me), Advil Liqui-Gels are tops—and I'm not just saying that because they gave me a free car! (I'm just kidding of course. My car, a mountain-beaten 1989 Honda Accord, looks like it was donated by Sanford and Son.) Aspirin, acetaminophen, or ibuprofen may work better for you. Mild AMS can occur anywhere between one and three days after arriving at altitude and usually lasts a few hours to two days, as symptoms gradually diminish. These conditions are generally harmless, but they do raise a yellow flag. If they do not subside, they could lead to more serious conditions.

Moderate cases of AMS are quite a bit worse. This is the worst condition I've experienced (read sidebar "The Bierstadt Incident," on page 27 for details), and even though it truly was a moderate case, I felt like I'd just gone 10 rounds with Mike Tyson in a room lit by 80,000-watt lightbulbs after eating a gallon of moldy mayonnaise. If you couldn't guess, moderate AMS is like a powerful hangover and is generally unaffected by most pain relievers (though antacids or Pepto-Bismol-type medicines may soothe your stomach). Moderate AMS is an amplified version of mild AMS: the headache is more intense, the nausea often results in vomiting, and even simple exertion can leave you out of breath. The only way to feel better is to descend. Going higher may be possible for stubborn souls, but it could cause the condition to worsen. Descending 1,000 to 3,000 feet will make a big difference and is recommended. (It may even rebalance the body enough for you to give the hike another go in a few hours).

Severe AMS is no joke. This life-threatening condition cannot be ignored, as it may be a precursor to cerebral edema. All the conditions of moderate AMS are present, along with the following symptoms: lack of balance and muscle coordination, confusion, or severe mood changes. At this stage, people may become unaware of their surroundings and may become angry, hostile, or unintelligible. A good test is having them walk a straight line, similar to the sobriety test issued by the police. Rapid descent is your only choice; get the afflicted person down anyway you can. Wait until the person is back to normal (which may take days, or not happen at all until you descend farther) to resume ascending, doing so with an eye on potential recurrence.

When diagnosing AMS, it is important to note that the symptoms may instead be signs of hypothermia (covered on page 34), fatigue, stress, dehydration, or nerves. A good rule of thumb: if the person isn't having fun (or can't tell you if they are or not), descend immediately.

HAPE and HACE are acronyms for altitude sickness in its most dangerous and deadly form. While both conditions are relatively rare in Colorado, both can happen as low as 8,000 feet above sea level. High-altitude pulmonary edema (HAPE) occurs when fluid from the blood leaks into the lungs. As blood struggles to adapt to altitude, pressure in the arteries (which is aggravated by exertion, dehydration, and cold) causes water and fluids to escape into the lungs. HAPE is a progressive condition. After several hours or days of undiminished AMS, the victim's condition may enter into HAPE. He or she will breathe rapidly, even when at rest. The smallest tasks will be exhausting and will leave the victim moody and tired. Often, even speaking becomes a laborious chore. If the condition is allowed to get worse, breathing becomes visibly frothy and audibly bubbly and is often accompanied by a dry cough that expels sputum from the lungs. The victim's lips turn permanently blue, due to the lack of oxygen traveling through the body. (Lips should be the same color as one's fingernail beds.)

HAPE is not a moderate condition; without immediate treatment at a medical facility, a victim can rapidly phase into unconsciousness and death. Descending will help, but professional medical treatment is paramount. Even with the best medicines, the decline is sometimes irreversible. It's serious business; luckily, it is fairly rare between 8,000 and 14,000 feet. In Colorado, most HAPE victims come from sea level and ascend to over 9,000 feet in a matter of hours (by plane or car), and stay there—or worse, go higher. Recovery from HAPE is normally a total return to the old self, though any occurrence may denote a propensity for HAPE.

High-altitude cerebral edema (HACE) is as scary and deadly as HAPE. HACE is a progression of severe AMS and is caused by excessive water swelling the brain. As cells dilate in a desperate effort to absorb more oxygen, the brain gets waterlogged. By the time your body is taking these extreme measures, it may be too late. HACE is characterized by severe confusion, inability to speak or function, inability to move, numbness or weakness on one side of the body, severe nausea, and severe headache. HACE shuts down a body at a terrifying rate: unconsciousness, coma, and death are the inevitable outcomes of untreated cases. Descent is imperative and medical attention must be found for the victim. Even with treatment, permanent neurological damage may result. This is a rare condition for Colorado's modest heights, but people have died from HACE at as low as 10,000 feet. Don't be scared of it, but be aware of it.

The X-Factor at Altitude: Psychological Strength

Performing well at altitude is not all in the legs and lungs. One's mental state can enhance or impede the experience of being at high elevations. Hikers who are relaxed, strong, confident, happy, and positive experience few problems at altitude—and when trouble does occur, they calmly deal with it. Part of this comes from knowing one's body and how it reacts: experience in the mountains is a big plus. Fear, anger, and apprehension increase the body's overall stress level and can actually accelerate and magnify the symptoms of AMS (or even induce "phantom" symptoms such as migraines, nausea, or weakness). Because emotions are extremely personal and affect us in very individual ways, there's no way to universally prescribe how one should balance the competing needs of the body, the mind, and the psyche when making decisions. A few things to consider:

- Highly emotional people are likely to have difficulty finding the balance between smart hiking and overthinking things. Hiking partners can make or break a day in the mountains. My advice: when you find a good hiking partner, hold onto 'em for life!

- Whenever an unexpected stressor (bad weather, irritable companions, exposure, etc.) happens, I take five slow, deep breaths. It sounds corny, but it helps me center my mind and focus on what needs to be done.

- Though we often escape to the mountains to clear our heads, burdening and troublesome thoughts may make it difficult to perform well at altitude. High-altitude hiking, scrambling, and climbing require an elevated state of concentration, which is sometimes a pleasant distraction from these issues. Some days, however, even the mountains can't purge these thoughts. Don't feel bad if you miss a summit because of a heavy heart; it happens to the best of us.

For some people, the mental side of hiking isn't an issue. For other more sensitive souls, a bad experience can make the prospect of returning to altitude an intimidating invitation. Take this into consideration when assessing why a hiking partner feels bad: sometimes a good joke or an encouraging comment can take the edge off, and make reaching the summit that much easier.

Fitness and Altitude

Research on fitness and altitude is a mixed bag. Some sources insist fitness has nothing to do with altitude sickness, though all agree obesity seems to be a catalyst for AMS. Fitness levels seem to have no impact on involuntary adjustments, so in a technical sense, it may be genetics or nutrition (or both) that determine the rate of acclimatization. That being said, stronger legs and lungs are undoubtedly a boon at altitude. Powerful muscles and leaner bodies will exert themselves less, thereby decelerating the affects brought on by tough physical efforts. Add in the psychological edge of knowing your body is "mountain ready," and it's safe to say fitness does play a part in adapting to altitude. The key for a newcomer to altitude is to keep a moderate pace, hydrate properly, and don't be a hero. Once you are adjusted, you can try all the pushups you want on the top of your favorite 14er. In the meantime, give your body the time it needs to adjust—no matter if you exercise infrequently or an Olympic marathon runner.

Sleeping at Altitude

Oh sweet sleep, how elusive you can be for those who seek slumber on high! A person's body continues to adjust to altitude, even if they're completely tuckered out. Even the most worn-out backcountry traveler may find sleep hard to come by. An increased rate of respiration inhibits deep sleep and promotes snoring—just ask your beleaguered tentmate. Also, having to urinate more will wake you from a sound sleep, often several times a night. In addition, you may feel your heart pounding for no good reason; other times you may feel like you are suffocating for no reason. The strange, sometimes scary, irregular patterns of a companion's breathing may also keep you awake. An odd breathing cadence, known as periodic breathing, is normal at high altitudes, and in most cases, is nothing to worry about.

The key to good sleep: climb high, sleep low. Don't attempt to sleep at elevations over 10,000 feet if you have just arrived from low elevation. Only increase sleeping elevation by 1,000 feet per night, once over 10,000 feet. Avoid caffeine and sugars before bed. As tempting as they may be, do not take sleeping pills. Over-the-counter pills decrease the rate of respiration and are detrimental to proper acclimatization. When you do fall asleep, you may have what the Sherpas of the Himalaya call the "sleep of the dead," a dreamless passing of time. More common are brief, incredibly vivid or erotic dreams, thought to be a result of REM sleep while your body stays in a near-waking condition. Remember, a good night's sleep is essential to good performance in the mountains. You can get away with a day or two of bad sleep, but once your body is more comfortable at altitude, make the time to get a good night's rest.

Prevention and Treatment of Altitude Sickness

The golden rule for treatment of altitude-related illnesses: descend, descend, descend! In Colorado, a difference of 1,500 to 2,500 feet will usually alleviate any symptoms of AMS. If HAPE or HACE is present, descend as low as you possibly can. (For people living in high-altitude places such as Leadville—elevation, 10,000 feet, this may require leaving town.)

For mild cases, ibuprofen, acetaminophen, and aspirin can help relieve discomfort without having to descend. Antacids and Pepto-Bismol can help settle queasy and gassy stomachs. Energy drinks such as Gatorade and Cytomax can help prevent dehydration and restore sugars and electrolytes to the body.

✳ ✳ ✳ ✳ ✳ ✳ ✳

It is my experience not to rely on prescription drugs—your body will naturally adjust, and perhaps, as is the case with muscle memory, get the knack of acclimating for the next time you visit high altitudes (this is a common belief amongst Russian mountaineers).

✳ ✳ ✳ ✳ ✳ ✳ ✳

Preventing altitude sickness is easier said than done. Ascend slowly and don't overexert yourself. Out-of-towners should spend at least one to two full days above 8,000 feet before heading out to the peaks in this book. Locals in Colorado may be able to ascend and descend quickly enough to avoid any ill effects of altitude. Dayhikes taken at a reasonable pace are often easier on the body than forcing a night's sleep at altitude. And one last axiom: never take a headache higher.

It is my experience not to rely on prescription drugs—your body will naturally adjust, and perhaps, as is the case with muscle memory, get the knack of acclimating for the next time you visit high altitudes (this is a common belief amongst Russian mountaineers). However, for those pressed for time or hoping to bag that one special summit, there are some doctor-prescribed options.

Drugs for Altitude Adaptation

Always consult your doctor before trying prescription drugs. The medicines used for altitude adjustments affect the heart, blood vessels, and respiratory systems. Never "borrow" a friend's prescription unless the situation is life-or-death (HAPE or HACE, for example).

Acetazolamide is more commonly known by the brand name Diamox. It is taken to ward off mild-to-moderate AMS and to help facilitate sleep at altitude. Basically, this medicine helps the body balance pH levels in the blood that can help regulate respiration and aid in acclimatization. Acetazolamide is taken in advance of heading to altitude as well as while one is there; it may also be taken if AMS becomes apparent. In that sense, it is both a preventative and a "cure." While it may not be useful in cases of severe AMS, it should be taken nonetheless to reduce the work the body has to do to get back to normal. For those coming to Colorado from lower elevations, acetazolamide is a good option that has proven to work well, especially at elevations of 12,000 to 14,000 feet.

Dexamethasone is a steroid that is usually reserved for severe cases of AMS and HACE. It is often carried by mountain guides for use in emergency situations. If you are heading to the remote backcountry for a number of days with unproven or weaker companions, it may be wise to take along "dex" (available by prescription only) in case of extreme emergencies.

Nifedipine is used specifically to curb the affects of HAPE. This drug is rarely seen in Colorado, though it may be advised for hikers who have had previous bouts of HAPE at altitudes up to 14,000 feet.

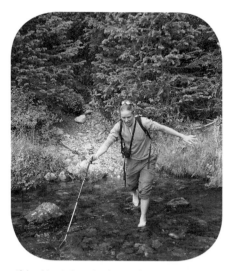

If the thin air doesn't take your breath away, the cold water might!

Use of narcotics of any kind should absolutely be avoided. Speaking frankly, marijuana should never be used at altitude—besides impairing judgment, marijuana decreases respiration and can actually promote or worsen AMS.

There are other drugs prescribed for those with specific conditions, including issues with vision, digestion, or prior illnesses. The scope of this book does not cover individual cases—consult your doctor.

What the Locals Know: Eight Tips for You and Your Out-of-Town Friends

1) Even if your friend is a superman or superwoman back home, don't push them too hard at altitude. Chances are they won't let on how tired they are. Be tactful and make it seem like you are the one who needs the rest, extra drink, or snack break.

2) Pay attention to your friend's moods. A jovial pal who becomes quiet may be starting to feel lousy. Don't take an angry or edgy friend too personally; acclimatization can make anyone grumpy.

3) Ibuprofen is a good preventative for altitude sickness, for those who rarely hike or who may be trying a difficult climb in Colorado.

4) Offer to carry a little extra weight (or do so without your friend's knowledge).

5) Never downplay the accomplishment of climbing a Colorado mountain. It may be easy for you, but it may be a life-changing experience for your friend.

6) Likewise, if a friend gets sick, don't make them feel bad about it. As soon as it's apparent going down is the best idea, concentrate on their well-being and try to get their mind on other things. Remind them altitude sickness isn't a sign of weakness, it's a sign of too little oxygen.

7) Offer to take photos for your pal. Not only is it cool for your friend to see him- or herself on top of a mountain, it's one less thing they have to worry about if they are struggling with the thin air.

8) And one from personal experience: don't ask them if they are alright 700 times on a single hike. They may be fine, and your insistent questioning may make them think they aren't. Most people will let you know if they aren't doing well, either by subtle hints or outright saying so.

Dogs at Altitude

Because animals are infinitely tougher than humans, it would be hard to tell if your dog was feeling bad at altitude. In general, dogs seem to be barely affected at altitude—many can be seen joyfully running up to the summits of Colorado's highest peaks. It's important to keep dogs hydrated and, of course, to keep an eye on their demeanor. If they become lethargic or struggle to keep up, it may be a good time to turn around. They aren't immune to altitude, but they are naturally better equipped to deal with it.

The Bierstadt Incident: A Personal Tale of Altitude Woe

My own experience with altitude sickness has given me sympathy for those who are feeling bad in the mountains. I have only had one incident of mild AMS, and it's one I'll never forget. I had just spent three full weeks at sea level in Maine. Upon returning to Colorado, my bravado got the better of me, and I figured I would be fine to hike a 14er the day I got back. I had always done fine at altitude, so I wasn't overly concerned.

I picked a mountain that has an easy standard route: 14,060-foot Mount Bierstadt. I made my first bad decision before even getting on the mountain. Instead of taking the easier standard route, I intended to climb an alternate way that started at 13,000+ feet from the Mount Evans Road. It dropped down a gully, crossed a basin, and then ascended the mountain. My entire day would be spent over 12,500 feet.

It was indeed a fun route, well within my ability, and I felt fine until I was about 300 vertical feet from the summit. I felt my whole body go shaky and I became nauseous. I lost sensation in my fingertips and got very dizzy. I yelled to my hiking partner (who was about 50 feet from the summit) that I was going down. At the time, I felt he could have summited without me and then caught up with me on the way down; he decided to abandon the top and help me down.

We dropped into the low basin and I still felt ok; not great, but I was moving under my own power. Unfortunately, I had to climb 1,000 feet uphill via a loose gully to reach the truck. The turning point was when I tried to eat a handful of totally unappetizing imitation M&Ms. I threw up at the smell of them, and I bonked.

The hike up was no picnic; waves of nausea and spinning black fuzz in my peripheral vision enervated my every step. By the time I topped out of the gully, I had been dry heaving for over an hour and didn't have the strength to walk across a flat section to the truck. My hiking partner (who had already taken my backpack) went to the truck, dropped off the packs, and returned to piggyback me to the parking area. Grateful, but still feeling awful, I fell asleep on the drive home. When I awoke an hour or two later, I was back in Boulder and I felt fine. Not even a hint of the breakdown that previously incapacitated me was present.

I had learned my lesson. Even strong climbers needs to respect altitude! From that day on, I was more aware of my body and took the time to reintroduce myself to altitude after visits to sea level. It was a rough lesson to learn (and it was only moderate AMS), but I'm a much wiser hiker, having learned it firsthand.

Weather: The Wild World Above the Mountains

If one needs to be assured that mountain environments are untamed, simply look to the sky. Mountain weather is a powerful element of backcountry travel that must be respected. Predicting weather at high altitude is a difficult science. The factors that contribute to storms may not be evident until the clouds are already forming. This isn't to say that mountain weather is completely random. Storm trends tend to be good heralds of what to expect in a given mountain range or at a specific time of the year. While clouds can build up quickly, how they do so can offer clues to the oncoming weather.

(Note: If you want to be a storm expert, see Appendix D for more comprehensive resources on mountain weather.)

Why So Many Storms? How Mountain Weather Builds

From late spring to mid-autumn (prime hiking season), afternoon storms should be expected to roll in between 1 P.M. and 4 P.M. every day. Storms and lightning are daily threats during this time because of the temperature variations from night to day and the available moisture present. Nights are cool and promote condensation of water vapor in the air; after sunrise, heat from the sun initiates evaporation. As hot and cool air collide, electricity forms in the condensed clouds and continues to build throughout the day. At the hottest part of the day (often around 2 to 3 P.M. in the high country), the balance is tipped, and the storms unleash brief but formidable torrents of rain, sleet, snow, and hail.

If no larger fronts have been forecast, these storms usually run their course by late afternoon. Be warned: these storms often display the violent power of lightning, making exposed travel above treeline especially dangerous.

General Weather Advice

The proven best advice for safe hiking in Colorado: start early! Beginning your hikes in the early morning (and in some cases, predawn) will ensure you are back into the safety of treeline if storms hit. For hikes in this book, consider the estimated time and distance along with your own pace to formulate the best time to start, summit, and finish a hike. Being off summits by 11:30 A.M. or earlier is a good guideline. As you get better at reading weather, you'll be better able to tell if you can push it back a little later. As a side note, with almost all hikes, if I can't be on the trail by 8:30 A.M. at the latest, I'll change the summit from a goal to an optional bonus.

I'm not a big fan of dawdling on summits unless the weather is near perfect. Some people like to snack, nap, or recharge on top of mountains—even when storms are looming. If you have gotten a later-than-expected summit, snap a few pictures, and then descend to a safer locale to eat and rest—preferably in treeline.

You can use the children's rule of counting the time between lightning and thunder to determine storm distance: count the seconds between the sight of lightning and the crash of thunder and divide it by 5; for example, a 5-second count means the storm is 1 mile away. Continue to count successive flashes and booms. If the time decreases, the storm is drawing near. If the time increases, the storm is moving away.

If you wake up the morning of a hike socked in by fog, it isn't necessarily a reason to call off the hike. If a cold front has moved in, it may rain and be foggy, but it can also ward off thunderstorms. If you are good at navigating in these conditions, it's worth giving it a try, but be warned: you run the risk of having storms build and having no real way of seeing them coming until that first flash and boom.

If you can feel or see electricity in your hair, the storm is forming right above you! This is an especially dangerous situation—if you're this close to the storm, it's advisable to drop metal items: hiking poles, snowshoes, ice axes, etc. and recover them later.

Local forecasts are good general indicators, but they do not apply to the variable conditions at elevation. The following sections discuss such conditions in greater detail.

Be prepared for bad weather. I bring a sturdy Gore-Tex shell and light rain pants on every hike, even when the weather looks clear.

Reading the Clouds

Many of Colorado's days start off sunny and clear, often with a small smattering of clouds harmlessly hanging in the sky. As the sun begins to heat up the atmosphere, radiation and wind cause moisture to evaporate and rise. Air becomes less dense as it warms, creating lower air pressure—the perfect canvas for storms. Moisture that rises with the warm air eventually cools and forms clouds.

The clouds that form over the course of a typical Colorado day can cue you into developing weather. Cumulus clouds look like puffy, cottony towers that initially form as individual mounds. Their presence indicates the cycle of weather has been set in motion, with moisture cooling on high. As long as they remain spaced out and their bottoms remain fluffy and white, you are in no immediate danger. When cumulus clouds begin to build and fuse together, the sky will become dense, with individual clouds being less distinct.

Be very wary of cumulus clouds if they begin to have dark, flattened bottoms and start to grow into towering pillars that reach high into the sky. When this happens, cumulus clouds transform into cumulonimbus clouds, which most people recognize as thunderheads. These powerful clouds are the bringers of lightning, rain, snow,

✳ ✳ ✳ ✳ ✳ ✳

Be very wary of cumulus clouds if they begin to have dark, flattened bottoms and start to grow into towering pillars that reach high into the sky. A wise safety rule: when puffy white clouds begin to turn an angry shade of gray, it's a good time to assess your position on the mountain.

✳ ✳ ✳ ✳ ✳ ✳

thunder, and hail—it is very important to pay attention to cumulonimbus clouds, especially if it is after noon. A wise safety rule: when puffy white clouds begin to turn an angry shade of gray, it's a good time to assess your position on the mountain—cumulus clouds can build very quickly, forming storms from clear skies in less than an hour.

Other clouds you may see in Colorado include:

- **Stratocumulus** clouds resemble darkened cumulus clouds lumped together. Unlike the epic, storm-nurturing cumulonimbus, stratocumulus clouds indicate a cold front and precipitation, often free of lightning and thunder (but not always!). These clouds are common in winter and during colder days.

- **Lenticular** clouds are the sleek, smooth clouds that arc like the bubbles in a lava lamp. These high-altitude clouds are indicators of strong winds and changing fronts; they often precede bad weather, which will generally arrive within 48 hours.

- **Nimbostratus** clouds form a uniform, gray cloud cover below 8,000 feet that creates fog and rain. It is often possible to climb above these moisture-laden systems to clear weather above.

- **Cirrocumulus** clouds are wispy, white, distant clouds that often form in flat sheets (such as the mackerel sky). These high-altitude dwellers form above 20,000 feet and are stabilizing clouds, meaning they carry no precipitation.

- Similar in form to cirrocumulus clouds are **altocumulus** clouds, which form from 8,000 to 20,000 feet. Altocumulus clouds have the same globular, wavy appearance as cirrocumulus clouds, but the white is interwoven with darker gray patches, indicating an oncoming cold front and potential storms later in the day.

Barometers. Many people who venture into the outdoors have barometers built into their watches, GPS units, or other electronics. Barometers measure atmospheric pressure; as a general rule, lower atmospheric pressure indicates bad weather, while higher pressure is a sign of clearing weather. Keep in mind that atmospheric pressure drops as you ascend, even on the clearest of days. I've learned to pay close attention to the fluctuations in my barometer when sketchy weather begins to blow in—a fast drop in pressure nearly always means storms are coming. Barometers aren't perfect in predicting storms, but they do give you one more clue in predicting mountain weather.

Lightning. Pressing your tongue against the terminals of a standard 9-volt battery creates a mildly uncomfortably shock that indicates how much charge is left in the battery. Multiply that voltage roughly 5,555 times and you have the power behind a normal lightning bolt! Anyone who has ever been caught in one of Colorado's brief but violent storms knows the fearful helplessness one feels when at the mercy of such a powerful and unpredictable adversary.

Lightning travels far too fast for a person to outrun and may strike several miles away from the visible center of a storm, even under clear blue skies. Many people only think about the most obvious danger from lightning: getting hit by a thunderbolt. While a direct strike is the worst thing that can happen, it's not the only threat. Splash strikes occur when lightning jumps from the initial strike target to surrounding areas. Ground strikes (or step voltage) hit the hiker from below as lightning dissipates into the surrounding ground. Contact strikes occur when a person is holding something that absorbs a direct strike, such as an ice axe or tent pole. Finally, shockwave strikes happen when a nearby bolt is powerful enough to generate a shockwave that can easily knock a large man off his feet.

Safety in Lightning Storms

Obviously, avoiding storms is the best practice in the mountains. Weather forecasts should always be referenced before heading out. However, even the most prepared and knowledgeable hiker can be caught in fast-building storms. I've seen storms metastasize from clear blue skies directly overhead in less than 15 minutes (and at all times of the day).

If you are caught in a storm, stay calm. You must assess the danger quickly, and act accordingly. Storms don't give you time to factor in all the variables: if you need to seek shelter, it must be done without hesitation. Following are a few rules for finding relatively safe places in lightning storms:

- Stay away from water, including the faux safety in gullies and streambeds.

- Always try to get as low as safely possible, hopefully back into treeline or the lowest areas in open meadows. Never stand under trees in open areas—keep moving to safer areas.

- Immediately get off summits and ridges, even if it means diverting to an off-trail pocket of safety.

- If you smell, hear, or feel electricity in the air (examples: your hair stands up or your snowshoes start to hum), move down quickly! Even if your lungs are burning, move as fast as you can to safer places. Sometimes you have to suck up the pain and just keep moving.

- Space out a minimum of 60 feet from your companions (think of this as the distance between a pitcher and catcher on a baseball field). If one member should get injured by lightning, maintaining this distance will keep other party members from being hurt.

- Stay away from metal objects such as hiking poles, ice axes, and climbing gear. Tent poles are especially dangerous—if you are stuck in your tent, make sure you are not in contact with the poles and you are insulated from the ground on a foam pad or backpack.

- If you are stuck in the storm with nowhere to go, assume the "safety position." Sit on a backpack or foam pad to protect yourself from ground-traveling electricity. Crouch down, but do not lie down (the idea is to minimize your surface area with the ground). If in the heart of a storm, sit on your pack and pull your knees close to you. Interlock your hands and put them over your head, resting your elbows on your knees. This last resort is known as the "Oh, s***!" position in most circles. Should lighting strike, it will course through your hands and into your legs, terminating in the ground. It sounds painful, but this position channels electricity through your body without it coursing through your vital organs. Lightning is especially prone to exit through the eyes or ears...not pretty stuff. For additional safety, feel free to consult the god of your choice while in this posture.

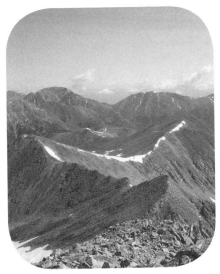
Avoid ridges when storms are brewing.

- The best shelter can be found in low-lying shrubs or trees. Avoid the highest patches or trees, and assume the crouched position while sitting on a backpack or foam pad. Stay a safe distance from companions. Pay attention to the progress of the storm and wait until it has passed for at least 20 minutes to proceed up or down.

- Caves obviously make great shelters, but be wary of "spark plug gaps" (gapped rocks that have an exposed or open top). These gaps actually attract lightning—look for better shelter if you can.

Lightning Strike First Aid

In the awful instance a companion is struck by lightning, it is imperative to act quickly. A body hit by lightning is not holding an electrical charge, so it will be safe to touch them. Any type of strike will often induce cardiopulmonary arrest—quickly check the "ABCs" of first aid: airway, breathing, and circulation. CPR (cardiopulmonary resuscitation) should be performed if the victim has stopped breathing or has no pulse. CPR is an invaluable technique that should be known by anyone heading into the backcountry.

In a case of a "light strike," in which the victim does not lose consciousness or vital functions, there will still be extensive burning that may not show up for many hours after the initial injury. Any tangle with lightning requires an immediate exit from the mountain and a visit to a hospital or medical facility. Call for help if possible, and evacuate the victim from the area as soon as you can.

Weather Trends by Season

Weather can blow in from any direction, any time of the year. I've seen lightning in January, snow in July, and hail on 80°F days. While anything is possible, there are some general patterns Colorado weather follows each season. These patterns can help you assess weather trends and make an informed decision when field forecasting.

Spring conditions (March through early to mid-June). Spring weather is often cool, bright, and free of thunderstorms. Days start cold and only warm up slightly, making early spring less prone to lightning storms. A bigger threat in spring is the danger of avalanche and rotten snowpack. As the sun heats up the snow, cornices become especially vulnerable to breaking off and triggering snowslides. Hiking conditions in spring often require winter mountaineering gear such as crampons, ice axes, helmets, and ropes. This is also the ideal time to attempt couloirs and other steep snow routes, depending on the stability of the snowpack. Late spring is a great time to hike, as many of the mountain flowers and trees are in bloom.

> ✳ ✳ ✳ ✳ ✳ ✳ ✳
>
> *Start early (pre-dawn on longer hikes) and be off summits by 11:30 A.M. There are only a few multiday storm fronts that hit Colorado each summer, so you should have a weather window most mornings to reach your summit.*
>
> ✳ ✳ ✳ ✳ ✳ ✳ ✳

Summer conditions (mid-June through September). Summer is the season of storms—but also of the best mountainside conditions! Nearly every day is punctuated by thunderstorms that roll in from approximately 1 P.M. to 4 P.M. Trails will be clear of most snow and the days are long. Start early (pre-dawn on longer hikes) and be off summits by 11:30 A.M. There are only a few multiday storm fronts that hit Colorado each summer, so you should have a weather window most mornings to reach your summit. Night hiking is also a nice option in the summer.

Autumn conditions (late September to late October). Autumn is a very brief "season" in Colorado. As the weather cools off, storms become less common. Another benefit of cool air: it does wonders to keep a hard-working hiker from overheating. Beautiful colors emerge in the foliage during this season. There is less daylight and a better potential of snow (and of the rare but dreaded snow-thunderstorm). Autumn is perhaps Colorado's most enjoyable and safest time of the year to climb mountains.

Winter conditions (late October to March). Winter in Colorado is a beautiful and dangerous world. Summits are hard-fought prizes that require in-depth mountaineering experience to attain. Trailheads often require a monumental effort to reach. The skills required for winter conditions take years to develop and demand a hearty constitution. Avalanches, hypothermia, frostbite, and fatigue are constant threats. Personally, I love winter adventures, but they must be undertaken with caution and courage. This book mentions a few good "starter" peaks for winter hiking in Appendix A. For those robust enough to challenge the outdoors in the harsh months, a unique and hidden world is yours to discover!

General First Aid

Mountains in Colorado, even the "easy" ones, are rife with natural booby traps and hidden hazards. Seemingly stable talus fields roll under your feet when you least expect it; solid-looking snow patches will swallow your legs in shin-bruising postholes; rocks will careen down from above like Randy Johnson fastballs. Bumps and bruises are part of the game in the mountains. Minimizing your risks and beefing up your knowledge in case of injury are important factors to safely enjoying the mountains.

Note: This overview is not a substitution for outdoors-related first-aid training. I would highly recommend all backcountry hikers take a wilderness first-aid course and be certified in CPR.

Blisters

Nothing ruins a good hike quite like painful blisters (or a hiking companion who won't shut up about their blisters). Ill-fitting boots are the primary blister-causing culprits, especially new boots that have not been properly broken in. It's a good idea to wear your new boots around town before setting out into the backcountry. Leather boots in particular require a suitable break-in time to mold to the shape of your foot.

Water and moisture also play a role in blister formation. When feet are wet, the skin is softer and easier to blister. Bulky or bunched socks can cause friction blisters. Irritants such as pebbles, twigs, or debris in your boots can also be to blame.

Blister prevention starts with well-fitting boots. The toes should be a little less than half an inch from the end of the boot. Many blisters occur in boots that are too loose or improperly laced during descents. A single-layer, lightweight noncotton sock (such as Smartwool light hiking socks) helps keep feet cool and dry. Wool and wool-synthetic-blends will wick moisture away from the feet. Cotton acts like a sponge, keeping moisture in the fibers and against the skin. I like to bring an extra pair of socks and a small towel in case I splash into an unexpected puddle. For hikes where there will be river crossings, I make sure to bring sandals or water shoes so my boots don't get soaked. For swampy or muddy hikes, a pair of Gore-Tex (or similar waterproof material) gaiters will prevent water/rain from seeping in above the top of your boots. If you are prone to blisters in a specific spot on your foot, adding a piece of moleskin or molefoam can prevent abrasion before it generates a blister.

Blister treatment should be administered at the first sign of discomfort. Most blisters start off as hotspots, which are pink or red disks of irritation on the skin. Applying moleskin or waterproof, plastic tape can ward off blister formation. Avoid using Band-Aids, as the non-adhesive part of the bandage will continue to rub against the skin. If a blister has already developed, do not pop or drain it. Ruptured blisters are breeding grounds for infection! Keep the blister intact; as long as it is not punctured, you will not risk infection. Cut a small circle out of moleskin and pad the area around the blister, leaving the actual blister exposed but below the level of the moleskin material (in other words, make the blister the middle of a moleskin donut). Tape the moleskin in place (covering the blister hole if you wish) with medical tape.

Only if the blister has already ruptured or is too large to comfortably continue hiking should you try to drain it. This should be a last resort. Clean the area thoroughly. Heat a needle with a match or stove flame to sterilize it. Once you have done so, poke a small hole in the bottom of the blister and gently squeeze the fluid out, top to bottom. Immediately clean the wound and apply a sterile pad. Wash the area out several times a day to ward off infection.

Dehydration/Overhydration

Dehydration is the most common ailment suffered in the mountains. Because hikers often don't drink until they feel thirsty, dehydration may not be apparent until the individual feels excessively tired or cranky. It is important to drink before a hike—about 8 to 10 ounces—and continue to drink roughly 8 ounces every half hour.

Dehydration is a catalyst for other more serious problems, such as cramping, hypothermia, and AMS. Signs of dehydration include a loss of energy, dark urine, and moodiness. A well-hydrated hiker should urinate frequently in the mountains, and the liquid should be clear and copious.

Sports drinks such as Gatorade, Cytomax, and Endurox will help replace salts and electrolytes; adding in a mildly salty snack such as pretzels or nuts can help replace salts, which in turn help the body process water. (Electrolytes are electrically conductive ions that help balance fluid levels on the cellular level in the body. This not only means feeding the cells water but also preventing overhydration.)

I like to bring 70 to 100 ounces of water in a hydration pack along with 32 ounces of Gatorade when I hike. I sip from the hydration pack all day and enjoy the Gatorade as a treat on layer breaks, summits, or snack breaks.

Overhydration is rare but something to look out for. Humans cannot process much more than 1 liter (32 ounces) of water per hour; excess water will usually be filtered out through the body. This process can dilute the nutritional absorption of food in the intestines. In other words, if you are dehydrated, there is no need to chug two bottles of water in five minutes; 8 to 16 ounces will be adequate. In extreme cases (usually during marathons or other high-endurance sports) water intoxication can occur. For most hikers, this isn't a threat.

Hypothermia

Hypothermia is a dangerous condition that results from a loss of body heat to the extent that core temperatures fall below 95°F. Prolonged exposure to wind, rain, snow, and chilly temps can bring about hypothermia. Many cases of hypothermia occur on rainy days, when the temperatures can be anywhere between 35°F and 55°F—so this is not just a winter weather malady.

Dehydration can speed up the onset of hypothermia. The initials signs of mild hypothermia include uncontrollable shivering, loss of coordination, and change in mood. Hypothermic hikers may not be able to zipper a coat or put on gloves, and they may not realize where they are. In their confusion, hypothermic victims may insist on continuing to hike or will agree to wait for other members of the party. Never leave a hiker you suspect is hypothermic alone. In severe cases, the victim may become completely disoriented and collapse, unconscious. If core temperatures continue to drop, the victim may lapse into a coma, which can cause permanent damage or death.

Hypothermia must be assessed and dealt with immediately. First priority is to get the victim out of wet clothes and, if possible, out of the wind and weather. Often, layers of dry clothing, adequate shelter, and warmer settings will be enough to reverse mild

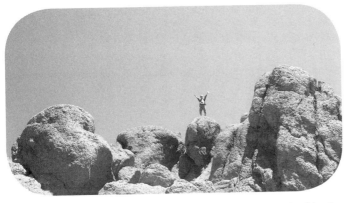

Storm-free days are a reason to celebrate in Colorado!

hypothermia. The victim should consume liquids, preferably those with a sugar base. The liquid does not need to be heated, though a warm mug may feel good in the person's hands. The important thing is to get water into the body. If camping, get the victim into a sleeping bag and heat up water in watertight bottles to place in the bag. In an emergency, body-to-body contact will help, but care must be taken that it doesn't chill the person helping to a state of hypothermia. Warming should be done gradually.

Remember, hypothermia affects judgment and coordination—do not climb higher until you and your partner are certain the effects are gone. On a personal note, I once got mild hypothermia on a 60°F, sunny and windy day, thanks to a very steep snowslope and a poorly wicking first layer (which was brand new). My hiking partner noticed I was shivering, and moreover, that I was complaining—which is not characteristic of me in the mountains. When I peeled off the offending layer, it was soaked with sweat. Before the condition got worse, I put on dry layers and drank Gatorade until I felt better. We finished the day without further incident, but it goes to show, hypothermia can occur in unlikely conditions.

Intestinal Ailments, Giardia, and the Importance of Water Filtration

As the body adjusts to altitude, it often produces more acids in the stomach. Most stomachaches and nausea in the mountains are a direct result of the body responding to changes in elevation. Nerves can also play a role in upset stomachs. For these instances, it is wise to bring along antacids and to avoid fatty foods and alcohol on hikes. More severe nausea that does not respond to antacids can be a sign of AMS; if these are accompanied by vomiting, head down.

Diarrhea may occur if a person is overhydrated, nervous, or experiencing mild AMS. It is important to drink enough to replace liquids in cases of diarrhea; sports drinks and salty snacks will help replenish the body's balance. Because energy bars can be hard to digest (or enjoy) at altitude, I suggest bringing along palatable gels (I prefer chocolate Gu) to help replenish lost electrolytes and sodium.

All water in Colorado should be treated with a filter, purification tablets, or by boiling. That seemingly fresh mountain stream is prime habitat for the pesky protozoan Giardia lamblia, more commonly known as giardia. Giardia has a long incubation period, anywhere between one week and one month. Once infected, an individual will experience awful bouts of explosive diarrhea, flatulence, cramps, vomiting, and dehydration. These symptoms will settle down but still be apparent after an initial period of flu-like symptoms. Giardia will continue to cause trouble until it is properly treated by a medical doctor.

Hygiene and Sanitation

Keeping clean in the outdoors can be a challenge, but staying hygienic is imperative. Good Leave No Trace practices (covered a bit more in the next section) mean you'll have to pack out any nonbiodegradable hygiene products, but staying clean is worth it. Alcohol-based hand-cleaning gels should be used after going to the bathroom, as well as before eating any snacks or preparing meals. Keep those hands clean!

On camping trips, I always bring along baby wipes (such as Wet Ones) to keep myself clean and avoid that "crusty" feeling. These wipes have to be packed out, but they can keep your butt cleaner than wiping with leaves or snow. Women may also want to bring similar wipes for staying clean during their menstrual cycle.

Be cautious when accepting snacks or drinks from strangers; the food is probably safe but the hands of your new friend may not be.

When brushing your teeth, bathing, or washing your hair, make sure to use eco-friendly toothpastes, soaps, and shampoos.

Sunburn/Snowblindness

At high elevation, radiation from the sun is extra powerful and needs to be taken seriously. High in the mountains is not the place to work on your tan. Ultraviolet rays from the sun are more concentrated, the closer you are to the atmosphere, causing untreated skin to burn quickly. Avoid sunburn by applying sunblock with a minimum UV rating of 15 every 90 minutes. In real life, hardly anyone keeps to this schedule while hiking. I like to use a less precise but equally effective system. I keep a small bottle of sunblock in my pocket and put it on every time I stop for snacks, to pee, or to adjust my layers of clothing. Sometimes I'll end up putting it on three times in an hour, but it's better than getting burnt. Keep in mind that even cloudy days shower your body with UV rays.

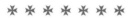

Although you may not have an obvious lobster-red sunburn, even a subtle burn will make sleeping difficult, keep you from hydrating (as the body is repairing the damage), and make you feel achy all over.

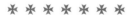

Wearing a wide-brimmed hat, visor, or baseball cap will help keep the sun off your face. Although you may not have an obvious lobster-red sunburn, even a subtle burn will make sleeping difficult, keep you from hydrating (as the body is repairing the damage), and make you feel achy all over. Pain relievers will help you feel better and make sleep come a little easier when a sunburn is keeping you awake. Drink enough liquids to help your body heal. Lotions will help soothe burns and relieve the infernal itching that comes with peeling sunburn.

Note that hiking on snow doubles the amount of radiation being aimed at your body. It's not unusual to get burns on your palms, the roof of your mouth, under your chin, or other less noticeable places from reflected light. Make sure to apply sunscreen everywhere vulnerable.

Trip Outtakes

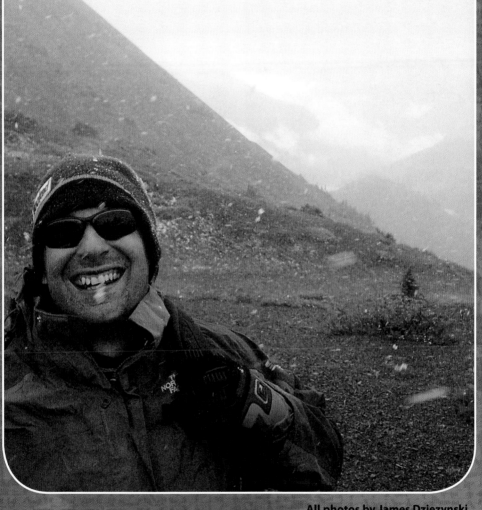

All photos by James Dziezynski
unless otherwise noted

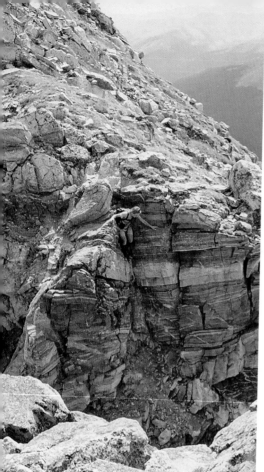

The **Citadel's** twin summits offer fun scrambling to reach their lofty pinnacles. This slot is the easiest way to descend the east summit (photo taken from the west summit).

This mountain goat means business! Remember to respect wildlife, especially those who have a propensity for head-butting hikers off narrow ridges.

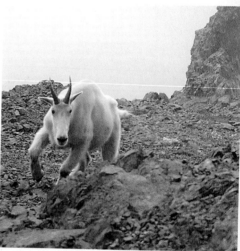

Photo by Jody Pratt

Mount Sniktau starts from the high point of Loveland Pass and offers great views for not a lot of work (relatively speaking!).

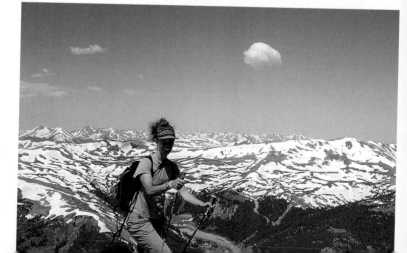

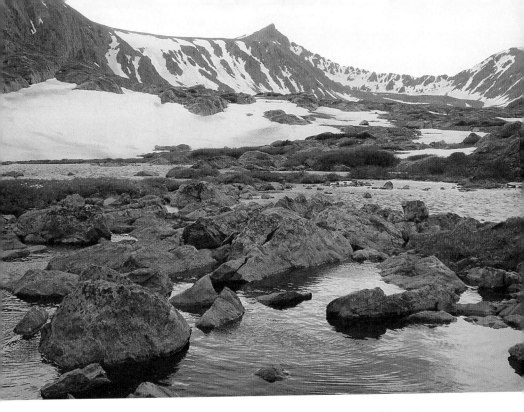

Spring thaw comes to the Mohawk Lake Basin with 13,950-foot **Pacific Peak** looming in the distance.

This inflatable clown suit was the perfect way to celebrate the summit of 14,309-foot **Uncompahgre Peak** and a fine homage to Billy and Benny McCrary of *Guinness Book of World Records* fame.

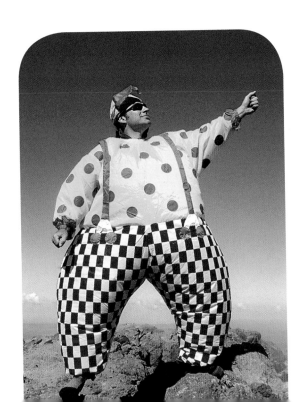

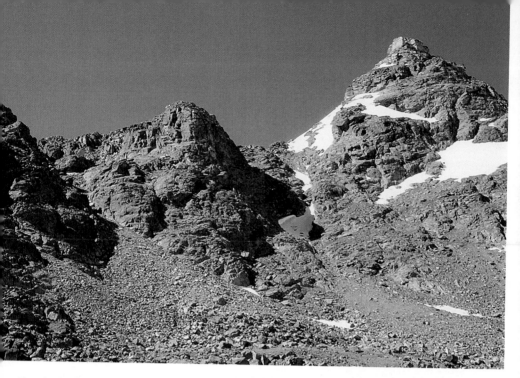

Navajo Peak's classic pyramid resembles an ancient Mayan temple. Airplane Gully is located to the right of the shadow from the pinnacle on the far left.

Breakfast at the **Treasury Peak** Trailhead as storms brew in the background

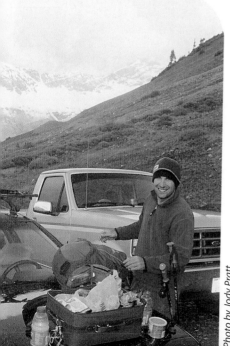

Photo by Jody Pratt

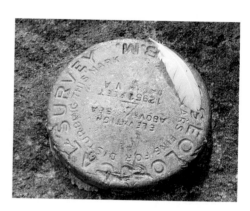

An avian visitor has artistically decorated the summit marker of **Mount Richthofen**.

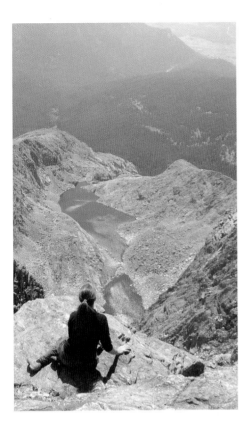

An amazing look at the aptly named Spectacle Lakes from just below the summit of **Ypsilon Mountain** in Rocky Mountain National Park

A gorgeous pasture of wildflowers erupts at the base of the southern **Sawatch Range** peaks.

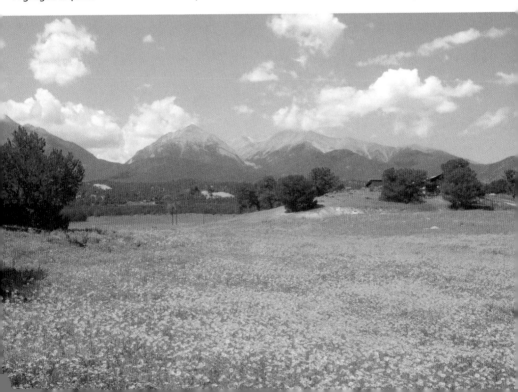

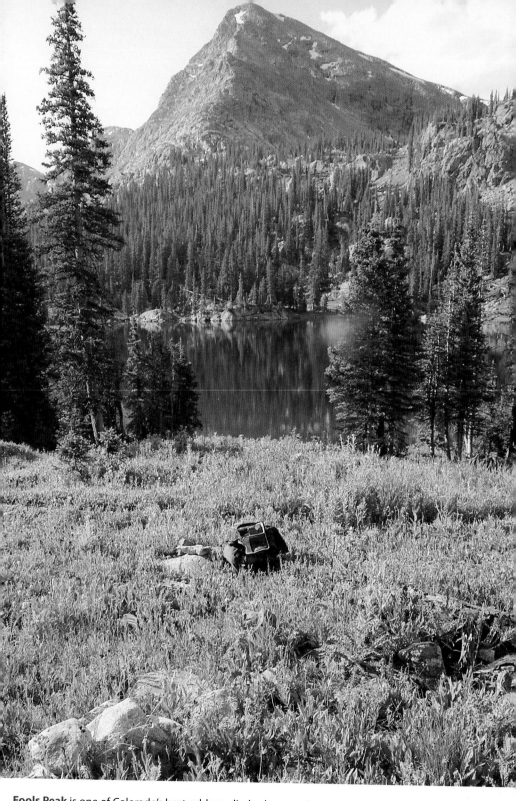

Fools Peak is one of Colorado's best seldom-climbed mountains, and an aesthetically pleasing picture when viewed from Lower Lake Charles.

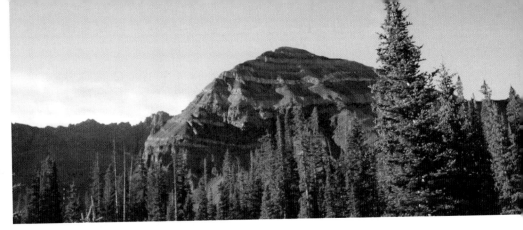

The stripes of **Hesperus Mountain** make me wonder if this is the real Big Rock Candy Mountain.

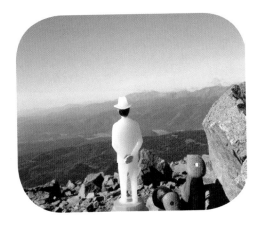

The gully up to the summit of **Mount Sneffels** offers a great look at the colorful palette of the San Juan Mountains (and yes, that's a Hartford Whalers baseball cap on my head).

Señor Misterioso calmly appreciates a stunningly clear day from the summit of **West Spanish Peak.**

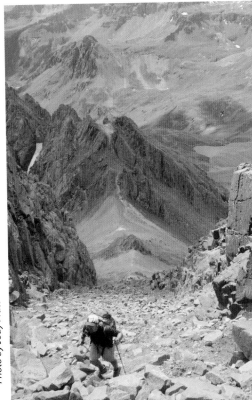

Photo by Jody Pratt

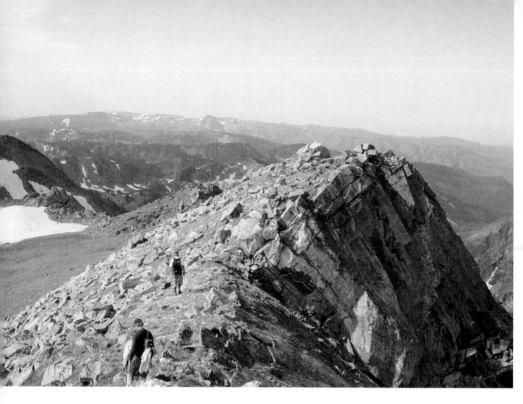

Hikers begin the descent from **Mount Zirkel**. This unique northern panorama looks out onto Steamboat Springs on the horizon.

Bobblehead Goofy is looking the wrong way on the summit of **Eureka Mountain**—he's missing a stunning view of the Sangre De Cristo Mountains!

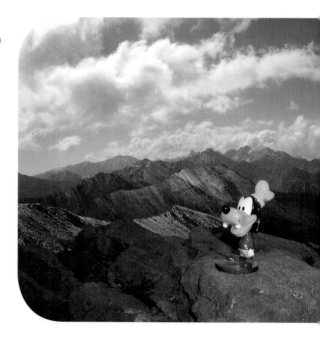

From the Lake Xanadu Basin en route to Jasper Peak, one is treated to this nifty view of **South Arapahoe Peak** and the notable Skywalker Couloir carved into the face of the mountain. May the force be with you!

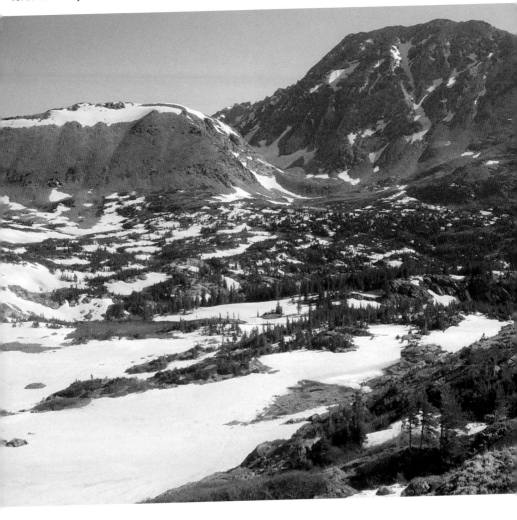

Colorado's sweeping alpine plateaus are perfect for those who love big sky country. The northern valleys extend for miles below the shoulder of **Mount Chapin** in Rocky Mountain National Park.

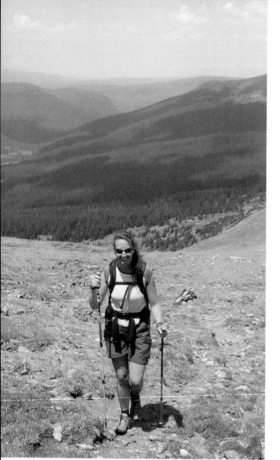

I'm not one to wear a tie to the office, but this was a special occasion. The first hints of autumn are visible from **East Beckwith Mountain**, my 50th and final hike for this book.

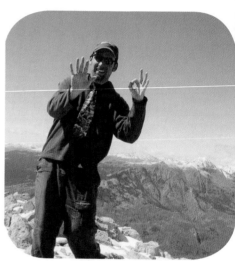

A twilight rainbow neatly frames Telluride's Sheep Mountain, as seen from the trailhead for the **Cross Mountain-Base of Lizard Head Traverse** hike.

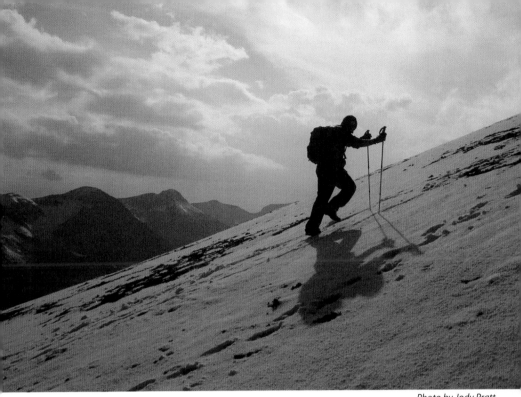

Photo by Jody Pratt

An ephemeral dreamscape of colors following a barrage of storms during the push up **Treasury Mountain**, just outside of Crested Butte

Lead Mountain's exciting ridge is a little-known gem in the Never Summer Range. Bring a helmet and sturdy boots for this airy class 3 ascent.

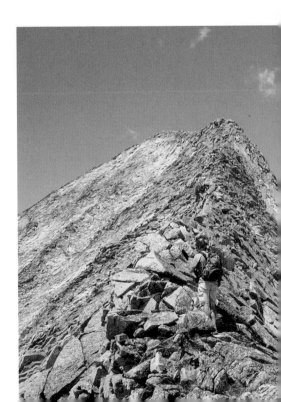

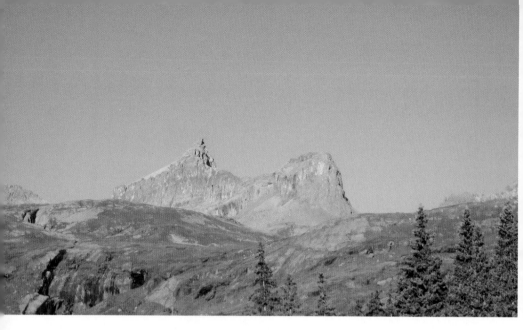

Golden Horn's impressive summit spire rises from the ebony-streaked walls of the Ice Lakes Basin.

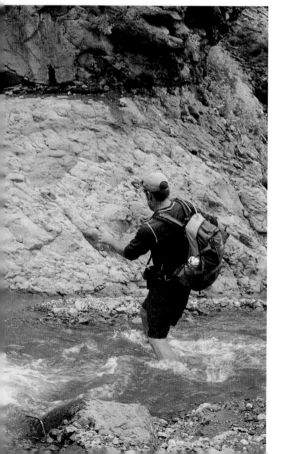

The trickiest part about getting to **Summit Peak** is this chilly stream crossing at "Confusion Rock." The hard-to-spot trail goes uphill to the right of the light grey rock.

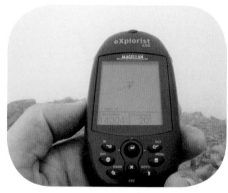

A scandalous elevation reading from the summit of **Mount Ouray**, officially listed at 13,971 feet. The big question: is the accuracy of this GPS unit *plus* or *minus* 20 feet? Could there be one more 14er?

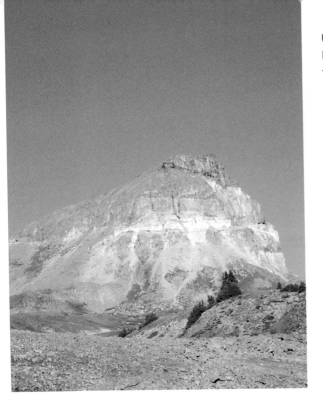

Uncompahgre's "sinking ship" profile on a perfect day in the San Juan Mountains

Sunset as seen from the **Mount Sopris** Trailhead

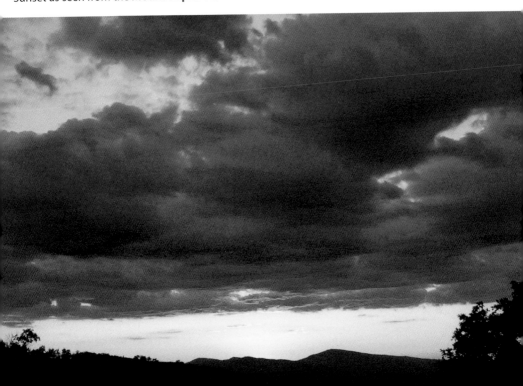

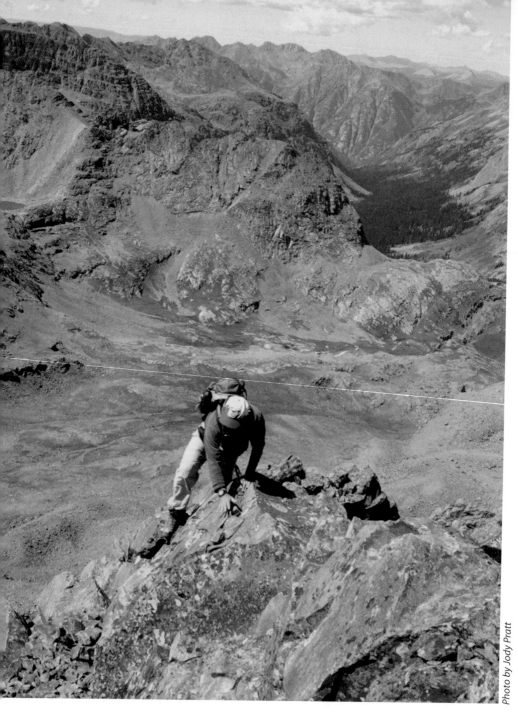

The Whalers hat makes another appearance on the exposed shoulder of **Storm King Peak** in the fabled Grenadier Range.

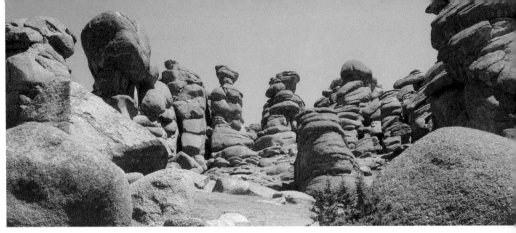

A courtyard of fantasy awaits you on **Bison Peak**. Hundreds of dramatic rock towers comprise this unique summit, which could truly be called the garden of the gods.

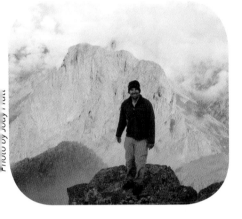

You can be forgiven if you think this photo was taken by Zeus himself; the view is from just below the summit of **Mount Eolus** during a break in the weather.

The locals above Herman Lake en route to Fortress Saddle on the **Citadel**

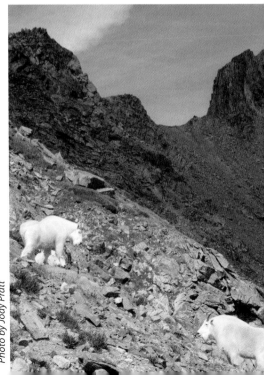

Photo by Jody Pratt

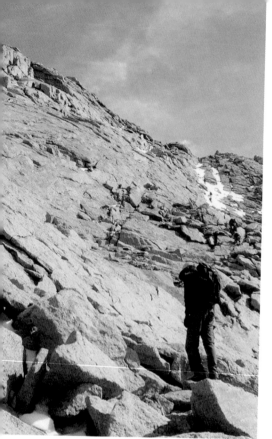

Hikers scale **Longs Peak's** final section, known as the "home stretch." Longs Peak's keyhole route is arguably the best class 3 scramble in Colorado.

The seemingly perilous path to the summit of **Belleview Mountain** is not as tricky as it initially looks. The crumbly consistency of this ridge is similar to what you'll find on the famous Maroon Bells.

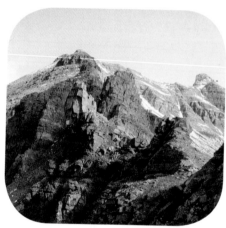

Mount Ida's apex offers superb views of peaceful meadows and alpine lakes. Herds of elk can often be seen grazing in the distance from Ida's spacious summit.

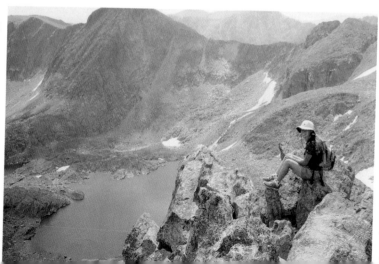

Snowblindness is a painful, often debilitating condition where the cornea of the eye becomes inflamed; put simply, it is sunburn of the eyes. Once afflicted, the condition takes several days to go away. The victim will experience severe headaches, sleeplessness, and general fatigue. There's not much one can do to expedite healing, other than staying in a dark room and keeping up a steady dose of ibuprofen. I will say this several times in this book: do not skimp on good eye protection. Make sure your glasses are large enough to cover the entire area around your eyes, including the sides and bottom. Lenses must block out 95% to 100% of all UVA and UVB radiation. Prevention of snowblindness is easy; recovery is not.

Heat Exhaustion

Heat exhaustion occurs when the body works up excessive heat that it cannot effectively dissipate. Dehydration is the first symptom of heat exhaustion; most cases are triggered by exertion in hot, dry environments. A victim will have cool and clammy skin, weakness, nausea, and may even faint. In extreme cases (known as heat stroke), the pulse will be rapid and the victim may become seriously disoriented.

Cooling the victim down and providing fluids are important steps in reversing this condition. Cease any strenuous activity, and rest, preferably with the feet elevated. Work on cooling the face, head, and body. Find shelter in the shade, or set up a tent (with the doors open) to provide shade if you are above treeline. Many cases of heat exhaustion occur when there is snow on the ground; use it to your advantage to help cool the victim. Once the person feels better and can hold down liquids, assess the situation. Unless the person is feeling 100%, descend and try for your summit another day.

Frostbite

Frostbite is a painful and serious condition in which the blood vessels in the body freeze and crystallize, causing damage to body tissue and circulation. Injury from frostbite can cause permanent impairments, and in severe cases, loss of appendages. Most frostbite will occur on the nose, ears, fingers, and toes. When the body gets cold, it prioritizes the areas close to the heart, leaving body regions distant from the core vulnerable to the cold. Initial symptoms include a bluish discoloration of the skin, sharp pain, numbness, and a burning sensation. If caught in the early stages (considered "frostnip"), warming the injured body part will prevent further damage. Note that frostbite rarely appears without hypothermia, so make sure to treat your victim for all conditions.

In severe cases, the skin will become blue or black, and hideous blisters may swell up. Never rub or try to massage frostbitten skin; this will only further damage tissue. Only a slow and painful thawing of the injury in lukewarm water will regain sensation. In these cases, evacuate the victim and seek medical attention. If the foot is severely frostbitten, do not attempt to thaw it in the field; once rewarmed, it will be too painful to walk on.

Note that women are more prone to frostbite than men. Poor circulation, diabetes, or overly tight clothing and footwear can also promote frostbite. Alcohol should also be avoided in cold conditions, as it can dehydrate a body and make the limbs less sensitive to the warning signs of frostbite as it develops.

Fractures, Sprains, and Broken Bones

Twisted ankles and sprained wrists are amongst the most common injuries in the mountains. Any swollen or bruised limb should be tended to immediately. SAM splints (soft aluminum splints lined with foam) or inflatable splints are lightweight and can be used to set and immobilize injuries. In a pinch, you can use hiking poles, sleeping pads, or an ice axe to set an injured limb. Anti-inflammatory medicines should be taken by the injured hiker, and evacuation should begin as soon as possible.

Shock

Shock occurs whenever the body experiences a sudden loss of blood pressure. Normally, blood loss from an injury causes this sensation, but people can incur shock (in the medical term) from witnessing a disturbing event or from sheer panic. Loss of blood pressure can disrupt the circulatory system, and if prolonged, can cause permanent damage to vital organs or death. A victim of shock may display any of the following symptoms: confusion, rapid pulse, clammy skin, dull or distant eyes, and rapid breathing. Additionally, the victim may feel nau-

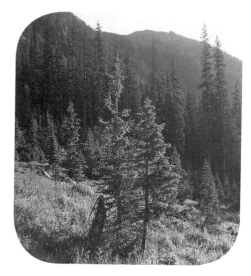

The piney deeps near Deming Mountain

seous, weak, and frightened. If shock occurs, do everything you can to keep the person warm. If they are conscious, provide liquids. Talk to the victims and reassure them they are not alone. Be calm and help ease them by tactfully apprising them of the situation. Seek medical attention if victims experience shock—and always in the case of blood loss.

Panic

Mountains can be intimidating places, and for good reasons. No matter how experienced the hiker, the bottom line is that Mother Nature holds the trump card when it comes to control. Storms, stress, exposure to heights, witnessing an accident, or unexpected illnesses can induce panic. A panicked individual can "lock up," both physically and mentally. Fear can literally make one weak in the knees and impair balance and judgment, often in the places where concentration and focus are imperative. If you begin to panic, focus on taking at least five deep breaths. Remember, your body is reacting to a perceived risk—one that must be dealt with using logical thought. If you are on tricky terrain, breathe deeply and flex your fingers slowly a few times—assure your body that your mind still has control. Figure out your safest option and follow through with confidence. This advice is easy to dispense from the comfort of my warm office, but it's a bit more difficult to execute in the heat of the moment. My own experience has been that when you control your breathing, you control your mind, and thus control your body.

If you are with companions who begin to panic, talk to them calmly and reassure them of their options in simple, supportive language. Offer suggestions in a positive tone. Once the moment of panic is over (for example, a tricky move has been accomplished) continue to be reassuring and positive. Panic is one of those ailments that is really all in the head—which proves that mountain climbing is just as much about mental strength as it is powerful legs and lungs.

Suggested First-Aid Kit

Every hiker should carry an individual first-aid kit. In addition, groups heading into the backcountry should also carry a group kit with extra supplies or individual-specific drugs. Keep in mind that pre-existing conditions should be known before heading into the backcountry and appropriate medical treatments should be included in your kit. Here is sample list of what every basic first-aid kit should have:

- Adhesive bandages (Band-Aids or similar brand): Minimum of 10 standard 1-inch bandages

- Butterfly bandages: to serve as temporary stitches for minor wounds

- Sterile pads: at least two medium and two large pads for larger wounds

- Antibiotic ointment packets or tubes (Neosporin or similar brand): to help wounds heal

- Roller bandages: to wrap around wounds and hold dressings in place

- Medical tape: to secure dressings or to tape up fingers and hands when climbing

- Moleskin: used to pad blisters or as a blister preventative

- Alcohol pads: used to clean small wounds. For large wounds, use soap and water with a syringe (alcohol will damage exposed tissues). Make sure to replace these pads in your kit every six months, as they can dry out even when left in the package.

- Iodine: used as antiseptic to clean out wounds

- Thermometer: used to gauge body temperature

- Medical scissors: used to cut medical tape or dressings

- Aspirin: used as a painkiller and also as a blood thinner (which may help with altitude adjustment). Avoid giving aspirin to children; instead administer acetaminophen-based pain relievers such as Tylenol.

- Ibuprofen: good old "vitamin I." Ibuprofen is an anti-inflammatory that is available under brand names such as Advil, Motrin, and Nuprin.

- Sugar packets or sugar candies: used for low blood sugar, notably when diabetes is present

- Elastic bandage (ACE or similar brand): used to compress sprains or similar injuries

- Sanitary pads: not only useful for female hygiene, but they also serve to absorb blood in larger wounds

- Rubber gloves: used to prevent infection from body fluids or wounds

- Sterile tweezers: used to remove debris, slivers, ticks, or glass from skin

- Syringe: used to wash out wounds

- Safety pins: various uses, including holding dressings in place

- Resealable plastic bags (Ziploc or similar brand): used to pack out contaminated materials

- Foam-lined aluminum splint (SAM or similar brand): used to mobilize a broken or fractured limb

- Antacids (Tums or similar products): used to neutralize stomach acids
- Laxatives: used to help with bowel movements
- Pen and paper to record accident vitals

Besides these things, I keep a small LED light in my first-aid kit; these lights are inexpensive and can come in handy when fumbling through your kit at night. Make sure you get one that doesn't "squeeze" to light up—it's hard to dress a wound while keeping a squeeze light on. I keep two packets of energy gels for instances when a body needs fast, easy-to-digest energy. I bring an emergency reflective blanket to keep myself or a victim warm. I also leave two to four extra batteries of the appropriate size to fit my headlamps or GPS units in my first-aid kit.

A few other items to consider:

- Sunscreen
- Lip balm with sunblock (such as ChapStick)
- Hand warmers
- CPR mask/shield
- Small backup knife or multitool (such as a Leatherman)

People who have allergies to bee stings should carry epinephrine pens, which are available through your doctor. Other prescriptions drugs such as Diamox (to deal with altitude) should be acquired as needed from your doctor. Note that sleeping pills are not tolerated well at altitude and should be avoided.

Nutrition: Eating Smart

Most outings into the mountains will take several hours, so you'll need an extended form of energy to perform well throughout the day. Carbohydrates are vital for extended energy, while simple sugars can give you a boost of short-term energy. Fatty foods are difficult for the body to digest and should be avoided at altitude. Snacks should be eaten throughout the day to keep from "bonking," a term usually used to describe the effects of low blood sugar or lack of fuel for the body.

What Works

Easy-to-digest foods, such as bananas, granola, nuts, dried fruits, peanut butter, and simple sandwiches on wheat/grain breads are all good energy sources.

Eat what tastes good to you. If you like a turkey and mustard sandwich in "normal life," it's a good idea to take it on your hike with you. Palatable foods are just as important as healthy foods.

Pasta and potatoes give a good boost of carbohydrates and serve well as a meal the night before a big hike. Breads, crackers, and dried fruits (raisins, for example) are good sources of carbohydrates the day of the hike.

Breakfast can be a tricky issue for hikers. Since your body is probably not used to getting up at the early hours required to get a safe start on the trail, breakfast may be unappealing. My trick for such mornings: if I am driving to the trailhead and my stomach doesn't feel like eating when I awake, I'll make a point to eat a peanut butter and jelly sandwich when I am 45 minutes or so from the trailhead. Delaying breakfast gives me time to wake up and actually enjoy the food instead of forcing it down.

Fruits are always good choices at altitude. Many have natural ingredients that help active bodies; for example, bananas have high potassium levels that help ward off cramps. Besides tasting good, they are good sources of natural sugars and there is even speculation that some fruits, like pineapple, may help bodies adjust to altitude.

My Personal Food System

I like to start every hike with a peanut butter and jelly sandwich on whole wheat bread, a few snack crackers such as Goldfish, and two packets of Gu chocolate energy gel. As an added bonus (or a psychological boost), I traditionally enjoy a two-pack of Hostess Sno-Balls, preferably pink. Throughout the day I munch on crackers, hard candies (Jolly Rancher are my favorite), salty nuts, dried peaches, and additional peanut butter and jelly sandwiches (I usually bring two for the hike). Before heading up tough, steep terrain (or if I feel my energy waning) I'll have another Gu packet. I avoid energy bars, as I personally cannot stand the texture and taste, though that's a purely personal opinion—they do provide good energy if you can swallow them down! Because I snack throughout the day, I generally won't stop for a formal lunch. I also make sure to keep snacking on the way down, when it's easy to forget your body needs fuel even though you aren't exerting yourself as much as on the way up. I

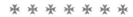

I'm probably not going to chomp down hot dogs and chug Mountain Dew when I'm over 12,000 feet. Finding the balance of foods that taste good to you and provide adequate energy comes with time and by listening to your body.

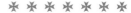

often keep hard candy or gum in my mouth throughout the day to keep it from drying out in the thin air. When I have concluded my hike, I make sure to eat a little extra to help aid my body in the recovery process.

What's important is that I like all the foods I eat when I hike. It sounds obvious, but if I were to switch to handfuls of granola and tofu treats, I simply wouldn't eat as much—and I'd have much less energy! Likewise, I'm probably not going to chomp down hot dogs and chug Mountain Dew when I'm over 12,000 feet. Finding the balance of foods that taste good to you and provide adequate energy comes with time and by listening to your body.

What to Avoid

As previously mentioned, fatty foods are tough to digest at altitude. Most junk food won't seem palatable at higher elevations, since saturated fats and oils won't be prioritized by your body. Not only can fatty foods make your stomach churn, they can slow active hikers down by providing inefficient energy sources.

Coffee is a diuretic that can promote dehydration, though the psychological boost (not to mention the caffeine) makes a cup of joe a morning ritual for many hikers. Don't drink too much coffee on the morning of a hike. One cup should do the trick.

Alcohol is an obvious no-no during the hike, as it not only promotes dehydration but can also impair judgment. Save those celebratory beers for after the hike! In general, the effects of alcohol at altitude, both good and bad, are amplified. Consider this before partying too hard the night before a big hike—if you get a hangover, it's going to feel twice as bad at altitude and last twice as long.

Note that you may come across delicious wild berries on your hikes. These are generally safe to eat, but it's a good idea to wash them off with filtered water if you are unsure of their cleanliness. Remember, however, you may be doing yourself more harm than good if you rinse them off in rivers or lakes, as such water can carry giardia.

Gear

As much as I appreciate a good pair of lederhosen, I can't blame modern hikers for outfitting themselves in more practical (if less stylish) attire. Modern mountain fashion has evolved to be both functional and fashionable. Gone are the days when your average alpinist resembled a threatening, grizzled version of Jim Henson (with fewer teeth). Advances in gear technology are a big reason why more and more people keep heading to the hills.

You don't need to have the latest and greatest in everything to enjoy the mountains, but I highly recommend not skimping on two vital items: boots and sunglasses. Boots are going to be what physically connect you with the mountain. Since you will be on your feet for many hours, you owe it yourself to get the most comfortable and functional footwear you can. Likewise, high-quality sunglasses will keep your eyes safe in the optically hostile environment of high-altitude sunlight. As a hiker on a budget, I'm reluctant to spend big bucks on trendy new gear, but keeping my eyes and feet in top shape is worth every last dollar.

Footwear/Boots/Gaiters

Boots are the most important pieces of gear for hikers. Proper fit, durability, and grippy outsoles (the tread) are essential qualities in a good boot. Different boots perform well in different settings, though with enough time on the trail, you'll begin to develop a penchant for a particular type of boot. Here's a rundown of mountain footwear:

Trail Runners. Pros: Trail runners are running shoes that have been beefed up to handle trail duty. These shoes are lightweight and offer a bit more "foot control," thanks to their lack of bulk. Many hikers (including me) like to use trail runners on mountains where there are established trails, dry terrain, or semitechnical scrambling. Cons: Trail shoes fare poorly in snow, mud, or other wet conditions. Avoid off-trail hiking and bushwacking in trail runners. Talus fields and rocky gullies can awkwardly twist ankles; trail runners do not provide good support on such uneven and loose terrain.

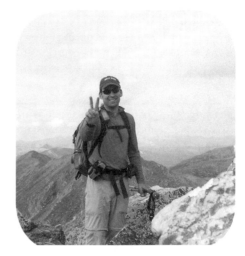

Light Hiking Boots. Pros: Light hikers are the perfect "all-around" boot: light enough to keep your feet from getting fatigued, tough enough to stand up to burly mountain conditions. A good light hiking boot starts with a solid outsole (such as Vibram or similar rubber blends) and is flexible yet supportive. Some brands use a Gore-Tex lining to

Good gear makes for happy hikers.

make the boot waterproof without adding excess weight. Cons: Many light hiking boots compromise on outsoles; imitation or cheap outsoles wear out quickly and slip on rocks. Look for good outsoles and you'll be in good shape. Light hikers lack support when you're carrying a heavy backpack, and like trail runners, they may not be adequately protective on rocky scree slopes or in snowy conditions.

Backpacking Boots. Pros: Backpacking boots are obviously great when you're lugging heavy loads; their sturdy design is intended to offer superb durability and excellent support. Traditional backpacking boots are made of hard-wearing leather, though newer models have cut off a few ounces by using ultraresilient synthetics such as Kevlar. Backpacking boots have great ankle support and are perfect for off-trail terrain as well as loose rock slopes and talus fields. Cons: Backpacking boots can be heavy, slow to dry, and tough to break in. Some hikers feel clumsy when trying to scramble or climb in bulkier boots, though climbing rock in boots is a skill that comes with practice. Ventilation is compromised, and hikers with hot feet may feel uncomfortable as their little piggies roast on long trails.

Mountaineering Boots. Pros: These specialized boots are made for the harshest conditions! Most models are leather, leather blends, or plastic. They are extremely stiff and protective, thanks to sturdy shanks that reinforce the foot bed. Nearly all models have notches to accept crampons. Their rigidity is essential when climbing ice or technical snow with crampons. Plastic boots include insulated liners and many leather boots have built-in insulation to keep feet warm. Cons: Mountaineering boots are made for snow, ice, prolonged mixed routes, and cold weather. As a result, they are very bulky, heavy, and require extended break-in periods. They are also quite expensive. These specialized boots are only required if you plan to attempt winter or early-spring ascents. Note that many backpacking boots and even some light hiking boots will accept certain crampons for basic snow travel. Ask at your local outdoors store if you'd like to try a lighter solution for simple snowfield travel.

Along with good boots, you're going to need a quality pair of socks. Your socks should fit without bunching and have padding in high-friction areas, such as the toes. Avoid cotton socks because they absorb moisture and keep sweat against your skin. Most hiking socks are made of high-quality wool such as merino wool, or a wool/synthetic blend. There is no need to layer socks—modern socks wick moisture from the feet and dry relatively quickly, eliminating the need for a liner. As a hot-footed hiker, I use thin wool running socks for most hikes.

A neglected piece of "footwear" is a useful pair of gaiters. Gaiters are knee-high leggings that fit over boots and keep snow, water, and debris from leaking in above the cuff of the boot. Gaiters are ideal in muddy or snowy conditions, which are typical in early spring. The ever-stylish shorts-with-gaiters look is a telltale sign of a transplanted New England hiker.

Since I am often asked about the footwear I use, here are the facts, current as of the writing of this book. I wear Salomon X-A Pro trail runners, Tecnica Vento Mids as my light hikers, and a pair of beautifully crafted, all-leather, lined-with-Gore-Tex Aku Utah Lite GTX backpacking boots.

Eyewear

High-altitude sun is especially harmful to our eyes, which is why I highly recommend tossing that adorable pair of Hello Kitty shades for something a bit more mountain worthy. Good mountain sunglasses will have lenses that block out 95% to 100% of UVA and UVB rays. Make sure your lenses don't distort your depth perception, a common feature of cheap sunglasses. Also ensure that peripheral light is adequately shielded. Frames should fit comfortably on your head; glasses that are too tight can form friction sores behind the ears (ouch!). Finally, secure your glasses with a tether (such as Croakies) to prevent them from falling off in case of a slip.

Layers

Dressing in layers instead of a single garment is standard practice in the mountains. Temperatures fluctuate at various points in a single hike, from the hot sun in the parking lot to the chilly gusts on summit ridges. A simple system of layers will help keep you comfortable in every weather condition.

Technical hiking clothes aim to keep you dry and warm. The ability of fabrics to wick and draw moisture away from the skin allows garments to dry quickly and prevent chills from your own sweat. Here's a rundown of a good layering system:

First layer: Thin, lightweight, and nice to the touch. Your first layer rests against your skin, so it should fit well and dry quickly. Cotton is a no-no for the upper body (read the sidebar, "Cotton Kills?," below); it does not wick and can make you very cold. An adequate quick-drying shirt is usually made of synthetic fibers, such as Bergelene, polypropelene, or Capilene. Old-school hikers may prefer silk, which is functional but gets very smelly after a few uses. For the lower body, go with underwear that is comfortable. Synthetic, wicking underwear is available in both short and long versions. If you are not donning long underwear, cotton briefs are acceptable (especially for women, who find that cotton ventilates better). Or you can always go "commando" and not wear any undies at all!

Second layer: This is your insulating layer. Fleece jackets are a great choice, especially microfleece and Windstopper garments. Vests can help keep your core warm and are easy to stuff in your backpack. For the lower body, nylon or synthetic fabric shorts or pants will do just fine. Zip-off pants that convert into shorts are popular and practical. Avoid cotton jeans and other cotton pants, as they will keep moisture next to you body.

Third layer: In colder weather, bringing along a down or thick fleece jacket is a good idea. Keep in mind that it can snow in any month in Colorado, so if there are storms forecasted, it's not a bad idea to bring an extra layer of warmth any time of year.

Outer shell layers: Complement your layering system with a waterproof, windproof shell. Gore-Tex or equivalent shell fabrics will keep you dry while allowing heat and water vapor from the inside to vent. For pants, lightweight, water-resistant garments are acceptable unless you intend to glissade on snow, in which case, you'll want something tougher. Gore-Tex pants with reinforced knees and butts are perfect for glissading.

Cotton Kills?

Perhaps "cotton kills" is a bit overdramatic, but it's not entirely off the mark. Cotton is hydrophilic, meaning it loves to absorb water. This makes it a poor choice to wear when you're working up a sweat in the mountains. Heat loss is rapid when moisture is present, and cotton garments keep sweat against your skin, making your body work harder to heat up and stay warm. Cotton garments that get saturated can chill a body, even in mild temperatures, bringing on dangerous hypothermia. In this regard, cotton can indeed be a catalyst to life-threatening conditions.

Cotton should be avoided as an upper-body layer in all cases, especially against the skin. The same goes for cotton jeans, pants, and shorts. The only place cotton is acceptable on a hiker's body is over your naughty bits. Cotton briefs and panties are fine, since you won't be sweating excessively in these areas. (Or, as many hikers prefer, don't wear underwear at all). Finally, avoid wearing the classic cotton "waffle" long underwear so popular in the Midwest; you'll essentially be wearing a skintight sponge.

Backpacks

Backpacks for dayhikes should be able to carry all your gear and food. A volume of 1800 to 2500 cubic inches will give you enough room to stuff everything in. A good pack will fit comfortably on the back. Most will have adjustable shoulder straps, a waist belt, and a chest strap. Another good feature of many packs: an inner hydration sleeve to hold a water bladder (such as a CamelBak). A backpack made of high-quality, abrasion-resistant material will be more wear-resistant, and may even give curious marmots a challenge when they try to gnaw their way to your M&Ms!

Hydration Systems

I'm a big fan of hydration systems. CamelBaks and similar systems let you hydrate without stopping, meaning you can take small sips throughout the day without much effort. Water bladders of 70 to 100 ounces should suffice for dayhikes in Colorado. The one drawback with hydration systems is that they freeze easily. When hiking in temps at or near freezing, blow water from your straw back into the bladder to keep the tube from freezing solid. Tube and bladder insulators are available, but for extremely cold weather, you're better off using water bottles and insulated holders.

Headwear/Neck Gaiters

Baseball caps, visors, and wide-brimmed hats are great for keeping sun off your face and are recommended at elevation. Cotton baseball caps and visors are ok, but for winter-style caps, go for fleece, wool, or wool blends. Soft fleece neck gaiters are a secret weapon in staying warm. While it's true you lose a great deal of heat through your head, you also lose a good percentage of warmth through your neck. Keep it warm with a neck gaiter

Gloves

Gloves can be layered for effective warmth. Thin liner gloves are often warm enough to keep your hands comfortable on windy days. Shell gloves are needed for colder weather or when traveling on snowfields. For really chilly conditions, use a mitt instead of a glove (keeping the fingers together keeps them warmer), along with a waterproof, windproof shell. Convertible mitts that pull back to allow the fingers to perform dexterous tasks are useful as well.

Navigation and GPS

Paper maps are a must for every hike, as well as basic knowledge in using a compass. Because electronics can fail, you need to have a reliable manual system to navigate vast landscapes. Dense forests and barren tundra are prime venues for people to become disoriented. That said, I am a huge proponent of GPS navigation. Today's GPS systems are accurate, affordable, and most have improved battery life and satellite locking. Integrating a GPS with your computer can help you track out hikes or examine your stats when you are finished. This book is very "GPS-centric." For tracking the hikes in this book, I used two Magellan eXplorist 600 units, an older Magellan Meridian Platinum for backup, and a basic Magellan eXplorist 100 for super backup. When fully equipped, I resembled a deranged, bird-watching cyborg. More detailed explanations on using GPS with this book are given on page 50.

Besides triangulating your position on Earth, many GPS units offer additional helpful information such as elevation, distance traveled, barometric pressure, time of day, elevation maps and contours, temperature, bearing, and heading. More advanced units also have accurate compasses and storm-warning features. GPS units are fun, functional, and add a margin of safety to the hiker who knows how to use them.

Watches

Keeping track of the time is important to ensure you elude the inevitable afternoon thunderstorms. Most watches will function perfectly fine at altitude. If you are using a watch that measures altitude and barometric pressure (most watches use barometric pressures to determine altitude, so you will probably have both functions), make sure to calibrate your watch at the beginning of your hike. All hikes in this book have an accurate starting elevation you can use to set your watch's altimeter.

Useful Extras

Here's a short list of a few additional items you may find helpful in the outdoors:

Trekking poles: Amazingly, the most-asked question I've gotten on hikes is whether or not I like using my trekking poles. I love 'em! I know they aren't for everyone, but they suit me well. Besides stabilizing my hiking, they help me set a good cadence. I use them to test snow and water depths, and in a pinch, I've used them to scare away animals. Some people find them cumbersome, but I recommend giving them a try—I rarely hike without mine.

Cell phones: We are all aware of the egregious faux-pas of calling your friends and family from the summit—"Guess where I am!"—right? Ok, maybe I'm being a bit harsh. Actually, cell phones are good to have in case of emergencies, though getting signals in the backcountry can be spotty. For solo hikers, calling to report you are safely off a mountain will alleviate the worry of your anxious friends.

Sandals or watershoes: Bring these along if you anticipate water crossings. The last thing you want is to slog around for hours in waterlogged boots.

Minitripods: For exquisite mountain photography, tripods are the way to go. Small, inexpensive, and lightweight tripods are perfect for summit shots. These smaller 'pods fit easily into the side pouches of backpacks.

Extra cords/straps: I like to carry a small length of cord on the topmost loop-strap on my backpack. In scrambling situations on sketchy terrain, I'll use it to lower my backpack. In can be unnerving when an outcropping of rock nudges you outward while you're attempting a tricky move! Taking off the pack and sending it down first is a safe and smart idea. There are countless other situations where extra cord is useful, especially when camping in the backcountry.

Cameras

With the digital revolution in cameras, it is easier than ever to get great shots while on the mountain. Knowing how to operate your camera is obviously beneficial, and digital cameras let you fool around with settings without the prohibitive cost of film development. I'm no expert when it comes to photography, but I can offer a few basic tips. Use a low-speed film setting on bright days to capture colors more vibrantly. Bring along tripods for landscape shots or summit pictures. Remember, when it comes to mountain photography, the first key to taking great pictures is simply being there.

To learn how to take really great shots, take an outdoor photography course or buy an outdoor photography book.

Hiking Ethics

The 10 Essentials

This longstanding list has withstood the test of time. These survival items should be in your pack every time you head into the backcountry:

1) Complete basic first-aid kit, with items updated every six months

2) Map and compass

3) Pocketknife and emergency whistle

4) Matches and firestarter

5) Emergency bivvy sack/blanket/shelter

6) Flashlight or headlamp

7) Clothing for warmth and for rain protection

8) Extra food

9) Extra water

10) Sun protection

The ever-important 11th Essential is a hiking companion (although I wouldn't recommend trying to stuff him or her in your pack!).

Leave No Trace

Leave No Trace ethics promote a system of keeping wilderness areas pristine by minimizing human impact. There are eight basic tenets in Leave No Trace travel:

1) Plan ahead and prepare.

2) Travel and camp on durable surfaces.

3) Dispose of waste properly.

4) Leave what you find.

5) Minimize campfire impact.

6) Respect wildlife.

7) Be considerate of other visitors.

8) Pack out what you pack in.

In addition to these rules, I would suggest picking up any trash you find along the trail and pack it out.

Trail Ethics

When out on the trail, you'll meet all manner of man and beast. It's important to be respectful of the land, the wildlife, and other hikers. Here's a simple list of 10 things you can do to maintain courtesy in the backcountry:

1) Greet other hikers with at least a smile. On crowded peaks, you may be smiling a lot, but there's nothing wrong with that, is there?

2) Be tactful before offering unsolicited advice. Most people will ask for help if they need it when in the mountains.

3) No matter how friendly your dog is, if he jumps on strangers or insists on thrusting his snout into their groins, keep him on a leash!

4) If someone needs help, help them. It sounds logical, but I've seen many people refuse to help others in need for whatever reason. Of course, if you are traveling solo (especially if you're a woman), use your best judgment before committing to helping others. Unfortunately, that's the way of the world.

5) Always yield to uphill hikers and don't be offended if they don't say hi. It's tough work climbing at altitude—give them room to maintain their pace.

6) Yield to horses and bikers. And don't step aside with a scowl; they'll pass in a few seconds.

7) Don't be afraid to tell new "trail friends" that you would like to hike alone (or with your partner). Likewise, respect the wishes of others you may meet on the trail. Remember, many people embrace the solitude found in the mountains.

8) Encourage other hikers and keep a positive tone.

9) Never downplay other hikers' accomplishments, and never speak in condescending tones. Boasting that you hike Mount Elbert as a warm-up is obviously going to deflate the hiker who trained all winter to reach the top. We all climb for different reasons.

10) Finally, don't take out your frustrations on your hiking partners. If you don't feel good, or if it's not your day, say so. Alert your partners if you are starting to feel "off" or ill. Good communication will make every outing a better experience.

Using This Book

My goal in writing this book was simple: provide accurate information for the best summit hikes in Colorado in an enjoyable-to-read format. All of the standard routes in this book are nontechnical and may be climbed without ropes or protection, though some sections may require scrambling and exposed moves. Although I provide a difficulty rating system, I always say there are no "easy" mountains in Colorado. Because of the variable nature of weather and the influence of altitude, even a short hike with mild terrain can be difficult for the uninitiated hiker. Likewise, a technical scramble may be less taxing on your legs, and therefore be easier on your body. Be ready to sweat, no matter where you hike…and bring your camera. These are truly the best summit hikes in Colorado!

Driving Directions

I find clear, concise driving directions of the utmost importance—starting a day late and frustrated because you couldn't find the trailhead is not only annoying, it can take you out of a safe weather window. I put extra time and effort into writing my directions, and I hope they will get you to the trailhead with ease. Because backcountry roads can change, I encourage readers to call ahead to see if conditions are suitable for your vehicle.

Vehicle Recommendations

In describing the types of vehicles that can reach certain trailheads, I've added notes for those of us who don't have 4x4, high-clearance trucks (48 of the 50 hikes in this book were driven to in a front-wheel-drive Honda Accord). When I mention the types of vehicles needed to reach the trailheads, here is what I mean:

Passenger Car (PC): Passenger cars are any vehicle with low clearance and without off-road modifications. In this regard, minivans are often included in this class. Trailheads that have easy access via a paved road or well-maintained dirt roads are perfect for cars.

Tough Passenger Car (TPC): This is a politically correct way to describe a "beater," a vehicle you aren't afraid to sacrifice a few parts of to reach a trailhead. My car fits this bill perfectly! Trailheads that TPCs can reach are generally passable but may have a few areas where your car will bottom out or have to blast through mud and water. My Accord made it up some wild roads during the research for this book, including the access roads to Pacific Peak and the "shelf of horror" on Mount Sneffles. I'm not saying you should drive your car as if it were a TPC, but the odds of reaching the trailhead are in your favor if you have the guts (and don't mind a few bangs and bumps). Good luck and Godspeed!

Sport Utility Car (SUC): Sport Utility Cars describe any light-duty, off-road vehicle with decent clearance. All-wheel-drive (AWD) or 4x4 or transmissions are standard for most of these vehicles. (Note that AWD drive is inferior to true 4x4. AWD uses power transfers to relegate a certain amount of available torque to whatever wheel can best use it, while 4x4 spreads an even amount of torque over all four wheels, giving them each power and traction at all times.) SUCs can handle mildly rutted roads, relatively steep terrain, and some rocky roads, though those without a "low" 4x4 option may have trouble. I've seen SUCs at trailheads where I am convinced they must have been dropped off by helicopter (such as on Uncompahgre Peak). Examples of this type include: Subaru Outback, Toyota RAV4, Honda CRV, Honda Element, Ford Escape, and small pickup trucks.

Sport Utility Vehicle (SUV): It may be odd to see these lawyer-pleasing behemoths beyond the familiar confines of the Starbucks parking lot, but most SUVs actually perform well in the backcountry. SUVs can tackle most rugged terrain, though many lack the high clearance to navigate tougher or more remote roads. Examples: Ford Explorer, Honda Ridgeline, Jeep Grand Cherokee, Nissan Pathfinder, Chevy Blazer.

4x4 High-Clearance Trucks (4x4): These are vehicles specifically designed for the rigors of rocky, rough, and steep roads. These trucks or Jeeps have high ground clearance, true 4x4 transmissions (usually with both four high and four low settings), rugged suspension, tough tires, and strong engines. These vehicles can make it up almost every road and are required for one of the best hikes in this book, Storm King Peak in the Grenadiers (Hike 45). (There is only one hike in this book for which a 4x4 would not be able to get to the end of the road: Mount Blanca.) Examples include: Toyota Tacoma, Jeeps of the CJ series (Wrangler, Rubicon, etc.), Dodge Ram trucks, Nissan Frontier, Nissan Xterra, and Chevy Silverado.

Modified 4x4: These amazing machines have been customized with huge tires, reworked suspensions, powerful engines, roll cages, and increased torque to get over anything in their way. Clever adaptations such as winches and independent tire-control mechanisms help these modified monsters succeed on 4x4 roads. Most of these vehicles are purely recreational, and very few are street legal. They are the only vehicles that have a shot of making it up the awesome test piece road that leads up to Mount Blanca.

GPS

Just thinking about the complexity of satellites in space beaming information down to a cool little handheld receiver makes me feel like James Bond. While Global Positioning System (GPS) units are undoubtedly valuable tools for tracking eclectic super-villains, I tend to use mine purely for wilderness navigation.

The hikes in this book have all been tracked and mapped using GPS. You don't need a GPS to use this book, but you will find them a nice complement to the information provided in each chapter. One thing to consider: even the best GPS units have a slight margin of error that may conflict with the data collected on your personal GPS. (Note that this same margin of error is noted in many traditional cartographic techniques as well). When using GPS, it's important to give the technology leeway for slight differences. Government standards on GPS satellites create an intentional margin of error for commercial units, though this discrepancy has been reduced in most modern receivers to plus or minus 30 feet.

Ratings

Round-Trip Distance: This is the total mileage you will be hiking over the entire route. Remember, hike distance is not an indicator of how easy or difficult your trip will be—some of the hikes in this book that are a mere 5.0 miles are many times more difficult than those double that length.

Hiking Time: The low end of estimated hiking times (for round-trip distances) are my personal hike times, including time taken for photography, snack breaks, and bathroom breaks. My estimates are meant to provide a good idea of what the average hiker can expect as a time investment: they are not meant to judge ability or fitness. Less experienced hikers should expect to complete the hikes in the upper range of the times given, while strong hikers will probably complete the hikes in less time than the estimates.

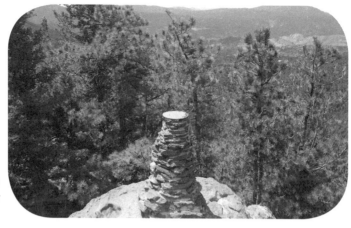

The summit of Green Mountain in Boulder

Difficulty: I have rated the hikes on a scale of 1 to 10, with one being the easiest. None of the hikes in this book requires ropes, so the difficulty is relatively based on the challenge of nontechnical scrambles and hikes. Elements that contribute to the difficulty include: steepness, route finding, distance, terrain, on-trail/off-trail, scrambling difficulty, and exposure. Not included in difficulty ratings are seasonal tribulations such as ice, snow, and high-river crossings (though such conditions are noted when the prime hiking time is during a specific season).

Class: I'm not a huge fan of the class rating system, due to variations of opinion on what defines a particular type of terrain (not to mention the structure of these ratings is more beneficial to technical rock climbers than hikers). Class ratings were first introduced by the Sierra Club in the 1930s to offer a relative scale for gauging hikes in the Sierra Nevada Range; rock climbers' influence has since changed the title of the system to the "Yosemite Decimal System." While the system has been universally adopted, it is most useful when defined in relation to the region it covers.

To make this system useful for Colorado's hikes, I've modified the ratings to accommodate Colorado's varied terrain. Here's how the class system works for this book:

Class 1: Easy, on-trail hiking terrain with few obstacles and minimal exposure. Class 1 trails are well-maintained and easy to follow (they may even be dirt roads). Many hikes begin with class 1 terrain that gradually gives way to sections with more difficult ratings.

Class 2: This is your standard hiking trail. Terrain may be rocky or muddy, and may require use of the hands for very short segments. On-trail class 2 routes are festooned with rocks and may be steep, with minimal exposure. Off-trail class 2 includes stable rock and talus fields, wide open tundra, stable ridgelines, and easy-to-navigate fields.

Class 2+: This designation defines class 2 terrain that has sustained, simple scrambling, or steep, strenuous trails that offer low-technical challenges. A 2+ rating may also cover off-trail terrain that is rife with obstacles such as fallen trees, swamps, and river crossings. Additionally, 2+ covers loose talus fields, rocky ridges, and off-camber paths.

Class 3: This is the fun stuff! Class 3 terrain utilizes handholds and is often steep; in other words, class 3 is true scrambling. Route finding is important on class 3 terrain, as a majority of it is off-trail or on rocky ridges. Exposure is more noticeable, though under normal conditions, you shouldn't need ropes (though if you're climbing off-season, they might be a good idea). Helmets are a good idea on class 3 terrain.

Class 3+: The hardest hikes in this book are 3+; these are advanced routes that require skilled scrambling and difficult route finding, and may require tricky moves in highly exposed areas. Class 3+ routes have solid handholds, but you will need to commit to your moves. Some moves on class 3+ routes may be unnerving, though fall potential is low (think high-risk moves with a very low probability of failure). Helmets are recommended on 3+ terrain.

Class 4: None of the standard routes in this book are class 4, though by some definitions, the class 3+ routes may be considered low class 4 in other regions. Class 4 goes beyond scrambling and gets into low-level climbing; slipping or falling on class 4 terrain may be fatal, so the stakes are fairly high. Often, class 4 routes are found on rock that is too loose to be protected, or on ridges that have sustained, highly exposed sections with good handholds.

Class 5.0 and up: Used to designate technical rock climbing utilizing protection, ropes, harnesses, and belay devices.

Examples of class designations for hikes on some familiar Colorado peaks:

Class 1:   Bison Peak, Longs Peak (from standard trailhead to the boulder field), Mount Thomas

Class 2:   Mount Elbert, James Peak, Uncompahgre Peak

Class 2+:   Mount Sneffles, Windom Peak, Blanca Peak

Class 3:   Longs Peak (from boulder field to summit), Mount Eolus, Mount Ricthoffen

Class 3+:   Mount Lead, Fools Peak, Storm King Peak

Class 4:   The finishing move on Mount Sunlight Peak, North Maroon Peak

Class 5:   The Diamond on Longs Peak, bolted climbs, vertical routes

Start Elevation: This one is obvious: it's the elevation above sea level at the beginning of your hike.

Peak Elevation: Also obvious: this is the elevation of the summit.

Total Elevation Gain: This is the total amount of elevation you will gain on both your ascent and descent; it is not the difference between start and summit elevations. Elevation gain is graphically displayed in the elevation profile graphs provided for each hike.

Terrain: Terrain features may not be obvious on maps. Knowing what will be under your boots lets you equip yourself accordingly.

Best Time to Climb: Almost all of the hikes will be most enjoyable from late June to mid-September, though some peaks are best scaled in early spring, when snowfields provide optimal terrain. A few peaks are great to climb year-round.

Gear Advisor: These are suggestions about gear that I found very helpful for a given hike. This includes footwear suggestions and terrain-specific gear such as helmets, ice axes, gaiters, crampons, or sandals for water crossings.

Crowd Level: If you're looking for solitude, check the crowd level. Traffic levels will always be higher on weekends during hiking season. Following are definitions for the four levels of crowds.

High: This designation refers to popular trails that see a lot of traffic. Such trails are good for social hikers or those wanting the comfort of others on the mountain—a very common occurrence on 14ers, since they are Colorado's "glory peaks."

Moderate: You probably won't be alone on hikes with a moderate crowd level, but you won't be overwhelmed by the masses. Such hikes are often somewhat well-known. A moderate crowd level can be expected on the easier-to-access 13ers.

Low: You'll probably have the summit to yourself, but you'll likely see a few others out and about on low-traffic peaks. You can expect low traffic on hidden gems or on mountains with remote trailheads.

Hermit: These are peaks where you have a great chance of being all alone, save for a few resident animals. These are the true secrets of Colorado (though some of these peaks may have initial access areas where you'll encounter hikers headed to alternate destinations).

Don't expect summit registers; if there are logbooks, expect them to have a short list of exclusive signatures. These hikes are great for solitude, but I'd still highly recommend bringing along a companion for hermit hikes.

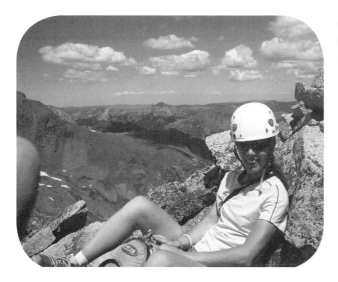

There's nothing better than a good day in the mountains!

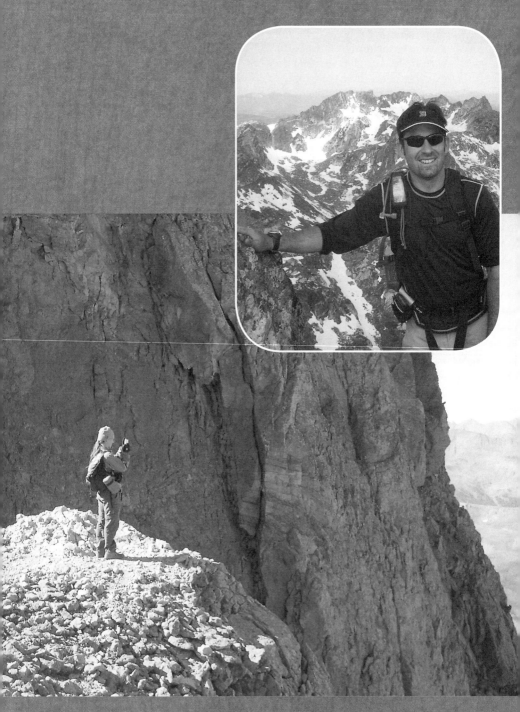

Top: The summit of Mount Zirkel with Big Agnes Peak in the background; *bottom:* Lining up the perfect photo on Uncompahgre Peak

The Hikes

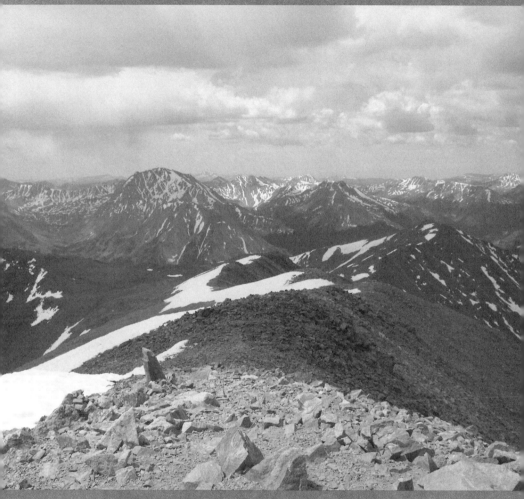

Looking out on a mountainous world from the summit of Colorado's highest mountain (Mount Elbert, 14,433 feet)

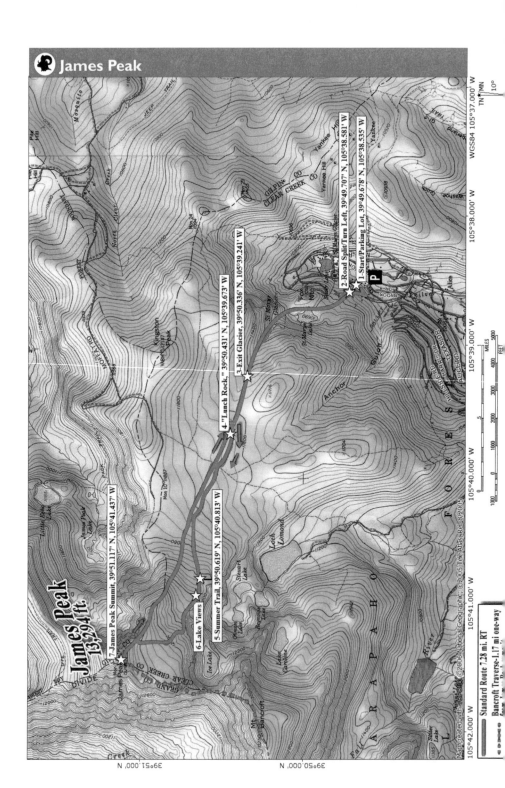

James Peak

James Peak 13,294 ft.

7-James Peak Summit, 39°51.117' N, 105°41.437' W

6-Lake Views

5-Summer Trail, 39°50.619' N, 105°40.813' W

4-"Lunch Rock," 39°50.431' N, 105°39.673' W

3-Exit Glacier, 39°50.336' N, 105°39.241' W

2-Road Split/Turn Left, 39°49.707' N, 105°38.581' W

1-Start/Parking Lot, 39°49.678' N, 105°38.535' W

Standard Route 7.28 mi. RT

Bancroft Traverse–1.17 mi one-way

Map created with TOPO!® ©2006 National Geographic; ©2005 Tele Atlas, Rel. 8/2005

1 James Peak

James Peak offers stunning alpine scenery and glacial goodness. Start your hike on St. Marys Glacier, traverse an alpine meadow, and then ascend an aesthetic dome to the top.

Round Trip Distance	7.28 miles
Hiking Time	4 ½–6 hours
Difficulty	4/10
Class	2
Start Elevation	10,300 ft., at St. Marys Glacier Trailhead
Peak Elevation	13,294 ft.
Total Elevation Gain	2,950 ft.
Terrain	Year-round glacier, alpine plains, rocky slopes on the descent ridge
Best Time to Climb	Early June–September
Gear Advisor	Crampons and ice axe in early spring
Crowd Level	Moderate on the peak/ High on the glacier

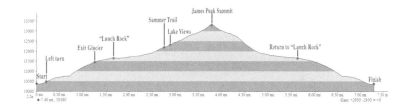

Location   Indian Peaks Range in the James Peak Wilderness/Arapahoe National Forest near Idaho Springs

Intro   James Peak is the centerpiece of the 14,000-acre James Peak Wilderness, a relatively new wilderness area designated in 2002 (prior to that, James Peak was part of the Indian Peaks Wilderness). James stands as the highpoint of Gilpin County, and its prominent "half-dome" profile is visible from the east, especially when viewed from the foothills of Boulder County. Relatively speaking, James is one of the easier 13ers to climb, yet it has all the incredible scenery and majestic feel of Colorado's highest mountains.

Why Climb It?   James Peak is a year-round attraction, thanks in part to St. Marys Glacier, a permanent ice field that graces the base of the standard ascent route. The glacier offers a great training ground for snow travel and is a short, steep warm-up for the southern slopes that lead to James's summit. Cresting the horizon at the upper terminus of the glacier, James Peak's impressive profile comes into view at the far end of a spacious alpine meadow. The flats leading to the final rise are great places to catch your breath while keeping an eye out for dozens of flowers and the occasional troop of ptarmigans.

Pushing for the summit can be done on a well-maintained, switchbacking trail, or by a direct climb of the rolling southeast ridge. Summit views include a unique perspective of the front-side runs at Winter Park and Mary Jane ski areas. Best of all, when James Peak holds snow, it's possible to have some rip-roaring fun glissading down the summit slopes and the glacier.

As a bonus, James Peak's Trailhead is easily accessed from Interstate 70 and is a relatively short drive from Denver, Boulder, or Golden.

Driving   James Peak is easily accessible by passenger car. The trail begins off a paved, maintained road.

How to Get There   From Interstate 70 (east or west), take the Fall River Road exit (exit 238, which is also labeled ST.MARY'S/ALICE). In Gazetteers, this is listed as "275 RD." If you are westbound on I-70, this exit is roughly 1.5 miles from the town of Idaho Springs. Follow Fall River Road northwest 8.6 miles. Be ready for some steep switchbacks as you get closer to the trailhead. At approximately 8.3 miles, you'll pass the well-hidden town of Alice on your left; a bit farther up you'll see the general store off the main road on your right. You're almost there! Continue to the top of the hill, bypassing a rusted-out ski lift and a parking area blocked off by boulders on the left (this is the old parking area). At the top of the hill, you'll see a fenced-off mining shack and a well-traveled dirt road with a ST. MARY'S GLACIER sign. This is where you start your hike. Drive past the trail approximately 200 yards to a parking area on the left-hand side of the road. Note that this lot gets very crowded on weekends, so arrive early, or else you'll have to park farther down the road. Also, please walk up to the main trail you passed; do not scramble up the improvised (and eroded) trails that are cut into the hill directly from the parking lot.

Fees/Camping   There are no fees required to enter the James Peak Wilderness Area. Backpackers can hike in and camp in the wilderness for free, though the St. Marys Lake area tends to get crowded in the summer.

Route Notes   None.

Mile/Waypoint   **0.0 mi (1)**   From the parking lot, walk 200 yards uphill (southwest) on the paved road to reach the wide, well-worn dirt road that leads up to St. Marys Glacier. You'll see a sign pointing out the glacier.

0.2 mi (2)   The wide road splits. Head left and uphill. (The road going to the right simply leads to a parking area for people who feel like driving their 4x4s up the 0.1 mile from the road.) Follow the well-worn and rocky path as it winds up to the woods toward St. Marys Lake.

0.5 mi   Pass by St. Marys Lake. The enormous, curving profile of St. Marys Glacier will be before you. Cross a small metal bridge and continue to the glacier. It doesn't matter if you take the higher path or the lower path; they both lead to the glacier (though the lower path can be mucky in spring).

0.7 mi   Get on the glacier and continue your ascent. Follow the icy snow to the top of glacier. This is a half-mile, steep ascent, with wonderful photo

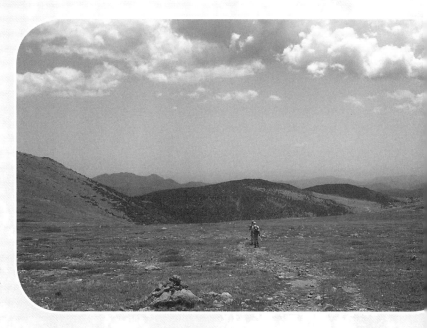

Hikers cross the alpine meadows below James Peak.

opportunities. The alleyway is notorious for funneling fierce winds, especially in the colder months.

1.2 mi (3) Top out and exit the glacier. Where the snowfield ends depends on the time of the year. A semi-maintained trail fades in on the left (west) side when there is no snow. This is a good waypoint to mark on your GPS; in bad conditions, it's easy to miss the entrance of the glacier. From here, you'll see the expansive flat plains with James Peak dominating the horizon. Continue along the plains to "Lunch Rock."

1.7 mi (4) Lunch Rock is a battleship-shaped formation that is the only distinguishing feature on the otherwise flat traverse to the base of James's slopes. There are some small, natural caves and manmade wind shelters in Lunch Rock. This is another good reference point. The faint, "sort of there" trail to the base of James, which is the left fork on the map at waypoint 4, is the easiest way to make your ascent. From here, continue along the flats, crossing a 4x4 road en route to the south slopes. The trail from the top of the glacier begins to fizzle out, but you can see where you need to go.

2.7 mi (5) Once the snow has melted off, a cairned, switchbacking trail is evident on the southeast slopes. This trail will lead you to the top. Alternatively, you can head directly up the steep hills to James's summit. When there is snow, this is a good option, but be sure to test the snowpack; these slopes are at a prime avalanche angle. Note that when dry, the rocky hill makes for rough climbing (but is a good descent route).

2.9 mi (6) Don't miss the stunning views of the alpine lakes dropping off to the south! Continue to follow the cairns and well-worn trail. There is something of a false summit at 13,000 feet, where you gain James's southeast ridge. A glance north looks down into the impressive couloirs stretching down to James Peak Lake.

3.8 mi (7) Reach the flat summit of James Peak! From here, you can return the way you came or descend directly down the rolling southeast ridge. Following the ridge gives you some new views to the north and is quicker, especially when the snow allows for glissades. When there is no snow, it's a rocky class 2 descent, so if you don't feel like banging up you knees, return via the standard trail.

4.7 mi When you get to the bottom of the southeast slopes and resume the flats, aim for Lunch Rock. You can pass it on either side; on the return, the main trail is to the right of Lunch Rock.

5.7 mi (4) Pass Lunch Rock.

6.1 mi (3) Return to the glacier, and follow it back to St. Marys Lake. Follow the well-worn trail to the road and parking lot. Don't shortcut down the hill to the parking lot just off the top of the trail.

7.28 mi Finish at the parking lot.

Options From the summit of James Peak, you can try a 1.17-mile traverse south-southwest over to Bancroft Peak. This is a class 3+ scramble that's a lot of fun in good conditions. You can descend Bancroft east into the Three Lakes Basin (Stewart Lake being the most prominent) and regain the flats toward Lunch Rock with a short, steep climb.

Another option is to ascend modest Kingston Peak (12,147 feet), north of the flats. The 4x4 road you cross on the plains goes directly to its mellow summit.

Finally, note that James Peak's northeast face has several moderate-to-hard couloirs that offer excellent snow routes in early spring. Sky Pilot is a great, moderate snow gully when in season (normally March through early June); Shooting Star and Super Star are more technical and offer fantastic ascent options for mountaineers.

Quick Facts James Peak is named for mountaineer, botanist, and historian Edwin James, who served on Stephen Long's Colorado expedition. James's claim to fame was his historic first ascent of Pikes Peak, which initially was dubbed James Peak. Zebulon Pike had surveyed the mountain in 1806 but never climbed it; James and two companions did the trick in 1820. Cartographers used both names—James Peak and Pikes Peak—on early maps, eventually favoring the more phonetically pleasing Pikes Peak for the 14er.

James Peak was officially named in 1866, five years after the death of Edwin James. A fine mountain in its own right, this peak is a respectable consolation for a pioneering Colorado climber.

Contact Info Arapahoe National Forest
Boulder Ranger District
2140 Yarmouth Avenue
Boulder, CO 80303
(303) 541-2500

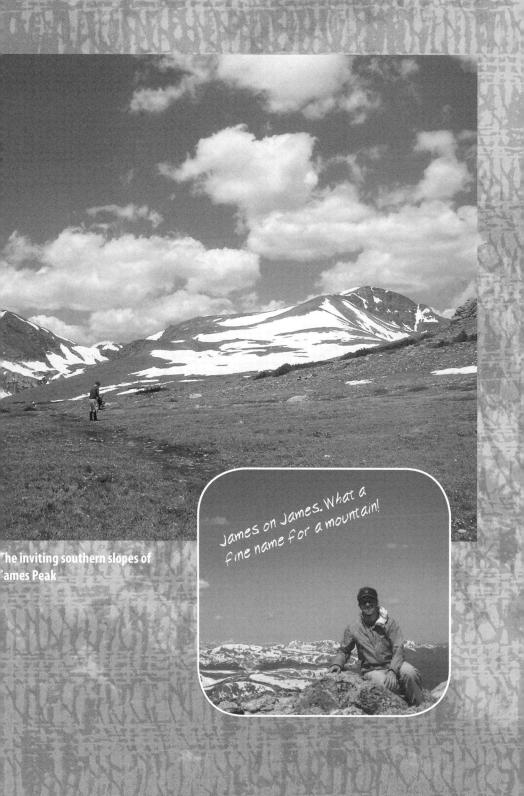

The inviting southern slopes of James Peak

James on James. What a fine name for a mountain!

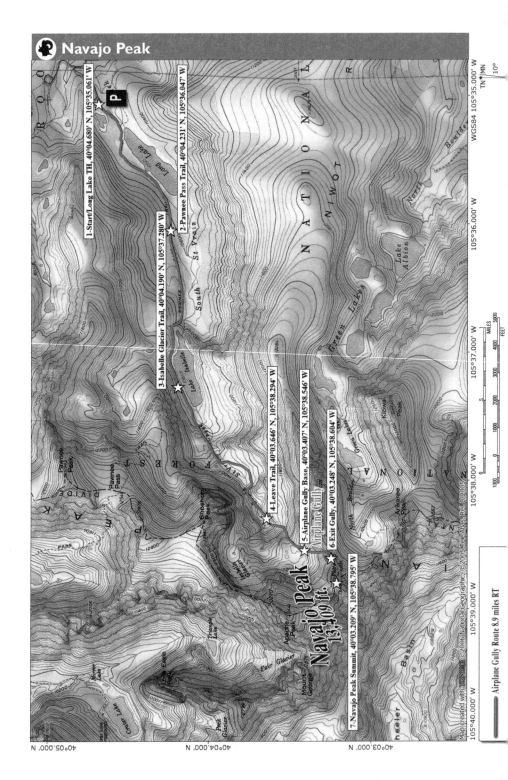

1-Start/Long Lake TH, 40°04.680' N, 105°35.061' W

2-Pawnee Pass Trail, 40°04.231' N, 105°36.047' W

3-Isabelle Glacier Trail, 40°04.190' N, 105°37.280' W

4-Leave Trail, 40°03.646' N, 105°38.294' W

5-Airplane Gully Base, 40°03.407' N, 105°38.546' W

6-Exit Gully, 40°03.248' N, 105°38.604' W

7-Navajo Peak Summit, 40°03.209' N, 105°38.795' W

Navajo Peak 13,409 ft.

Airplane Gully Route 8.9 miles RT

2 Navajo Peak

A trip to the glacial basin below Navajo leads you to the base of Airplane Gully, where ghosts of the past await. A thrilling scramble is the grand finale to Navajo's airy summit.

Round Trip Distance:	8.9 miles
Hiking Time:	6½–8 hours
Difficulty:	8/10
Class:	3
Start Elevation:	10,500 ft., at Long Lake Trailhead
Peak Elevation:	13,409 ft.
Total Elevation Gain:	2,825 ft.
Terrain:	Steep, loose gully, and airy but solid scrambling on summit block
Best Time to Climb:	June–September
Gear Advisor:	Gaiters, stiff boots, ice axe in spring, helmet, GPS
Crowd Level:	Low

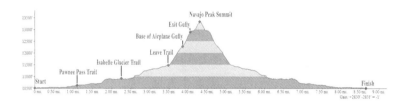

Location   Indian Peaks Range in the Indian Peaks Wilderness/Roosevelt National Forest outside the town of Ward

Intro   From a distance, the clean, four-sided pyramid block that sits atop Navajo Peak brings to mind ancient Mayan temples. Amongst the peaks that grace the skyline from Brainard Lake Recreation Area, Navajo offers the most challenging standard route. Half of the hike is off-trail, culminating in a gully climb and an exciting class 3 scramble to the summit. Along the way, you'll have a chance to examine the wreckage of a C-47 aircraft that crashed in January of 1948 en route to Grand Junction. Parts are strewn throughout the gully, and a huge piece of the bulkhead rests near the gully exit.

Why Climb It?   Shipwrecks and ghost towns fascinate humankind. We are drawn to relics, the very shells of history, which hold stories of hardship and bravery and are at the same time symbols of mortality. The wreckage on Navajo Peak is half of the appeal of this hike. Debris from the crash is strewn throughout the gully; small, rusty gears are so numerous they seem like bizarre, metallic sunflowers pushing through the rocks. Besides serving as an archive of aviation history, the scramble to Navajo's summit is exciting itself. Beginning on-trail in the beautiful Long Lake area of Indian Peaks, an easy start leads to an off-trail adventure, where you'll pass two of Colorado's permanent glaciers (Isabelle and Navajo). After a loose scramble up the gully, the remaining ridge climb to the summit concludes with an exposed but very solid scramble 35 feet to the summit block.

Driving

Passenger cars can make it to the trailhead with ease: the road is paved all the way.

How to Get There

Take Colorado Highway 72 (Peak-to-Peak Highway) to the Brainard Lake Road, which is above the town of Ward. From Nederland, it is 12 miles to this turnoff; from Lyons, it's 10.2 miles from the junction with Colorado Highway 7. If you are approaching from Boulder, it's quicker to take US Highway 36 north out of town approximately 6.0 miles and take a left onto Left Hand Canyon Drive. Stay on this road 17 miles, all the way through the car graveyard/town of Ward. At the top of the road, take a right on

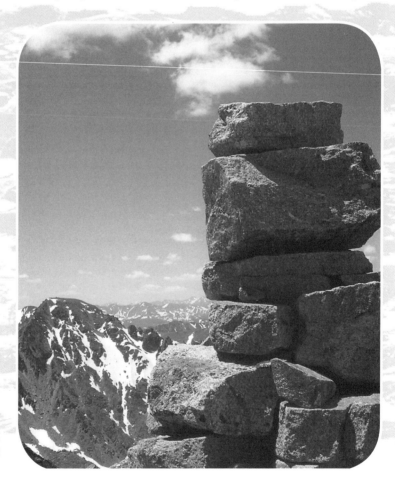

Cairn on the summit
of Navajo Peak

Highway 32 and then a quick left to Brainard Lake Road. Follow this road 5.0 miles (you'll pass a pay station and Brainard Lake), and follow the well-marked signs for half a mile to Long Lake Trailhead.

Fees/Camping   As of 2006, the permit for the Brainard Lake Recreation Area is $7 for a seven-day pass. You can buy an annual pass for $25. Pawnee Campground fills up very quickly; if you're able to get a site, it's $12 per night. Backcountry camping requires a permit and a small fee ($5) from June 1 through September 15. Note that you'll have to go over the west side of Pawnee Pass to reach the designated backcountry camping zones.

Route Notes   The off-trail portion of this hike is a little easier in spring, when snow covers the boulders in the basin above Lake Isabelle. Snow in Airplane Gully melts out early, so you shouldn't have to bring crampons after early May. The moves to reach the summit are exposed, but the rock is very solid. The crux of the climb is the short downclimb off the summit.

Mile/Waypoint   **0.0 mi (1)** Start at the Long Lake Trailhead and go west. Enjoy the flat trail, which is a great warm-up. At the west end of Long Lake, stay right and follow the trail to Pawnee Pass (for the time-being).

1.1 mi (2) Pawnee Pass Trail. Continue west to Lake Isabelle.

1.9 mi (3) After hiking up some switchbacks and crossing a cool waterfall, you've arrived at Lake Isabelle and the Isabelle Glacier Trail. Follow the lake on its north side; do *not* go up the trail to Pawnee Pass. Instead stay on the trail to Isabelle Glacier. This trail climbs above Lake Isabelle, eventually coming to a flat, marshy section with a small lake at 11,500 feet.

3.5 mi (4) You will need to get off-trail at the marshy section. However, do *not* follow the steep switchbacked trail to the north going to Isabelle Glacier. Instead, head southwest to the dry basin at the foot of Airplane Gully. It is best to stay on the left (west) slopes instead of dropping down to the flat part of the basin, as the tracks indicate.

3.9 mi (5) This is the base of Airplane Gully (12,280 feet). Finding the right gully can be tricky. Looking up at Navajo Peak, you'll see the Navajo Glacier on the right, the lumpy north face, and a steep gully that ends where the summit pyramid joins the ridge—this is *not* your gully. To the left of this gully is an outcrop of rock; Airplane Gully runs to the left of this rock. There is a minor talus fan of large boulders at the base (as well as a silver wing from the plane, with identification numbers). When you go over to the base of the gully, it will seem very climbable.

There are many loose rocks in Airplane Gully, so be careful if you are scrambling above people. It's steep, but I'd still only rate the gully class 2+. More difficult than its grade is its total of 900 vertical feet. About halfway up (at approximately 12,550 feet), the gully forks. Take the right fork, despite the fact the straight south route offers a keyhole of blue sky through the rocks topping its exit. The correct fork climbs southwest. At 12,900 feet, just before the exit, lies the largest part of the wreckage. A major section of the bulkhead, motors, gears, and wires are everywhere. Do not touch or take any of the wreckage! It's illegal to take pieces of the plane, as it's a recognized crash site. Furthermore, the heavy metal pieces sit in a loose, unstable gully—they may shift at any time. Above the wreckage, a grassy slope exits onto Navajo's east ridge.

4.2 mi (6)   At the gully exit, the final pyramid looms before you. To reach the summit, hike up to the base of the block, favoring the south (left) side of the slope. Head west until you reach about 13,260 feet. There is a perilously balanced rock on the west side, known as the "Monkey Fist." This is your cue to begin scrambling north on exposed but solid rock. It's a short push, maybe 30 to 40 feet with several class 3 moves. Note that more experienced climbers can find a way up the face to the right (east face) via several class 3+ and class 4 sections. Novice or inexperienced hikers may find the exposure a bit unsettling.

4.4 mi (7)   Navajo Peak's tiny summit has a register tube and a cairn. It can accommodate two people, though there are places for others to sit just below the summit. The downclimb back to the east ridge can be tricky. The safest and easiest way is to retrace the way you came, even though it looks like the rocks drop off into oblivion. There are several slightly more direct exits you can take by going down the southeast side; if you take them, you'll have short sections of face-in downclimbing, with some fall potential—class 4 stuff.

Once you are safely on the ridge, return via Airplane Gully. The loose rock makes this descent tough; I'd recommend using an ice axe/trekking poles for stability, even when there is no snow. Once you're out of the gully, return to Lake Isabelle, regain the well-worn trail, and enjoy the hike out.

8.9 mi   Finish.

Options   Hiking Navajo Peak makes for a fairly demanding day, so linking to other routes isn't really an option for a dayhike. There are some good views if you explore northeast on Niwot Ridge, which would require a left turn at the top of Airplane Gully (waypoint 6). Navajo's southeast ridge looks as if it would provide an exciting class 3+ traverse over to nearby 13,150-foot Arikaree Peak, but Arikaree has the unfortunate fate of being in the off-limits Boulder watershed. The impressive standalone peak you see from atop Airplane Gully to the east, 13,276-foot Kiowa Peak, is likewise forbidden. Fines are strictly enforced for trespassing in this area.

Quick Facts   Ellsworth Bethel advocated naming a series of peaks to honor native peoples; that series is now known as the Indian Peaks. Navajo Peak is one example; others include Apache, Shoshoni, Arapahoe, Pawnee, and Arikaree peaks, as well as Niwot Ridge. A mountain was named in Bethel's honor also, though not in this range. You can spot Mount Bethel when driving east on I-70 just past the Eisenhower Tunnel, thanks to the snow fences high on its slopes, which are its trademark.

The airplane wreckage is from a crash that occurred on January 21, 1948. Three men were killed when the C-47, en route from Denver to Grand Junction, was caught in bad weather and was pushed into the ridge by strong winds. The crash site was not discovered for several months. There are some who believe that the wreckage should be left alone. It is my opinion one should not feel guilty or morbid for wanting to see the crash debris. The accident was tragic, but it serves as an example of how man and mountain are intertwined by the threads of fate. Like many scenes that remind us of our mortality, such an experience can also manifest itself as an affirmation of life.

Contact Info   The good news: the Brainard Lake Recreation Area is free from sometime in October to early June. The bad news: the road is closed at the pay station, roughly 2.0 miles from Brainard Lake. You can park there and bike, ski,or hike in if you want to try an off-season ascent. This area is very popular in the winter for snowshoeing and cross-country skiing.

Grand Country Wilderness Group
(This group helps the US Forest Service manage the Brainard Lake
Recreation Area)
P.O. Box 2200
Fraser, CO 80442
(970) 726-4626
Recorded Voice Information Hotline
(303) 541-2519

Arapahoe/Roosevelt National Forest
Boulder Ranger District
2140 Yarmouth Avenue
Boulder, CO 80301
(303) 541-2500

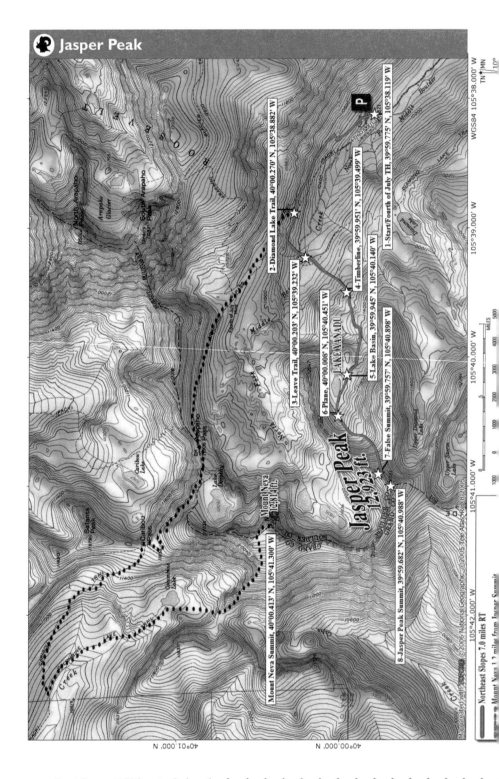

2-Diamond Lake Trail, 40°00.270' N, 105°38.882' W

1-Start/Fourth of July TH, 39°59.775' N, 105°38.119' W

4-Timberline, 39°59.951' N, 105°39.499' W

3-Leave Trail, 40°00.203' N, 105°39.232' W

5-Lake Basin, 39°59.945' N, 105°40.140' W

6-Plane, 40°00.008' N, 105°40.451' W

7-False Summit, 39°59.757' N, 105°40.898' W

Jasper Peak 12,923 ft.

Mount Neva Summit, 40°00.413' N, 105°41.300' W

8-Jasper Peak Summit, 39°59.682' N, 105°40.988' W

Northeast Slopes 7.0 miles RT

Mount Neva 1.2 miles from Jasper Summit

3 Jasper Peak

Jasper is such a secret, it doesn't even appear on the map! This great climb requires off-trail navigation and passes by the most beautiful unknown basin in Indian Peaks.

Round Trip Distance	7.0 miles
Hiking Time	5½–7 hours
Difficulty	7/10
Class	2+
Start Elevation	10,170 ft., at Fourth of July Trailhead
Peak Elevation	12,923 ft.
Total Elevation Gain	3,010 ft.
Terrain	Spongy, off-trail forests leading to snowfields and grassy rock slopes
Best Time to Climb	Late May–September
Gear Advisor	GPS, gaiters, ice axe, crampons in early spring
Crowd Level	Hermit

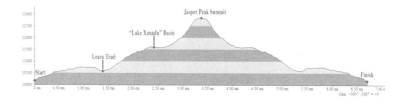

Location — Indian Peaks Range in the Indian Peaks Wilderness/Roosevelt National Forest north of Nederland

Intro — Jasper Peak (also known as Mount Jasper) has held its name informally for years, despite not appearing on official maps. It is a hard mountain to spot from lower elevations. When the peak becomes visible at higher elevations, it has a very alluring pyramid shape, just begging to be climbed! It takes solid navigational skills to reach "Lake Xanadu Basin," a stunning alpine lake tucked away in the folds of the Indian Peaks. Prime hiking time for Jasper is in late May and early June, when snow on the northeast face is stable enough for an ascent and for blazing glissades on the way down.

Why Climb It? — It's good that Jasper doesn't appear on the map! The on-trail hikes in this area of the Indian Peaks see a lot of traffic, yet this mountain remains a mystery to most. Once you leave the trail, navigation through the trees is a fun challenge (without severe repercussions if you take a wrong turn). After finding your way through woods and meadows, you'll find yourself in a pristine basin with the small, sparkling Lake Xanadu as the centerpiece. There is also a small plane wreck at the west end of the lake, a curious relic in such a remote area. Climb to a false summit that hides the true apex a short distance beyond. Strong hikers can continue the fun by taking the optional trek over to Mount Neva.

Driving   Tough passenger cars can make it to the Fourth of July Trailhead. The road is rocky, with sections of washboards and ruts, but it is passable by cars. I've driven up in my Accord many times, and I've seen other similar cars in the parking lot. Road maintenance is performed every spring, so the road may be in better shape in mid-June.

How to Get There   To reach the Fourth of July Trailhead, start in the town of Nederland and go south on Colorado Highway 119 toward Eldora Ski Area. About 0.2 mile out of town, turn right and follow the signs for Eldora Ski Area (Road 130). At 1.4 miles down this road, there is a left turnoff for Eldora Ski Area—do not take this road. Instead, continue straight and at mile 2.9, pass through the small town of Eldora. At the end of town, the road turns to dirt. Continue on for 1.4 miles to a split; stay right (the left road goes to the Hessie Trailhead). The road gets rougher but still passable in normal conditions. Drive 4.4 miles farther and the Fourth of July Trailhead will be on your right, just past Buckingham Campground. The little access road into the parking lot may be the toughest driving of the whole trip.

Fees/Camping   There are no fees to hike in this area. Overnight camping trips in the Indian Peaks require a backcountry permit from June 1 to September; the cost is $5. Buckingham Campground charges $10 per night, as of 2006.

Route Notes   A majority of this hike is off-trail and you'll need to perform basic navigational skills to reach Xanadu Lake Basin. (Once you are there, the route is visually clear on good days).

Mile/Waypoint   **0.0 mi (1)** Start at the Fourth of July Trailhead. Get on the well-worn Arapaho Pass Trail and follow it for 1.0 mile to the junction with the Diamond Lake Trail. You'll get a preview of Jasper from viewpoints on this section of the trail.

1.0 mi (2) Bear left onto the Diamond Lake Trail. You will be going down hill and into deeper woods.

1.4 mi (3) Say goodbye to the trail once you reach Middle Boulder Creek. Cross the modest stream, and head southwest through the woods. The ground is spongy, but the trees are well spaced. If the weather is clear, in the clearings you'll have glimpses of where you need to go. The difficult navigation (in trees) is only for about 0.5 mile.

1.8 mi (4) You will reach timberline around 11,060 feet. There will be a large mountain ridge due west and a small bulge south of the mountain. The easiest way to reach "Lake Xanadu Basin" is to find the gap south of the small bulge (between the small bulge and a ridge to your left, farther south). Find a good route up to the basin from here; it's easier when snow covers the boulders.

2.4 mi (5) Soak in the views at the flat and accommodating Lake Xanadu Basin. The moderate slopes to the southwest become obvious.

Note on Alternate Route: Those who like ridge walks can make the steep scramble directly north of Lake Xanadu and gain Jasper's northeast ridge. Follow it on class 2+ terrain to Jasper's summit.

2.7 mi (6) On the west end of the lake is the wreckage of a small silver and red airplane. It's an interesting sight, especially in contrast to the beauty of the area.

Gain the northeast slope and find a good line up to connect with the northeast ridge. In early spring, you may need crampons for the snow. (I didn't need them the first week of June 2006.) Follow these slopes west and intersect with the northeast ridge.

3.3 mi (7) False summit! At 12,887 feet, you're almost there. The actual summit is just beyond, via an easy scramble heading southwest.

3.5 mi (8) Jasper's summit may surprise you. When the snow is melted, it's a grassy patch with small wildflowers. The Winter Park and Mary Jane ski areas can be seen to the west and Mount Neva is visible to the north. Return the way you came, or continue north on the optional route to Mount Neva.

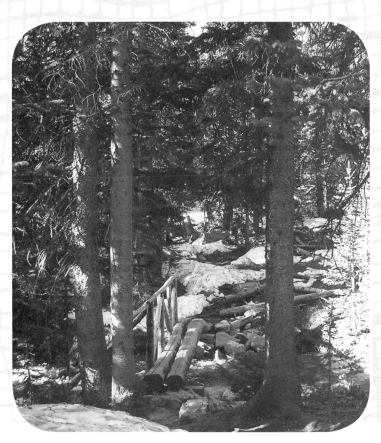

Enjoy your last glimpse of on-trail hiking; from here on out, you'll be off the beaten path.

If returning via the standard route, take care when navigating back to the Diamond Lake Trail (GPS is a huge help at this point).

7.0 mi Finish.

Options Mount Neva is 1.2 miles from the summit, along a class 2+ ridge. Head north to reach Neva. Once you are there, it's best to return to Jasper and descend via the standard route—Neva's north ridge to Arapahoe Pass is a class 4 route, which may require ropes

One option that looks like fun (though I have not tried it) is to do a "super loop" as a two-day endeavor. Camp the first night at Lake Xanadu, and go light, since you won't be coming back this way. The next day, climb Jasper and traverse to Neva, and then descend Neva's northwest ridge down to Columbine Lake. Pick up the Columbine Lake Trail and go north to the junction with the Caribou Trail. Return east over Caribou Pass to Arapaho Pass, where you can follow the Arapaho Pass Trail back to your car. From Lake Xanadu, this loop is about 10 miles (12 or 13 total, depending on your navigation skills). It would be difficult to do in a single day, due to afternoon storms, which could catch you high on Caribou Pass or Arapaho Pass.

Quick Facts Jasper is not the official name of the peak (technically, it is unnamed), but it has gone by the name for many years. Some previous maps and guidebooks have identified it as Jasper Peak or Mount Jasper; we'll use Jasper Peak. For that matter, Lake Xanadu is an unofficial name but one that seems to fit the area well. The only landscape feature with an officially recognized name around here, Mount Neva, is named after the brother of Arapahoe leader Chief Niwot.

Contact Info Arapahoe/Roosevelt National Forest
Boulder Ranger District
2140 Yarmouth Avenue
Boulder, CO 80301
(303) 541-2500

Recorded Indian Peaks Information Hotline
(303) 541-2519

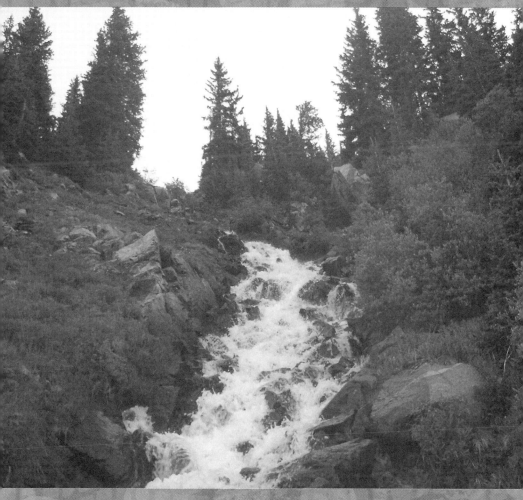

You'll cross this beautiful waterfall not long after starting off from the Fourth of July Trailhead.

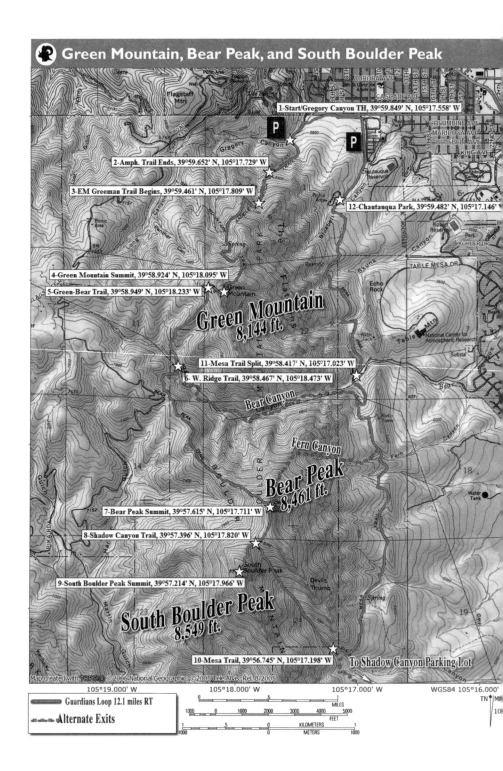

Green Mountain, Bear Peak, and South Boulder Peak

1-Start/Gregory Canyon TH, 39°59.849' N, 105°17.558' W

2-Amph. Trail Ends, 39°59.652' N, 105°17.729' W

3-EM Greeman Trail Begins, 39°59.461' N, 105°17.809' W

12-Chautauqua Park, 39°59.482' N, 105°17.146' W

4-Green Mountain Summit, 39°58.924' N, 105°18.095' W

5-Green-Bear Trail, 39°58.949' N, 105°18.233' W

Green Mountain 8,144 ft.

11-Mesa Trail Split, 39°58.417' N, 105°17.023' W

6- W. Ridge Trail, 39°58.467' N, 105°18.473' W

Bear Peak 8,461 ft.

7-Bear Peak Summit, 39°57.615' N, 105°17.711' W

8-Shadow Canyon Trail, 39°57.396' N, 105°17.820' W

9-South Boulder Peak Summit, 39°57.214' N, 105°17.966' W

South Boulder Peak 8,549 ft.

10-Mesa Trail, 39°56.745' N, 105°17.198' W

To Shadow Canyon Parking Lot

Map created with TOPO!© ©2006 National Geographic, ©2005 Tele Atlas, Rel. 8/2005

Guardians Loop 12.1 miles RT

Alternate Exits

105°19.000' W   105°18.000' W   105°17.000' W   WGS84 105°16.000'

4 Guardians of the Flatirons: Green Mountain, Bear Peak, and South Boulder Peak

This three-peak traverse is the pride of Boulder, giving you a deluxe tour of the local mountains and the slanted pinnacles of the Flatirons. A big hike that's right in town.

Round Trip Distance	12.1 miles
Hiking Time	7–10 hours
Difficulty	6.5/10
Class	2
Start Elevation	5,833 ft., at Gregory Canyon Trailhead
Peak Elevations	Green Mountain: 8,144 ft.; Bear Peak: 8,461 ft.; South Boulder Peak: 8,549 ft.
Total Elevation Gain	5,171 ft.
Terrain	On-trail tour of Boulder's Flatirons
Best Time to Climb	Year-round; may be very hot mid-summer
Gear Advisor	Normal gear
Crowd Level	Moderate overall; high on Green Mountain and the Mesa Trail

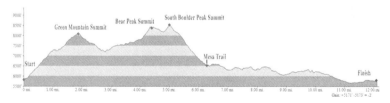

Location   Boulder Mountain Park in beautiful Boulder, Colorado

Intro   Who says you need have your head in the clouds to have an epic day? This three-peak traverse begins in the civilized confines of Boulder. First, wind your way through shady, vanilla-scented pine forests bracketed by towering rock formations to Green Mountain. Descend from Green into a hidden world of alpine flowers and grandiose valleys. It will seem hard to believe a city of 90,000 people is just on the other side of the ridge as you drop into Bear Canyon. Gradually ascend to the rocky summit of fashionable Bear Peak, and complete the traverse by visiting the less-popular (but slightly higher) South Boulder Peak. Descend via the rocky Shadow Canyon Trail, where the Devil's Thumb will be poised to your left, frozen midsmite. Complete the loop with a casual return hike below the impressive Flatiron rock formations.

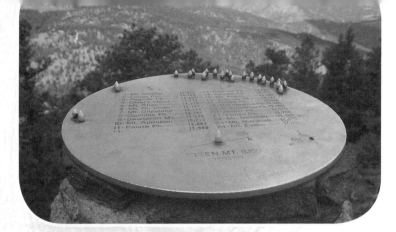

This metal disk atop Green Mountain shows you what mountains are visible on the horizon.

Why Climb It? The Flatirons serve as the mountainous backdrop to Boulder and denote the eastern terminus of the Rocky Mountains. Their abrupt angles and reddish hues make them the perfect ambassadors for the subsequent peaks that rise to the west. This hike gives you an extended tour of the area, offering great views of Boulder and Denver to the east, and the Indian Peaks and Front Range to the west. On clear days, you can see from Longs Peak to Pikes Peak. The western side of these mountains is surprisingly wild; standing on the summit of Bear Peak feels like you're on the dividing line between civilization and wilderness. As the trail drops down to the base of the Flatirons, it bypasses dozens of amazing rock formations. Even though it's in town, the elevation gain and mileage gives you a workout on par with one you'd experience on higher mountains.

Driving Any vehicle can make it to the trailhead; it is paved all the way.

How to Get There From US Highway 36 in Boulder, take the Baseline Road exit, turn west onto Baseline Road, and continue for 1.8 miles. You'll pass Chautauqua Park on your left. Just after the large signs for Boulder Mountain Parks and the fire danger warnings, turn off left as the road bends abruptly uphill to Gregory Canyon Trailhead. If this parking lot is full, you can park on the designated south side of the short access road or simply go 0.1 mile back to Chautauqua's parking lot. On weekends, these parking lots fill up fast.

Fees/Camping There is a $3 parking fee for cars at the Gregory Canyon Trailhead (this fee does not apply to Boulder Country residents). Free parking can be found at Chautauqua Park or along the side roads (such as 9th Street) to the north of Baseline.

    As for camping…you're in a major city. There's no real legal camping to speak of nearby, but there are plenty of nice hotels in Boulder.

Route Notes There are many trails that intersect this route, especially once you drop down onto the Mesa Trail. Read the description closely so that you don't take a wrong turn along the way. This route is very well marked, with signs at most junctions.

Mile/Waypoint 0.0 mi (1) Start at Gregory Canyon Trailhead. There are two trails you can take to start your hike; this route favors the Amphitheater Trail (on the east side of the parking area). Get on this trail (staying right at the early inter-section with the Bluebell-Baird Trail) and begin hiking upward, quickly reaching a section of steep "stairs." Bypass the Amphitheater Express Trail on your right (which leads to rock climbing routes). You'll know the junc-ture to avoid when you see a sign previewing the neat formations to come at the Amphitheater.

0.4 mi (2) The Amphitheater Trail ends and joins the Saddle Rock Trail, which comes in from the right (this is the other route that leaves from the parking area). Stay left on the Saddle Rock Trail and continue hiking uphill through the vanilla- and pine-scented forest. Continue to follow the Saddle Rock Trail. Do not turn off at the Saddle Rock climbing access trail on your left, at 0.7 mile.

1.3 mi (3) The Saddle Rock Trail ends and becomes the E.M. Greenman Trail, which comes in from the right. Bear left and continue your ascent on the E.M. Greenman Trail. This trail will lead you to the summit of Green Mountain. Note that there is one slightly tricky part at mile 1.45—the trail takes a turn to the left over some large tree roots. A worn but incorrect path to the right has been blocked off with rocks and sticks. Stay left over the roots and the trail will become obvious again. Follow it up to Green Mountain's summit.

2.0 mi (4) Green Mountain Summit. There is a register here and a neat metal plaque that identifies the mountains on the horizon to the west. You can see at least four other mountains that this book details hikes for: Mount Alice (Hike 9), Longs Peak (Hike 8), Jasper Peak (Hike 3), and James Peak (Hike 1). Continue south off the summit and down a well-worn, switch-backing trail.

2.1 mi (5) At this four-way intersection, turn left onto the Green-Bear Trail, which goes downhill to the southwest. Keep your eye out for any Green Bears! The trail feels worlds away from the city din of Boulder. Enjoy the wildflowers. There are also good views of the back sides of Bear Peak and South Boulder Peak.

2.9 mi (6) The Green-Bear Trail ends in Bear Canyon. At the well-marked sign, take a right onto the Bear Peak West Ridge Trail. This well-traveled and well-marked path starts out as a series of gentle switchbacks and then begins climbing more steeply up the rocky slopes of Bear's west ridge.

4.4 mi This trail ends just below the rocks that make up Bear Peak's sum-mit. The scramble up looks tough, but there is an easier way. Traverse a short distance left (north), where you can scramble directly south on a "ramp" to the top. (This is the most difficult scrambling on the hike, and it's only class 2.)

4.5 mi (7) Bear Peak Summit! These are the best 360-degree views on the entire hike. To the south is Pikes Peak; to the west, the Indian Peaks; to the north, Longs Peak and Fort Collins; and to the east, the sprawling metrop-olis of Denver and its suburbs. Exit the summit the way you came up, and return to the west side of the peak below the summit, where the Bear Peak West Ridge Trail ended. Pick up the connector trail, in the rocks, that goes south to South Boulder Peak.

4.9 mi (8)   A dip in the ridge between Bear and South Boulder peaks introduces the Shadow Canyon Trail on your left. Eventually, you will descend on this trail; for the time-being, however, stay on the South Boulder Peak trail heading southwest. You can tell from the growth in this area that this peak sees much less traffic than the previous two summits.

5.1 mi (9)   South Boulder Peak Summit! This is the highest point of your hike, even though it is blocked by trees on the east side. Keep your eyes open for wild raspberry bushes up here. Return to the junction with the Shadow Canyon Trail.

5.4 mi (8)   Take the Shadow Canyon Trail southeast and descend via this rocky road. There are a few brief sections where the trail passes over talus fields; follow the cairns to resume the trail after these interludes.

5.9 mi   In a slight clearing, look up to your left. The upturned Devil's Thumb gives you its approval.

6.5 mi (10)   At the bottom of the rocky trail, you'll enter a small clearing with a few trails intersecting. Turn left (north) onto the marked Mesa Trail and begin the "lower tour" of the Flatirons.

Mesa Trail: From here on out, you'll be on the class 1 Mesa Trail until you reach Chautauqua Park. You will have many great views of the Flatirons on your left. Several trails intersect with the Mesa Trail along the way. Stay on the Mesa Trail, and continue going north.

9.1 mi (11)   This is the only "tricky" part of the Mesa Trail, though it's still well marked. After passing the Fern Canyon cutoff, you'll pass a small stream on your right. The wide dirt trail you're on continues to the west; make sure you stay on the Mesa Trail which cuts off to the left (north) uphill and becomes a single-lane footpath again. Follow it north through a four-way intersection just below the National Center for Atmospheric Research (NCAR) to your right. After this, you'll drop in and out of Skunk Canyon and continue to the boundaries of Chautauqua Park. Several trails continue to come in on both sides of the Mesa Trail.

10.8 mi (12)   The Mesa Trail turns into a gravel path as you drop down into Chautauqua. Look west to see the loop you just made over the mountains. To return to Gregory Canyon Trailhead, you can hike west on Baseline Road or take a footpath that parallels the road in the open meadow.

12.1 mi   Finish.

Options   If you'd like to cut an hour or two off your hike (and still bag the three peaks), bring two cars (or a bike and a car). You can leave a vehicle at the Shadow Canyon/Mesa Trail Trailhead, accessed by taking Colorado Highway 93 (Broadway) out of Boulder and then taking a right onto Colorado Highway 170 at a stoplight (there's a convenience store on the right). Follow the road toward Eldorado Springs for 2.0 miles, and the marked trailhead will be on the right-hand side of the road. At waypoint 10, instead of turning onto the Mesa Trail after your descent of Shadow Canyon, follow the Shadow Canyon Trail 1.5 miles to this parking lot. You could also park a car at the NCAR lot (no fee), accessed by taking CO 93 and then turning west onto Table Mesa Drive and following it to

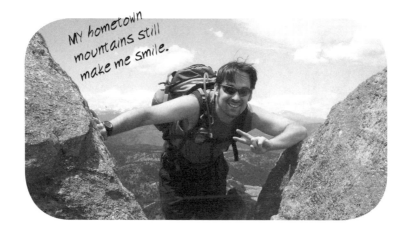

My hometown mountains still make me smile.

its terminus. You would end your hike at NCAR by taking the Mesa Trail past Fern Canyon and turning right at the well-marked sign at the top of a small hill (shortly after waypoint 11); this trail leads to NCAR.

If you want an early exit, it's nice to know there are a few cutoffs that return to the Mesa Trail. You can follow the Bear Canyon Trail (at the end of the Green-Bear Trail) or the Fern Canyon Trail (from the summit of Bear Peak) east. Both intersect with the Mesa Trail, shaving time off your hike but still giving you a fun loop.

Quick Facts These three peaks have very common names. Did you know there are more than 20 Green Mountains in Colorado? One twist on this Green Mountain: it may allude to E.M. Greenman, an early Boulder conservationist. Chautauqua Park was part of an educational movement at the turn of the 19th century that aimed to create communities in which members were encouraged to delve into the arts, sciences, and music as a part of daily life. Touring units of entertainers would visit Chautauqua communities in each state. While the concept was a positive, progressive alternative to mundane living, many of the Chautauqua communities soon became too expensive for normal folks, and the exclusivity stymied the movement, though the practice still exists to some degree in Boulder today.

Contact Info This hike is especially beautiful on a snowy winter day. If you're hiking in the summer, bring a little extra water, as it can get very toasty in Boulder from June to late September. And if you want a good view of fireworks on the Fourth of July, Bear Peak is a fun (and social) place to watch the displays from towns across the Front Range.

Note: This area is undergoing changes as Boulder Mountain Park aims to improve the trail system. Call for more information, as several issues are pending (such as making the E.M. Greenman Trail a no-dog trail).

Boulder Mountain Parks
P.O. Box 791
Boulder, CO 80306
(303) 441-3440

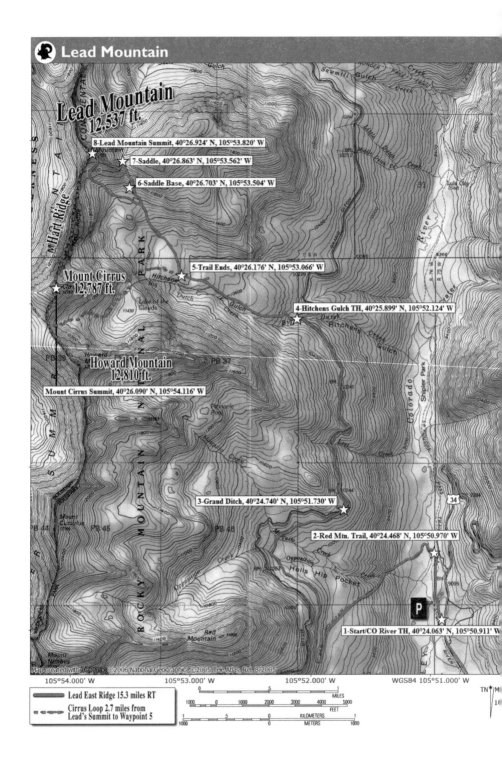

Lead Mountain
12,537 ft.

8-Lead Mountain Summit, 40°26.924' N, 105°53.820' W

7-Saddle, 40°26.863' N, 105°53.562' W

6-Saddle Base, 40°26.703' N, 105°53.504' W

Mount Cirrus
12,787 ft.

5-Trail Ends, 40°26.176' N, 105°53.066' W

4-Hitchens Gulch TH, 40°25.899' N, 105°52.124' W

Howard Mountain
12,810 ft.

Mount Cirrus Summit, 40°26.090' N, 105°54.116' W

3-Grand Ditch, 40°24.740' N, 105°51.730' W

2-Red Mtn. Trail, 40°24.468' N, 105°50.970' W

P

1-Start/CO River TH, 40°24.063' N, 105°50.911' W

Map created with TOPO!© ©2006 National Geographic; ©2005 Tele Atlas, Rel. 8/2005

105°54.000' W   105°53.000' W   105°52.000' W   WGS84 105°51.000' W

Lead East Ridge 15.3 miles RT

Cirrus Loop 2.7 miles from
Lead's Summit to Waypoint 5

5   **Lead Mountain**   *Good Overnight!*

This beautiful, airy ridge is great scramble that will keep you on your toes. The rock is solid, and the views are phenomenal. An optional loop to Mount Cirrus adds to the fun.

Round Trip Distance	15.3 miles
Hiking Time	9–14 hours
Difficulty	9/10
Class	3/3+
Start Elevation	9,100 ft., at Colorado River Trailhead
Peak Elevation	12,537 ft.
Total Elevation Gain	3,727 ft.
Terrain	Long prelude to exciting class 3 ridge
Best Time to Climb	July–September
Gear Advisor	Helmet, good grippy boots
Crowd Level	Hermit

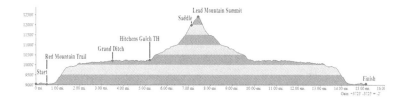

Location   Never Summer Range in Rocky Mountain National Park outside of Estes Park

Intro   Lead Mountain has one of the premier ridge walks in the state. The exposed, airy, class 3 traverse is short, but it certainly gets your attention. Rock is solid for the most part. Those hikers uncomfortable with hanging out on the spine have the option to drop down slightly to the south side, where terrain is less exposed. The Never Summer Range is a special treat for hikers looking to get away from the crowds. The loop over to Mount Cirrus may be Colorado's best class 3 route that's not in the Grenadiers!

Why Climb It?   The mileage looks daunting, but a good deal of this hike is the long and scenic approach. Trails are class 1 from the trailhead, all the way to the end of the Hitchens Gulch Trail, 6.2 miles in. The actual class 3 terrain is only roughly 1.3 miles on the standard route, but every foot is an exciting experience. Lead's east ridge is airy and exhilarating, with sheer drop-offs to the north. Rock is solid but the exposure will boost your concentration. A few moves may be considered class 4 or 3+ if you stay on the spine of the ridge. The holds are solid and obvious, but if you blow it, you'll be shuffling off this mortal coil with haste. If you aren't used to this kind of exposure, an alternate class 3 route on the south side of the ridge is just as good.

Driving   Any vehicle can make it to the trailhead; the entire drive is on paved roads.

How to Get There   From the east entrances (Beaver Meadows or Fall River), go about 4.0 miles (from either) to the intersection of US highways 34 and 36. Continue on Trail Ridge Road (US 34) 28 miles, up and over the highpoint near the Alpine visitor center. After the road exits the final hairpin turn downhill, it's about 1.2 miles to the Colorado River Trailhead on the right (west) side of the road. The turnoff is well marked. This trailhead is 11.5 miles north on Route 34 from the west entrance at Grand Lake.

Fees/Camping   It is $20 for a day pass to Rocky Mountain National Park. There are several drive-in campgrounds in the park that range from $10 to $14 a night; call for more information. A better option (and one that gives you the time to complete the Hart Ridge traverse to Mount Cirrus) is to camp at backcountry sites at Hitchens Gulch (Hitchens Gulch Campground and Dutch Town Campground—beware of mosquitoes in the summer!). It is $20 for a backcountry camping permit but well worth the price for this incredible optional loop.

Route Notes   I highly recommend the Mount Cirrus loop, starting with an overnight at Dutch Town and getting an early start to the day. It's a scrambler's delight.

Mile/Waypoint   **0.0 mi (1)** Start at the Colorado River Trailhead and head north on the very well-trodden trail (this is the La Poudre Pass Trail). You will only be on this smooth section for a short distance.

0.5 mi (2) Turn left (west) onto the well-signed Red Mountain Trail. The turnoff sign includes mileages to Hitchens Gulch, Grand Ditch, Dutch Town, and Thunder Pass. Stay on this pleasant trail all the way to the Grand Ditch. Along the way, you will pass the rather benign canyon called Hell's Hip Pocket.

3.3 mi (3) After a nice walk in the woods, you come to…a road? This is the Grand Ditch. Turn right and hike north on this easy-going road (don't worry that Lead Mountain is directly west; you have to loop around to reach it). Public access to this road is limited to foot traffic, so any vehicle sightings are rare. (And no, you can't drive up here as a shortcut!)

5.2 mi (4) Eventually, you'll come to the Hitchens Gulch Trailhead on your left (west), where the road crosses Dutch Creek. There is a sign here for Hitchens Gulch and Dutch Town. There is a good trail that heads northwest toward Lead's talus-filled basin. Hitchens Gulch Camp area is at mile 5.5; Dutch Town is at mile 5.9. Stay on this trail until it ends abruptly at a post near a mosquito-filled swamp.

6.2 mi (5) Luckily, there is only one small hill to climb after the trail ends (there may still be a faint footpath). Atop this hill, you're out of the trees, and the incredibly rock-filled basin is before you. Gradually ascend, first on rocks and then on grassy slopes, northwest to the scree slope that goes

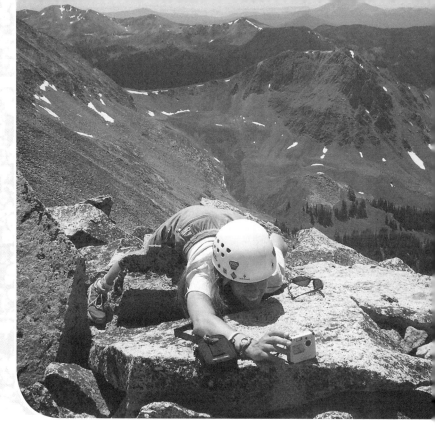

Getting the perfect shot can be tricky on Lead's rocky summit.

to the saddle between Lead and Point 12,438. There are some crazy rock formations on 12,438, and it looks like some large boulders have peeled off the mountain in recent times.

7.0 mi (6) You will come to the base of a loose, red scree gully. The grass on the right side is deceptive; the terrain there is just as loose as the middle of the gully. It's a bit of a knee burner. Make your way to the saddle and get ready to climb.

7.2 mi (7) You are now in the saddle. Don your helmet and get ready to head west on Lead's east ridge. To the north, there is a great view of another mountained featured in this book, Mount Richthofen (Hike 7). You can go a short bit on the north side of the saddle to gain the obvious ramp up to the ridge.

Climbing the east ridge: This ridge is quite short, only about 0.4 mile to the summit, but it will take awhile to get up. As mentioned, the route is all class 3 and 3+ stuff, with the easier sections coming at the lower parts of the ridge. The rock is quite solid but with some big-time exposure. Staying on the ridge all the way up is a thrill, with a few 3+ moves thrown in to keep your heart rate up. Take your time to find and test good holds—they are there. After the initial "connecting ramp" puts you on the east ridge proper, you have the option to drop down to the south side and traverse via rocky ledges just below the ridge. This terrain is still fun class 3, minus the exposure. Scramblers on the ridge will make it directly to the summit, while those on the south side will have a fun, solid rock gully leading to the top. This thrilling little scramble is a great way to wrap up your hike.

7.6 mi (8) Lead Mountain's summit! If you're going for the Hart Ridge Loop, your path awaits. If Lead was your objective (which is probably the case if you're doing this as a dayhike), you have two descent options. You can retrace the east ridge, which has some sketchy spots with exposed downclimbing but is the fastest way to get back. Experienced scramblers will prefer this route. The other option, which I've outlined on the standard route, goes south via the lower path's ascent gully. Drop down and head right (west) on ledges toward Hart Ridge. Going left onto Lead's face looks more direct, but it cliffs out with difficult and dangerous class 4/5 gullies to downclimb. Aim for the ground below the saddle between Lead Mountain and Mount Cirrus: the scrambling is class 3, but it is much safer than other routes. Once you reach the big talus field, head southeast back to where you came up. Return the way you came and bask in the afterglow of this fine summit.

15.3 mi Finish.

Options   Hart Ridge runs between Lead Mountain and Mount Cirrus (12,797 feet). This fun class 3 scramble is a great option, and may actually provide the safest descent route. It is 1.0 mile between summits. From the top of Lead Mountain, go south along the ridge. It begins with relatively easy terrain; at 0.5 mile, the scrambling becomes similar to stuff on Lead. Again, the holds are solid and the exposure is thrilling. Once you top out on Cirrus, keep going south to the saddle between Cirrus and Howard Mountain at 12,400 feet. (Howard is a quick diversion if you'd like to summit another peak.) Hike/surf down the broad gully of loose scree to Lake of the Clouds at 11,430 feet. From Lake of the Clouds, shuffle down the slopes back into the basin and return via the Hitchens Gulch Trail (waypoint 4), picking up the route that you began the hike with. This option is approximately 2.7 miles from the top of Lead, over Cirrus, down to Lake of the Clouds, and back to the basin where you hiked up—about 6.0 miles round trip from Dutch Town Campground.

Quick Facts   Lead Mountain earned its name in 1879. Lead wasn't a particularly coveted ore, and it served more to frustrate miners than to line their pockets.

In 1914, James Grafton Rogers named three sky-high peaks in the Never Summer Range for clouds: Cirrus, Cumulus, and Nimbus. Later, Mount Stratus was added to the mix. Howard Mountain may seem like an atmospheric outcast amongst these mountains, unless you consider that Luke Howard was the English meteorologist who first named and classified cloud formations. It's a good theory, but according to Rogers's own account, "Howard" appeared on maps prior to the naming of the "cloud mountains." Thus, the true identity of "Howard" is a mystery. Just for fun, I like to think it was named after Moe Howard, leader of the Three Stooges. (Harry Moses Horwitz, a.k.a. Moe Howard, was born June 19, 1897, making this theoretically possible, assuming he took his stage name early in life.)

Hart Ridge is named for Lt. Eldon C. Hart, who was killed while flying for the Kansas Air National Guard when his F-100C Super Sabre fighter jet crashed into Mount Cirrus on January 30, 1967. The wreckage is on the west side of the mountain, so you won't be seeing it on this route.

Contact Info Rocky Mountain National Park
1000 Highway 36
Estes Park, CO 80517-8397

General Park Information: (970) 586-1206
Visitor Information Recorded Message: (970)-586-1333
Backcountry Information (970)-586-1242
Campground Reservations (800) 365-2267

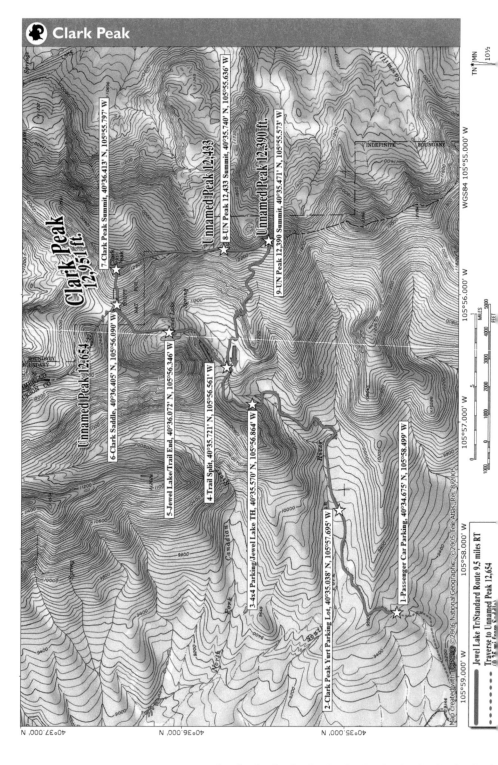

Clark Peak
12,951 ft.

7-Clark Peak Summit, 40°36.413' N, 105°55.797' W

Unnamed Peak 12,433

8-UN Peak 12,433 Summit, 40°35.740' N, 105°55.636' W

Unnamed Peak 12,390 ft.

9-UN Peak 12,390 Summit, 40°35.471' N, 105°55.573' W

INDEFINITE   BOUNDARY

Unnamed Peak 12,654

6-Clark Saddle, 40°36.405' N, 105°56.090' W

5-Jewel Lake/Trail End, 40°36.072' N, 105°56.346' W

4-Trail Split, 40°35.721' N, 105°56.561' W

3-4x4 Parking/Jewel Lake TH, 40°35.570' N, 105°56.864' W

2-Clark Peak Yurt Parking Lot, 40°35.038' N, 105°57.695' W

1-Passenger Car Parking, 40°34.675' N, 105°58.499' W

WGS84 105°55.000' W

105°56.000' W

105°57.000' W

105°58.000' W

105°59.000' W

TN ★ MN   10½°

MILES
FEET

Jewel Lake Tr/Standard Route 9.5 miles RT

Traverse to Unnamed Peak 12,654

N 40°37.000'   N 40°36.000'   N 40°35.000'

6   Clark Peak

Clark Peak is the highpoint of the Medicine Bow Mountains, a less-known but beautiful range in the Colorado State Forest. A good hike with a sky-walk ridge traverse.

Round Trip Distance	9.5 miles for cars; 4.2 miles from 4x4 parking
Hiking Time	3–6 hours
Difficulty	5/10
Class	2
Start Elevation	9,470 ft. on Ruby Jewel Road
Peak Elevation	12,951 ft.
Total Elevation Gain	4,087 ft.
Terrain	Nice trail, steep grassy slopes, great flat ridge walk
Best Time to Climb	June–September
Gear Advisor	Trekking poles
Crowd Level	Low

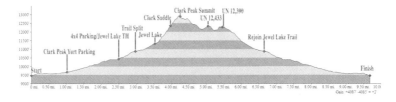

Location   Medicine Bow Range in the Colorado State Forest near the small town of Gould.

Intro   Clark Peak is the highpoint of the Medicine Bow Range (as well as the highpoint of Jackson County). Clark's setting in northern Colorado means you'll be hiking on unique topography, complete with dramatic basins and prolific peaks. Views from the top are awesome, especially the far-off view of the seldom-seen northwest face of Longs Peak. The Colorado State Forest borders the Rawah Wilderness, and both areas offer great backpacking.

Why Climb It?   Clark feels very different than most other peaks in Colorado—in a very good way. Those who have hiked in Wyoming's Wind River Range may find the atmosphere in the Medicine Bows familiar. This route goes by Jewel Lake, a dreamy alpine pool at the base of a dramatic basin. The stiff, off-trail hill that goes from Jewel Lake is flooded with flowers of all colors. From Clark's summit (which will be hidden until you actually ascend to the top), the southern skywalk to neighboring unnamed peaks is a tran-scendent traverse. Many who hike in this area return to backpack and camp (the terrain is similar to the Mount Zirkel Wilderness in Steamboat Springs).

Driving	Passenger cars—even tough passenger cars (TPCs)—will be fine on the well-groomed dirt of County Road 41 but can only reach 1.0 mile up Ruby Jewel Road before it gets too rough (read below for more info on the road conditions). High-clearance SUVs or 4x4s are needed to reach the trailhead; sport utility cars (SUCs) and AWD vehicles can make it most of the way up Ruby Jewel Road but will struggle with the last 1.5 miles. The road is steep and very rocky in sections, with smooth, flat sections between. There is a minor river crossing just before the parking lot.
How to Get There	From Fort Collins, turn west onto Route 14 (Poudre Canyon) and get ready for a long, twisty ride! You will be on this road for just under 70 miles, but expect the trip to take about two hours, thanks to the curviness of the highway. Go up and over Cameron Pass (those cool rock formations you see in front of you are the Nokhu Crags). Drop over the pass, and at mile 69.8, turn right onto County Road 41; this turn comes up quickly. The dirt road entrance to 41 has info kiosks, self-pay stations, and a campground; it's a gateway to Colorado State Forest. **Note:** there is a ranger station about a mile before this turn on the left side of the road, where you can get additional information.
	Stay on 41, passing the Michigan Reservoir (and its large concrete sluice) at mile 4.6. At mile 4.9, you'll reach a plateau where Ruby Jewel Road splits off to the right (there are signs). From here, it is 3.5 miles to the Jewel Lake Trailhead. Passenger cars can drive up 1.0 mile and park in a small lot on the right where Francisco Road splits from Ruby Jewel Road. SUCs, SUVs, and 4x4s continue straight uphill (do not turn left onto Francisco Road) on Ruby Jewel Road. At mile 2.0, the parking lot for Clark Peak Yurt appears—this is a good place for lower clearance and AWD vehicles to stop; 4x4s and tougher vehicles can drive 1.5 miles on the rocky, steep road to reach the trailhead. The road is well signed.
Fees/Camping	As of 2006, there is a $5 self-pay fee for day use in Colorado State Forest. You will need a permit to backcountry camp, but there is no charge other than the day-use fee. There are several developed campgrounds in the area that range between $7 and $16 per night.
Route Notes	You can do this loop either way, though dropping down to Ruby Jewel Lake is rough on the knees. Bring trekking poles!
Mile/Waypoint	**0.0 mi (1)** This is the passenger car parking lot at the split of Ruby Jewel Road and Francisco Road (1.0 mile from the split with 41). There are 3 to 4 spots here. Hike/drive/bike up the road to Jewel Lake Trailhead.
	1.0 mi (2) There is a large parking lot for the Clark Peak Yurt.
	2.5 mi (3) Reach the fenced-in 4x4 parking lot. The Jewel Lake Trail may not be marked, but it is the obvious footpath that starts north after passing over a footbridge. Stay on the worn path as it crosses a few streams; you'll eventually come to a clearing and have to follow the path across a talus field.
	2.7 mi (4) After the talus field, the trail splits. Stay left for Jewel Lake; you'll return to the main trail later from the right (of course, if you'd like to do the

hike in reverse, you can turn right here and loop north instead of south). The Jewel Lake Trail bypasses a lush meadow, which will be on your right. The trail may be overgrown or difficult to find in the mud, especially in early spring. If you get off-trail, remember Jewel Lake is above you to the north.

3.3 mi (5) Reach Jewel Lake. The trail ends here. Head northeast and pick a line up the steep, grassy slope that heads to the saddle between Clark Peak and Unnamed Peak 12,654. In the spring, this hill is flush with flowers; the route tracked here goes up a shallow gully I have dubbed "Flower Gully." Flower Gully is the path of least resistance. Climb straight up, roughly 1,200 feet, to gain the saddle.

4.0 mi (6) At the saddle, turn directly east and scale your second steep hill to reach Clark's summit (which won't be apparent until you are standing on it).

4.2 mi (7) Clark Peak Summit. The huge peak you see to the northwest is South Rawah Peak. You have the option to descend the way you came up, but it is murder on the knees. The more scenic option takes the same amount of time. Leave the summit and traverse the high plains south. This is the beginning of the "skywalk."

5.1 mi (8) Reach Unnamed Peak 12,433. You can drop down here if you like; however, this route carries on to one more unnamed peak.

5.4 mi (9) Reach Unnamed Peak 12,390. Descend the switchbacks to the pack trail below you and follow it to the Jewel Lake Trail (or simply bushwhack back down to the Jewel Lake Trail).

6.8 mi (4) Rejoin the Jewel Lake Trail near the talus field and return to your vehicle.

9.6 mi Finish at the passenger car parking area.

Options From the saddle above Jewel Lake (waypoint 6), it's a short detour (0.25 mile) over to Unnamed Peak 12,654. To get there and back only adds about a half mile to your trip. The back side (north face) of UN 12,654 looks like it would be a very cool ski descent (though it would drop you into the Rawah Wilderness).

Quick Facts Clark Peak is named for none other than William Clark, of the fabled Lewis and Clark Expedition. There are no mountains to the north in the state of Colorado that are higher than Clark Peak.

Contact Info Colorado State Forest
2746 County Road 41
Walden, CO 80480
(970) 723-8366
www.parks.state.co.us

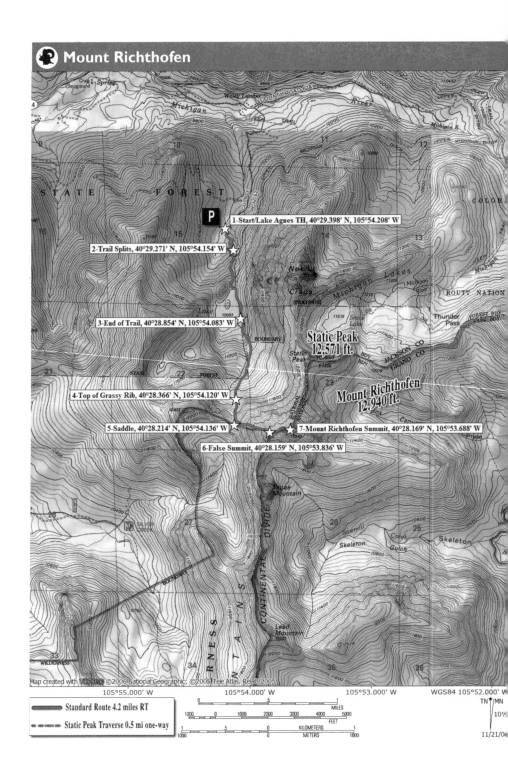

1-Start/Lake Agnes TH, 40°29.398' N, 105°54.208' W

2-Trail Splits, 40°29.271' N, 105°54.154' W

3-End of Trail, 40°28.854' N, 105°54.083' W

Static Peak
12,571 ft.

Mount Richthofen
12,940 ft.

4-Top of Grassy Rib, 40°28.366' N, 105°54.120' W

5-Saddle, 40°28.214' N, 105°54.136' W

7-Mount Richthofen Summit, 40°28.169' N, 105°53.688' W

6-False Summit, 40°28.159' N, 105°53.836' W

Standard Route 4.2 miles RT

Static Peak Traverse 0.5 mi one-way

Map created with TOPO!® ©2006 National Geographic; ©2009 Tele Atlas, Rel. 08/2005

105°55.000' W   105°54.000' W   105°53.000' W   WGS84 105°52.000' W

7 Mount Richthofen

Situated in the northern part of the Never Summer Range, Richthofen is a short but sweet scramble with great views. A secret passage grants you access to this impressive summit!

Round Trip Distance	4.2 miles
Hiking Time	4–6 hours
Difficulty	7.5/10
Class	3
Start Elevation	10,270 ft., at Agnes Lake Trailhead
Peak Elevation	12,940 ft.
Total Elevation Gain	2,627 ft.
Terrain	Rocky scrambling with some loose sections
Best Time to Climb	Mid-June–September
Gear Advisor	Helmets are a good idea if in a group
Crowd Level	Low

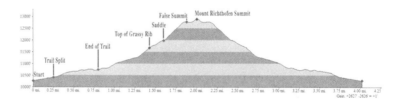

Location Never Summer Range; Richthofen's east and south faces are in Rocky Mountain National Park, while the north and west faces are in the Colorado State Forest. This route approaches from the Colorado State Forest side, just past Cameron Pass.

Intro Good scrambles always appeal to my inner mountain goat. The west ridge on this route starts off a bit loose but becomes increasingly solid as you near the summit block. Richthofen is the highest peak in the burly Never Summer Range, a special range with some of the most rugged mountains in Colorado. Talus is king in the Never Summers, but that doesn't detract from the great hiking and scrambling.

Why Climb It? If you've never been to the Never Summer Range, you owe it to yourself to check out the spectacular terrain that defines the region. Before you even set foot on the trail, you're treated to views of the sinister-looking Nokhu Crags, a collection of crooked spires and crumbling towers that loom west of the access trail. Lake Agnes is a glacial lake surrounded by an amphitheater of boulders. In direct sunlight, the water glows a translucent green hue. As you gain the west ridge, these sights become even more impressive. The final scramble to the top involves a "secret" notch on the north face.

Driving

This road to the trail is good for tough passenger cars; you'll probably scrape a low-clearance vehicle here and there, but cars can reach the trailhead without too much trouble. SUCs, SUVs, and 4x4s will be fine. The road is a little rocky and narrow, but it never gets too steep or too rocky.

How to Get There

From Fort Collins, head west on Colorado Highway 14 for 62 miles (this drive is going to take awhile, thanks to the curvy road). Once you are at Cameron Pass, it is 2.0 miles to the left-hand turn off to CR 62 (there are signs to Lake Agnes on the road). A self-pay fee station greets you at the turnoff; as of 2006, the day-use fee was $5. At 0.6 mile, the road splits. Stay right and continue to follow the signs to Lake Agnes (you'll be going uphill abruptly after this turn). Continue along this brief road; at mile 1.75 you'll reach the Lake Agnes Trailhead. There are signs that lead you to the trailhead; there are also a few jeep roads that intersect CR 62. Stay on the main road until the parking area, which is home to a weird, football-shaped bathroom.

Fees/Camping

It's $5 for a day-use fee at Richthofen. There's really not much in the way of camping near Richthofen, but there are several campgrounds beyond Cameron Pass in Colorado State Forest, where sites are between $7 and $12 per night.

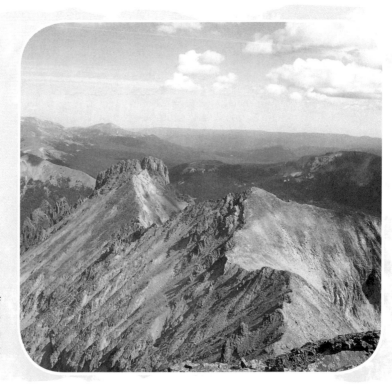

Amazing views of Static Peak and the Nokhu Crags from the summit of Mount Richthofen

The mileage here is low, but you'll have to earn every foot of elevation you gain. Your trail ends at the south side of Lake Agnes; from there, you'll need to use some basic navigational skills to reach the saddle between Richthofen and Unnamed Peak 12,942. Most of the hike is out of the trees, so visually following the lines of the mountain is not very difficult.

0.0 mi (1) Start at the Lake Agnes Trailhead and take the Lake Agnes Trail. You'll enter the woods and immediately hit a swath of switchbacks.

0.25 mi (2) Stay right (south) on the Lake Agnes Trail at this split. (The left trail goes north and skirts around the Nokhu Crags to the Michigan Lakes.)

0.6 mi Beautiful Lake Agnes, complete with a rocky island, greets you as you come out of the woods. Several trails appear here; you want to stay on the path through the talus on the east side of the lake. Follow it to the southern terminus of the lake. From there, the terrain gets steep: you'll cover 1,250 vertical feet in 1.0 mile to reach the saddle.

0.8 mi (3) The trail ends at the terminus of the lake. Richthofen will be looking down at you, a little bit left of your bearing. Your goal now is to reach the large, obvious saddle to the south. There is a creek (or creekbed in late summer) that can guide you to the easiest path up the saddle. Staying on the grassy sections makes this ascent easier. About halfway up, you can gain a grassy rib that will lead you to the base of the bowl leading up the saddle.

1.5 mi (4) At the top of the grassy rib, you can bear a little to the right and start the push up the saddle. There are some faint trails you can follow, which may help on the loose rock. This is least enjoyable part of the hike, but it isn't very long.

1.7 mi (5) Alright, you're at the top of the saddle! The elevation here is just under 12,000 feet. Only 940 vertical feet to go! I hope your legs are ready, because you're going to gain all of that elevation in a mere 0.4 miles. (Now you understand why this low-mileage hike takes so long.) Note that you'll have a good look at Lead Mountain (Hike 5) to the south. Even though it is close to Richthofen, the trailhead for Lead Mountain is a good three hours away, in Rocky Mountain National Park.

As you embark on the west ridge of Mount Richthofen, scramble along the spine. The lower rock is a bit loose but will get more solid as you gain elevation. In the morning, it may be tough to follow the ridge when the sun is breaking just over the top of the mountain (curse these west ridges sometimes!).

2.0 mi (6) There's nothing quite like a false summit. This one isn't too bad; once you're on it, the remaining climb to the summit isn't far. But how *does* one scramble up to the top? That block looks like it's going to take some tricky scrambling.

When you reach the "minisaddle" between the false and true summits, peek around the corner out onto the northwest face of the mountain to find the perfect access gully. This is a short, class 3 scramble that makes topping out on Richthofen a marvelous experience. A wind shelter and a gold USGS marker await you on the top.

2.1 mi (7) On top of the world, Ma! Mount Richthofen summit! To the south, Tepee Mountain connects Mount Richthofen to Lead Mountain. Orange-tinted peaks of the Never Summer Range twist southwest, where they merge with the Rabbit Ears Range. The Mummy Range and other peaks north of Trail Ridge Road are to the east. Far north, you can see the tips of the Medicine Bow Mountains and the top of Clark Peak, yet another great hike in this book (Hike 6). Return the same way you came up (unless you want to take a quick tour of Static Peak, to the northeast, listed in the "Options" section below).

4.2 mi Finish. That was quite a workout for a 4-mile hike!

Options   From the top of Richtofen, it's a clean 0.5-mile traverse to the northeast to reach the top of 12,571-foot Static Peak. This class 2 ridge is a good walk. If the weather (and your legs) allow, check it out. Return back the way you came. The scramble down from the saddle of Static and the Nokhu Crags is loose, dangerous, and prone to rockfall from above. Return back over Richthofen for the safest way home.

Quick Facts   Mount Richthofen is named for a famous German but probably not the one you are thinking of. Clarence King, director of the Fortieth Parallel Survey, named the mountain after Ferdinand von Richthofen, a globetrotting German geologist. Educated in Berlin, he began his world tour as a geographer and geologist in 1860 by joining a scientific outfit that explored Japan, Taiwan, the Philippines, and Burma. He made his way to the United States in 1862, staying here for six years. He helped discover several gold deposits in California before returning to explore China and other places in Asia. One of his discoveries in China was the dried-up lakebed of Lopnur, a feature visible from space. For his efforts, a mountain range in China is named in his honor.

Oh yes, and Ferdinand von Richthofen was the uncle of Manfred von Richthofen, better known to history as the World War I flying ace "the Red Baron." Manfred's other uncle, Walter von Richthofen, helped found the Denver Chamber of Commerce and is credited with founding the neighborhood of Montclair, Colorado. He modeled his home in Montclair after the Richthofen family castle in Germany. Admittedly, it seems a little out of the place in the Western frontier.

Contact Info   Colorado State Forest
2746 County Road 41
Walden, Colorado 80480
(970) 723-8366

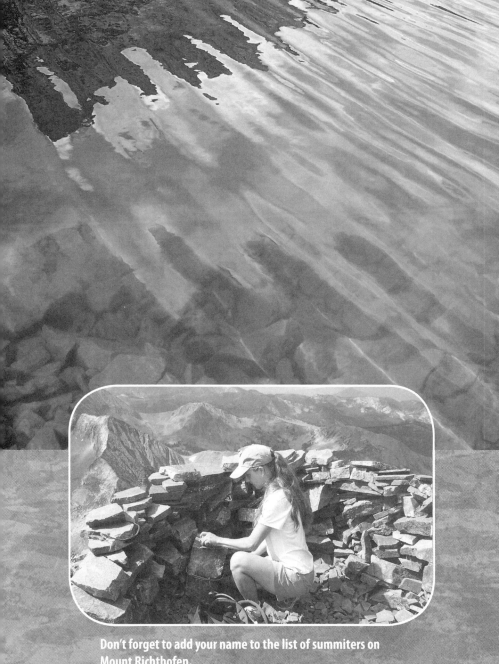

Don't forget to add your name to the list of summiters on
Mount Richthofen.

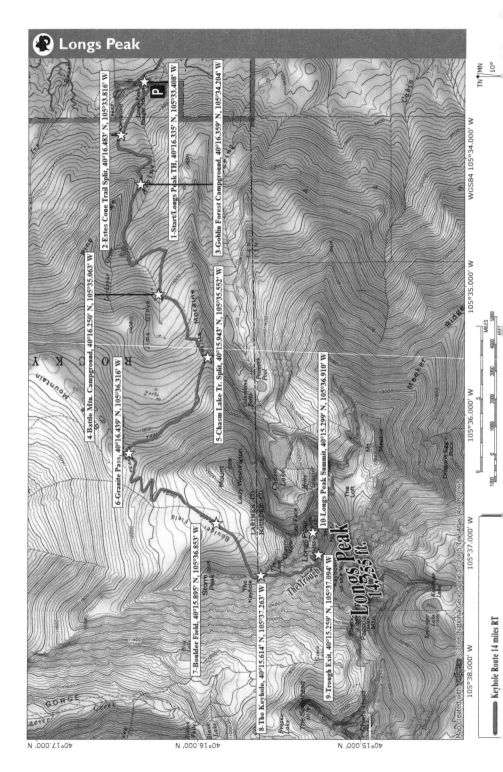

Longs Peak

1-Start/Longs Peak TH, 40°16.335' N, 105°33.408' W
2-Estes Cone Trail Split, 40°16.483' N, 105°33.816' W
3-Goblin Forest Campground, 40°16.359' N, 105°34.204' W
4-Battle Mtn. Campground, 40°16.250' N, 105°35.063' W
5-Chasm Lake Tr. Split, 40°15.943' N, 105°35.552' W
6-Granite Pass, 40°16.439' N, 105°36.316' W
7-Boulder Field, 40°15.895' N, 105°36.853' W
8-The Keyhole, 40°15.614' N, 105°37.263' W
9-Trough Exit, 40°15.259' N, 105°37.094' W
10-Longs Peak Summit, 40°15.299' N, 105°36.910' W

Longs Peak 14,255 ft.

Keyhole Route 14 miles RT

Map created with TopoFusion ©2006 National Geographic; ©2005 Tele Atlas; Rel. 8/2005

8 Longs Peak *Good overnight!*

Longs is the classic 14er. Despite the fact that it's a strenuous circuit, most people climb the keyhole route in a single day. The scrambling is amongst the best in the state!

Round Trip Distance	14 miles
Hiking Time	11–15 hours
Difficulty	8/10
Class	3
Start Elevation	9,375 ft., at Longs Peak Trailhead
Peak Elevation	14,255 ft.
Total Elevation Gain	5,580 ft.
Terrain	Long, easy approach trail to solid scrambling and a steep gully to summit; moderately exposed terrain
Best Time to Climb	Mid-June to September
Gear Advisor	Ice axe, helmet, crampons in early spring and after mid-September
Crowd Level	High

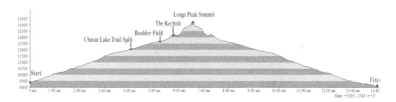

Location Front Range in Rocky Mountain National Park outside of Estes Park

Intro Get ready to make some new friends. Longs Peak is one of the most social summits in the state, even though it's a tough climb. For many, an ascent of Longs Peak is the culmination of their hiking "careers." It may be popular, but it's still tough. The classic way to climb the peak is to begin around 3 A.M. (to avoid storms) and summit in the early morning. No other 14er sees more traffic, nor does any other peak bestow everyday glory on the humble hiker more than Longs.

Why Climb It? Yes, you'll be dealing with all kinds of crowds on Longs. In my opinion, this is part of the fun. You'll see it all: families, gutsy weekend warriors, cocky climbers, teenagers, grandparents, guys, girls, the hefty and the slim, all aiming to stand on the flat summit of the mountain whose image is reproduced on the Colorado state quarter. Dreamlike phantom-trains of headlamps heading up in the predawn hours are a surreal sight. Passing through the Keyhole is like reaching the next level in a video game. A new world waits on the back side of Longs. Even veteran hikers and scramblers can appreciate the moderately exposed traverses and good class 3 terrain that leads to the summit. Longs is a must-do mountain. I could not in good faith write about the best summits in Colorado and exclude it.

Driving The road to Longs Peak Trailhead is paved and passable by all vehicles.

How to Get There The road to the trailhead is off Colorado Highway 7. From the south, this is 10.4 miles north of the junction of CO 7 and Colorado Highway 72; from the north, it is 9.2 miles from the junction of US Highway 36 and CO 7. Turn west onto the well-marked Longs Peak Road and drive approximately 0.8 mile to the ranger station and Longs Peak Trailhead.

Fees/Camping Longs is in Rocky Mountain National Park, but there is no fee for dayhiking the area. Camping requires a permit and a $20 fee. There are three campgrounds along the way: Golbin's Forest, Battle Mountain Group Site, and the Boulderfield. Call for reservations, as these sites fill up quickly in the summer. Longs Peak Campground is just below the trailhead and offers 26 sites for tents only. There is no overnight camping allowed in the parking lot.

Route Notes I've noticed my GPS tracks recorded a slightly shorter round-trip distance than official park publications proclaim (most say either 15 or 16 miles). I stayed on trail where there is a trail; however I made direct approaches in the boulder field and in the trough, which may have cut my mileage a bit. (I grew up hiking in New England: we don't believe in switchbacks!) As a result, I had a mileage of 6.91 miles to the summit, and 6.89 miles on the descent. My elevation profile includes the up and down in the keyhole, the boulder field, and the slight ups and downs around Chasm Lake. I explain these discrepancies because there is so much literature available providing statistics about Longs.

As mentioned, dayhikers should aim to start no later than 3 A.M. (early is better). A considerable amount of this hike is above treeline, with little shelter from the inevitable summer storms. Longs is a serious hike; many people have died on the "standard" route from falls, lightning, and other accidents. Don't underestimate it just because it is popular!

Note: The Keyhole Route is formally known as the East Longs Peak Trail.

Mile/Waypoint **0.0 mi (1)** Start at the Longs Peak Trailhead, gaining the East Longs Peak Trail just behind the ranger station. There's a good chance you'll be hiking in the dark (as you should!). The trail is wide, well worn, and easy to follow.

0.4 mi (2) Don't make a rookie mistake in the early morning. At this fork, the Longs Peak Trail goes left, so stay the course. The trail that cuts off to the right goes to Eugenia Mine and Estes Cone. Once you clear this intersection, you have a long approach to the Keyhole. Set a good pace and enjoy the sunrise.

1.1 mi (3) Goblin Forest Campground.

2.4 mi (4) A short distance above timberline, Battle Mountain Campground is off to the right. Stay left on the well-marked trail.

3.1 mi (5) Great views of "the Diamond" are evident from the flat section that serves as the junction between the Longs Peak Trail and the Chasm Lake Trail (there's a toilet here, too). The Diamond on Longs Peak's northeast face is a test piece for advanced rock climbers; practically every line you can see on the sheer face has been scaled. *Do not* descend to Chasm Lake. Continue northwest to Granite Pass and the boulder field.

4.0 mi (6) Granite Pass. Stay left on the trail to the boulder field at the trail junction. In the case of a fast-moving storm, the rocky caves to the north of Granite Pass provide emergency shelters.

5.6 mi (7) This is the heart of the boulder field. There is a toilet here. Gaps in the rock at the west end of the boulder field form the fabled Keyhole. The trail fades out on the rocky slope up to the Keyhole, but your short-term goal is obvious. At the Keyhole is a storm shelter, complete with glass windows. Get ready to climb once you pass this gateway to adventure.

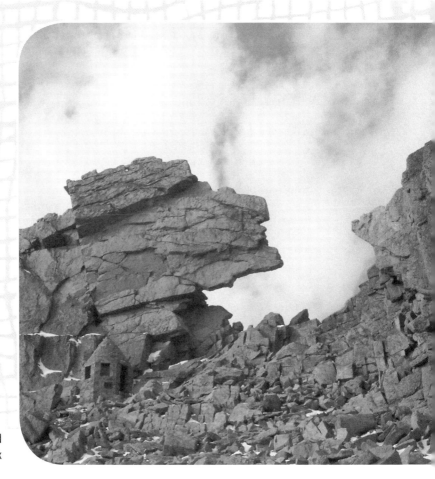

The fabled keyhole and shelter on Longs Peak

5.8 mi (8) Behold the world beyond the Keyhole! Your route goes left (south) and follows a 0.3-mile trail marked with spray-painted bull's eye markers. This traverse is slightly exposed and gives you the first real taste of the challenge of Longs.

6.1 mi You are now at the base of a long gully known as the Trough. The base of the Trough is roughly 13,100 feet, so you'll be doing the steepest climbing at dizzying altitude. It's 900 feet to the top of this cardiovascular-pumping chute. Watch out for rocks dislodged by climbers above you, and try not to knock any on the climbers below you.

6.5 mi (9) The Trough tops out just below 14,000 feet. There are great views of another mountain featured in this book, Mount Alice (Hike 9), from this gap. The next short section is known as the Narrows. The exposure may be unsettling for inexperienced hikers. The path is cut into the slope and there are plenty of good handholds along the way. These sections are short and well marked, so the map of this route will not include them as individual waypoints.

6.7 mi Drop down about 30 feet to 13,980 feet and the beginning of a section known as "the Home Stretch." To the southeast, long chimneys of rock are worth looking at while you take a water break.

The Home Stretch entails the most difficult scrambling of the hike. The holds are very good and the route is marked. Push your way through "Victory Gap" to the surprisingly mellow, flat summit.

6.9 mi (10) Longs Peak Summit! You're halfway done! A rock outcrop to the west has the USGS marker, the summit log, and the best views. Allow me to describe the top using an all-American measuring system: the summit of Longs is three football fields long.

On the descent, return the same way you came. Take your time when there is snow. Be courteous as you pass other hikers. Many will have the blank stare of exhaustion with a glimmer of determination in their eyes. Be positive! In case of bad weather, remember there are shelters at the Keyhole and in the rocks at Granite Pass. It's a very long walk down; the last few miles in the trees get tedious. With luck, the afterglow of such a great hike will keep you moving.

14 mi Finish the hike and give yourself a pat on the back; you've just completed Colorado's classic 14er.

Options This hike is a big commitment. If doing this as a dayhike, you're probably not going to want to add to it. Some people will make the short traverse over to Storm Peak, north of the Keyhole…the showoffs! If you really have the legs (or you're camping in the area), the Estes Cone hike is a nice diversion; it's 4.8 miles round trip (from the trail intersection at waypoint 2) on a good trail.

Quick Facts There is far more history to report about Longs than I can cover in a paragraph. I would suggest reading *Longs Peak: The Story of Colorado's Favorite Fourteener* by Dougald MacDonald, published by Westcliffe Publishers. It is an excellent account of the history of Longs Peak.

A few quick facts: the peak is named for Stephen Long, who surveyed the area in 1820 but never climbed the mountain. He didn't formally name the peak after himself. Rather, he described Longs and its 13,911-foot neighbor as "the Two Ears," a name given to the peaks by French fur trappers. The sister peak would later be named Mount Meeker, in honor of Nathan Meeker, founder of Greeley.

The first official climb of the peak was recorded in 1868 by a group made up of John Wesley Powell (the famous one-armed Civil War vet), his brother W.H. Powell, William Byers (for whom a mountain was later named), L.W. Keplinger, and three Illinois college students who apparently forgot to sign the register. Upon reaching the summit, they discovered an Arapahoe eagle trap, clearly indicating others had been to the top before them. To his credit, Powell never disputed this fact.

Longs is the highest point in Boulder County and the Front Range. It is also the northernmost 14er. The correct spelling of Longs Peak does not include an apostrophe. Mapmakers agreed long ago that geographical features would not have apostrophes in their official names.

Contact Info Rocky Mountain National Park
1000 Highway 36
Estes Park, CO 80517-8397

General Park Information: (970) 586-1206
Visitor Information Recorded Message: (970) 586-1333
Backcountry Information: (970) 586-1242
Campground Reservations: (800) 365-2267

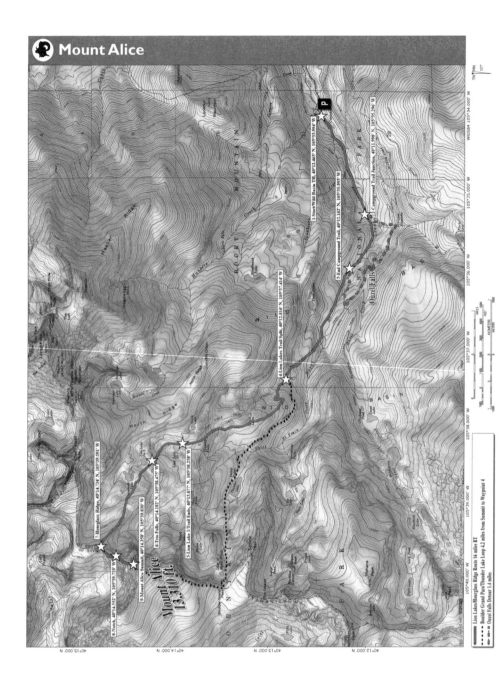

Mount Alice

Mount Alice 13,310 ft.

Labels on map:
- P
- 1 Stone/Wild Basin TH, 40°12.465' N, 105°33.994' W
- 2 End Campground Trail, 40°12.182' N, 105°35.992' W
- 3 Campground Trail Junction, 40°11.998' N, 105°35.296' W
- Ouzel Falls
- 4 Lion Lakes Trail Split, 40°12.816' N, 105°37.414' W
- 5 Lion Lake 1 Trail Ends, 40°13.577' N, 105°38.258' W
- 6 Ten Falls, 40°14.182' N, 105°38.479' W
- 7 Hourglass Ridge, 40°14.734' N, 105°39.591' W
- 8 Notch, 40°14.552' N, 105°39.728' W
- 9 Mount Alice Summit, 40°14.350' N, 105°39.830' W

Legend:
- Lion Lakes/Hourglass Ridge Route 16 miles RT
- Boulder/Grand Pass/Thunder Lake Loop 4.2 miles from Summit to Waypoint 4
- Ouzel Falls Detour 1.4 miles

9 ■ Mount Alice *Good Overnight!*

Mount Alice is like Longs Peak without the crowds. It even has its own "Mini-Diamond" on the east face. An epic adventure with robust scrambling.

Round Trip Distance	16 miles
Hiking Time	11–15 hours
Difficulty	8/10
Class	3
Start Elevation	8,515 ft., at Wild Basin/Thunder Lake Trailhead
Peak Elevation	13,310 ft.
Total Elevation Gain	4,825 ft.
Terrain	Long, smooth prelude trail to off-trail meadows and rocky summit scramble
Best Time to Climb	July–September
Gear Advisor	Trekking poles; ice-axe/crampons in spring and past September
Crowd Level	Low

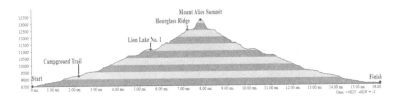

Location Front Range in Rocky Mountain National Park, Wild Basin Area, outside of Estes Park

Intro Wild Basin is one of the most beautiful areas in Rocky Mountain National Park. Like most places in the park, the crowds thin out the farther in you go. By the time you reach Lion Lakes at the foot of Mount Alice, there's a good chance you'll be all alone. The beauty of this area is unmatched in the park. Wildflowers and wildlife abound in the lakes area and all are watched over by the grand matriarch that is Mount Alice.

Why Climb It? The Mount Alice hike is similar to the Longs Peak hike: a long, moderate, on-trail approach leads to a class 3 ascent via an exciting route. Unlike Longs, however, Alice doesn't attract the masses—for most, it's not a "glory peak." The setting is beautiful and remote, a world apart from the rest of the park. Ascending the connecting ridge to Alice's northeast ridge is a wonderful way to start the challenging ascent. Once on the ridge, the class 3 scrambling is steep but solid (it's like an extended version of the scrambling on Pacific Peak, Hike 15 in this book). From the summit, you can

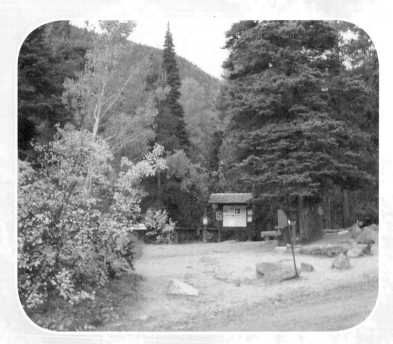

Mount Alice gives you the perfect tour of pristine Wild Basin.

return the way you came or make a loop down to Thunder Lake—a nice tour. After the exciting climb, you can further extend your trip by making an easy side trip to Ouzel Falls.

Driving All vehicles can make it to the Wild Basin Trailhead; the dirt road is very well maintained.

How to Get There The road to the trailhead is off Colorado Highway 7. From the south, this is 6.5 miles north of the junction of CO 7 and CO 72 after the town of Allenspark; from the north, it is 13 miles from the junction of US Highway 36 and CO 7. Turn west into the well-signed Wild Basin Area and continue along the road 2.6 miles, following the signs to the Wild Basin Ranger Station and the parking area at the end of the road. Try to get there early!

Fees/Camping The day-use fee for Rocky Mountain National Park is $20 for a seven-day pass. Camping at the several sites along the way requires a permit and a $20 fee. Contact rangers before you go, to make sure there is site availability. Much like Longs, this hike is feasible as a one-day outing if you get a very early start. The campsites along Campground Trail are good, backcountry sites. There is also camping at Thunder Lake.

Route Notes The route described here uses the Campground Trail to cut a mile off the hike (as well as a bit of elevation gain and loss) by bypassing the Ouzel Falls Trail. This explains the discrepancy between the mileages noted in this section and what you might find in other references (though the accuracy of the GPS plays into that a bit, too). I'd suggest seeing the falls on your descent, which adds a mile to your total trek. If climbing in spring, expect there to quite a bit of snow on the mountain.

0.0 mi (1) Start your hike on the Thunder Lakes/Ouzel Falls Trail from the Wild Basin parking area. This is a very easy class 1 trail that serves as a good warm-up. Stay on the main trail when it passes the junction for Copeland Falls.

1.4 mi (2) There is a signpost here pointing to several campgrounds. To save time (and cut about a mile off your hike), take the side Campground Trail to the right instead of taking the tour of Ouzel Falls. This trail is unimproved but still easy to follow, as it goes by four campsites.

2.8 mi (3) The Campground Trail rejoins the main trail at a bridge. The trails then split to Ouzel Falls and Thunder Lake. For now, go north on the trail toward Thunder Lake, which is listed as 3.3 miles away.

3.8 mi (4) At the signed junction, do *not* head toward Thunder Lake. Note that this sign marks the distance to the ranger station as 4.8 miles; this mileage is determined by taking the Ouzel Falls Trail. Stay right (north) on the trail that goes uphill to Lion Lakes. This trail is a bit faded but is still visible as you climb toward the lakes.

5.7 mi (5) After previewing a few small ponds on your left, you'll drop down into the clearing at Lion Lake No. 1. From this point on, consider this an off-trail hike. It's downright beautiful, and the views of Alice are impressive. Pass Lion Lake No. 1 on its east (right) side; a faint trail may or may not be underwater. From here, there are cairns that loosely lead to Trio Falls, a cool waterfall perched on a shelf of rock. If you are unable to follow the cairns, stay close to the stream that leads to the falls.

6.0 mi (6) At Trio Falls, you'll need to do some easy scrambling to get up to the next plateau, where Lion Lake No. 2 awaits. Just left (west) of the falls is a good spot to climb up. From Lion Lake No. 2, you'll be just below the connecting ridge that intersects Hourglass Ridge. Go northwest to the spine of this broad hill and meet up with your goal—Hourglass Ridge.

7.2 mi (7) You've gained Hourglass Ridge, and Alice's imposing north face looks down upon you. It's not as bad as it looks. Go south on the ridge and then downhill just a little to a notch in the ridge.

7.5 mi (8) At the notch (12,520 feet), you'll see your final 0.5-mile scramble as a jumble of blocky boulders. Scramble up, staying closer to the spine on the west side. Too far east, and you'll be on the side of the sheer Mini-Diamond (called the "Cubic Zirconium" by some). This is class 3 territory and is best climbed once the snow and ice have melted off.

8.0 mi (9) Alice's summit. The register here records very few visitors You have two equally good descent routes from here: return the way you came, or take the optional loop route southwest to Boulder-Grand Pass (read the "Options" section for info on this route). Both are good choices. The first route returns back via Lion Lakes. After scrambling back down the ridge, return exactly the way you came up. However, on the descent, you can take the Campground Trail again or loop over to Ouzel Falls. I recommend the Ouzel Falls Loop if you have the energy.

16 mi Finish.

Options From the summit of Alice, the loop down to Thunder Lake is roughly 4.3 miles to the junction at waypoint 4. Hike southwest along the Continental Divide to Boulder Grand Pass and drop down to Lake of Many Winds. Pass this lake on the south side, and follow the stream down to Thunder Lake, where a pack trail on the north side of the lake brings you back to waypoint 4.

As you return, you have the option at waypoint 3 to go 0.8 mile to Ouzel Falls (the mileages on the signs refer to this route) or to take the camp trail back to the trailhead. I'd suggest taking the Ouzel Falls Loop, even though you gain and lose a bit of elevation. The falls are great. The loop back to the main trail is about 1.4 miles.

Quick Facts The identity of the Alice for whom this peak was named is unknown. Most signs point to her being a "woman of ill-repute" who earned favor with the survey team. Perhaps a cartographer made a hasty promise to the lady to put her on the map, but when questioned about it later, played dumb in order to save his own bacon (metaphorically speaking). Since there is no known Alice on record, I say we dedicate this mountain to Alice Cooper, rock-and-roll icon and all-around interesting guy.

Contact Info Rocky Mountain National Park
1000 Highway 36
Estes Park, CO 80517-8397

General Park Information: (970) 586-1206
Visitor Information Recorded Message: (970) 586-1333
Backcountry Information (970) 586-1242
Campground Reservations (800) 365-2267

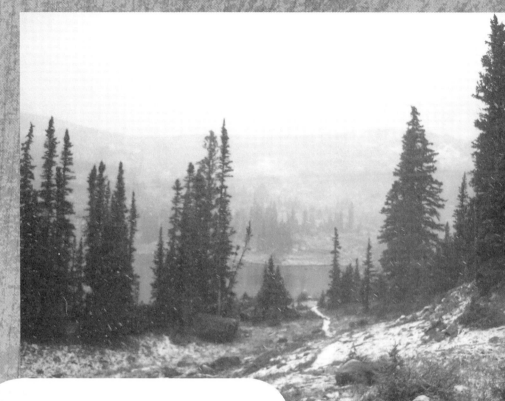

A snowy self-portrait somewhere near the second Lion Lake.

Mount Alice was pounded by a snowstorm during my ascent in early September.

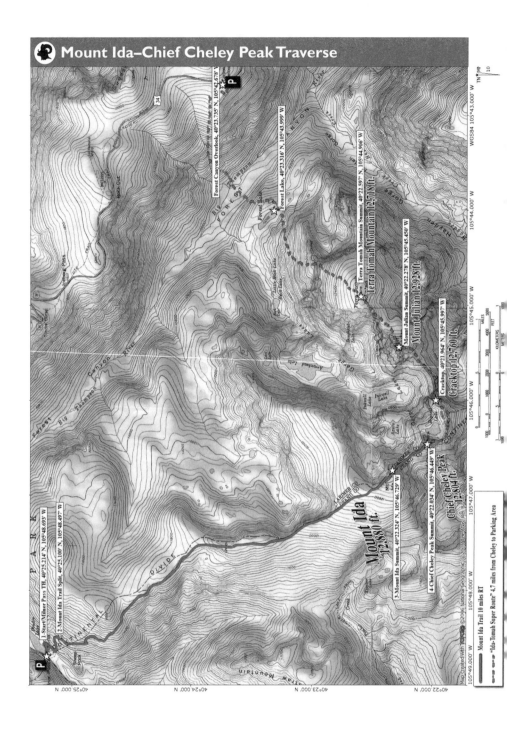

Forest Canyon Overlook, 40°23.735' N, 105°42.678' W

Forest Lake, 40°23.316' N, 105°43.999' W

Terra Tomah Mountain Summit, 40°22.597' N, 105°44.906' W
Terra Tomah Mountain 12,718 ft.

Mount Julian Summit, 40°22.278' N, 105°45.450' W
Mount Julian 12,928 ft.

Cracktop, 40°21.964' N, 105°45.997' W
Cracktop 12,760 ft.

Chief Cheley Peak
Chief Cheley Peak 12,804 ft.

4-Chief Cheley Peak Summit, 40°22.034' N, 105°46.449' W

Mount Ida 12,880 ft.

3-Mount Ida Summit, 40°22.324' N, 105°46.729' W

1-Start Miller Pass TH, 40°25.214' N, 105°48.693' W

2-Mount Ida Trail Split, 40°25.100' N, 105°48.497' W

PARK

Big Thompson River

Forest

CONTINENTAL DIVIDE

———— Mount Ida Trail 10 miles RT

- - - - "Ida-Tomah Super Route" 4.7 miles from Cheley to Parking Area

10 Mount Ida–Chief Cheley Peak Traverse

Mount Ida is one of the most beautiful, yet seldom visited, peaks in Rocky Mountain National Park. Cruise the Continental Divide and keep an eye out for the many "locals"!

Round Trip Distance	10 miles
Hiking Time	5–8 hours
Difficulty	6.5/10
Class	2 with long class 1 sections
Start Elevation	10,750 ft., at Milner Pass Trailhead
Peak Elevations	Mount Ida: 12,880 ft.; Chief Cheley Peak: 12,804 ft.
Total Elevation Gain	3,376 ft.
Terrain	Wide open alpine meadows with class 2 scramble on good rock on Cheley
Best Time to Climb	June–September
Gear Advisor	Normal gear
Crowd Level	Low

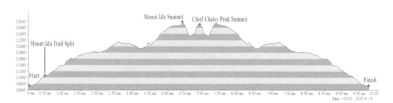

Location   Front Range in Rocky Mountain National Park, just below the northernmost point on Trail Ridge Road

Intro   With more than 3 million visitors annually to Rocky Mountain National Park (RMNP), it may come as a surprise that Mount Ida is relatively unknown to the masses. The trail to Ida is easy to reach and follows a particularly beautiful line along the Continental Divide. Because it is in the high country of the northern boundaries of RMNP, views of the Never Summer Mountains to the west and the "glory peaks" (such as Longs) to the south are quite impressive.

Why Climb It?   As soon as you leave the crowds behind at the parking lot, the walk along the Continental Divide opens up vast tracts of alpine meadows for your enjoyment. Views are spectacular throughout the hike, especially of the pockets of lakes to the east when you near the summits of these two mountains. Wildlife viewing is exceptionally good in RMNP, and this area is no exception. Elk, mule deer, marmot, pika, ptarmigan, and more mingle in the trees and on the tundra. After you have reached Ida, the solid scramble over to Chief Cheley may inspire you to continue east via the optional route to Cracktop, Mount Julian, and Terra Tomah Mountain.

Driving Passenger cars can make it to Milner Pass Trailhead, which is off the paved Trail Ridge Road. Perhaps the most difficult part of this drive is not getting rattled by the exposure on the thrilling Trail Ridge Road!

How to Get There If you are coming from the east side (Estes Park) of RMNP, enter the park at either Fall River or Beaver Meadows. From both of these points, it is roughly 4.0 miles to the junction of US highways 36 and 34. From this junction, follow the always exciting Trail Ridge Road 22 miles, past the Alpine visitor center, over the highest section of road (at 12,183 feet), and descend to the Miler Pass Trailhead, which is on the Continental Divide. You'll see Poudre Lake on your left just before the lot, which has a lot of informative signs.

Fees/Camping The entrance fee to RMNP (which gives you a seven-day permit) is $20 per car (not per person); an annual pass to the park is $35. A backcountry camping permit is $20. There are six drive-in campgrounds in the park; most operate at a first-come, first-served basis. You can make reservations at Moraine Park and Glacier Basin areas (call 800-365-2267). Fees are $20 per night, though once the water utilities are shut off in autumn, some sites drop to $14 per night.

Route Notes None.

Mile/Waypoint **0.0 mi (1)** Start at the Milner Pass Trailhead. Your adventure begins on the Ute Trail, which has a sign declaring MOUNT IDA 4.0 as well as distances to other destinations (apparently, everything is 4.0 miles!). Hike past the wheezing tourists and up a few modest switchbacks on the very well-worn trail. In the early morning, the reflections on tiny Poudre Lake make for good photographs.

0.5 mi (2) After climbing the switchbacks through the trees, you'll come to a trail intersection. Stay the course to Mount Ida by taking a right (south) and continuing along the well-worn trail as it breaks timberline. Once out of the trees, the trail stretches south as far as the eye can see. Follow it along the Continental Divide, soaking in the awesome views. The orange-tinted Never Summer Mountains to the west contrast with the black, green, and gray Front Range mountains to the south and east. You'll see Ida in the distance; simply continue your southern trajectory on the ridge to reach it. Eventually, the trail fades out (about 3.2 miles in), and you'll have to navigate easy, sparse boulder fields. Staying close to the rim on the western side of the ridge offers great views of the lake-filled basin to the northeast. The navigation here is easy, though the walk to Mount Ida may take a little longer than you think. When the spaces are this wide open, things are always a little farther away than they appear.

4.5 mi (3) The summit of Mount Ida! Depending on how you navigated the boulder fields, your mileage may be a little more or less than the mileage specified above. Alpine lakes, below to the east, shimmer in the sun and darken to ink black when the clouds move in. To continue to Chief Cheley Peak, drop down 400 feet via the southeast ridge to a saddle between the two mountains. (The scramble is not as hard as it looks from the top of Ida.) A class 2/2+ scramble up to Cheley is done on solid rock. I find it a nice change from the placid pace of the approach.

5.0 mi (4) Huzzah, the summit of Chief Cheley Peak! From here, you can return the way you came, along the Divide, to return to your vehicle. However, I have a sneaking suspicion you may be tempted to continue east

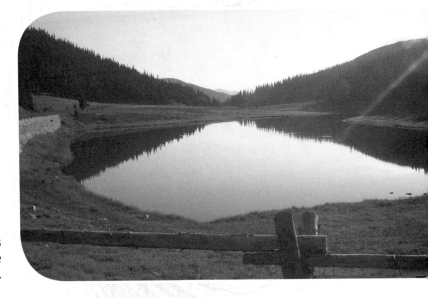

A still morning is reflected in Poudre Lake at the trailhead.

for a few more peaks; read the "Options" section below for more on this route.

10 mi Finish your hike by returning the way you came to the Milner Pass parking lot, which will probably be much more crowded than when you left it in the early morning.

Options The "Ida-Tomah Super Route" option can be done as an out-and-back or as a two-car endeavor, with one vehicle at Milner Pass and one at the Forest Canyon Overlook parking area. I suggest the two-car option. You'll need to start predawn to get a safe window of weather (getting to RMNP very early has its benefits). The hiking distance to the Forest Canyon Overlook is approximately 4.7 miles from the summit of Cheley and is a class 2/2+ traverse.

From Cheley, follow the ridge as it curves east and then northeast to Cracktop (0.6 mile from Cheley), and then to Mount Julian (1.2 miles from Cheley), and then over to the mammoth, glacially carved Terra Tomah

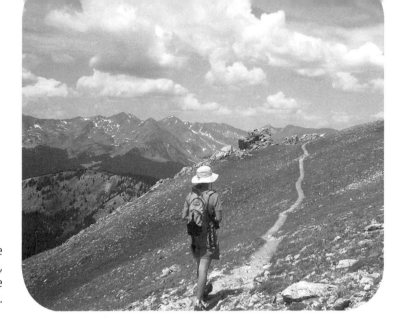

With nearly the entire hike above treeline, you'll have awesome views in all directions.

Mountain (2.0 miles from Cheley). There are no trails to the Forest Canyon parking area, but the land is very wide open. From Terra Tomah, head northeast to Forest Lake, and conclude your day with a 1,500-foot push up grassy slopes to the parking area, roughly 4.7 miles from Cheley. This is a good place to use your GPS and compass skills. If you complete the loop, you'll have bagged five of the best summits in the park! You can see all the peaks in this route from the highpoint on Trail Ridge Road.

Quick Facts   If Mount Ida was named after a specific woman, her identity is lost to history. The name "Ida" was probably transferred from Mount Ida in Crete, Greece. According to ancient Greek mythology, Mount Ida was the birthplace of Zeus, ruler of the Gods.

Chief Cheley Peak is named after Frank Cheley, who founded a pre-Outward Bound-style summer camp in the area in 1921, a program which is still active today.

Mount Julian is named after Julian Hayden, a civil engineer who lived in Estes Park.

Terra Tomah's name is a bit of a mistake on the map. In 1914, a hiker named George Barnard was inspired by the sight of a lake near this peak to break out in song, and chanted the Cohuila Indian classic "He northeast Terratoma, northeast Terratoma." "Terratoma" sounded good, and despite the fact no one knew what it meant, the word was proposed as a name for the lake and area around it. When James Grafton Rogers, chairman of the Colorado Geographic Board, sent his maps off for approval to Washington, D.C., he was shocked to find the name had mistakenly been used to identify the mountain. The lake that was to have borne the noble name Terratoma was instead dubbed "Doughnut Lake"(a name that might entice even Homer Simpson to make this hike!).

So what does "Terra Tomah" actually mean? The song was allegedly overheard by spying college students in California (and by "spying," they probably meant "drunk"), who heard the song performed at an authentic Cohuila Ghost Dance in 1892. The students took the melody back to their school, Pomona College, where it became an anthem, even though no one knew what the words meant. As with much of modern pop music, the words didn't make any sense, but the song had a good beat. When questioned, Cohuila Indians said they did not know what the words meant. Of course, they may simply have wanted to keep the meaning a secret from white men. Thus, what Terra Tomah means remains a mystery; except, perhaps, to a few Cohuila Indians who understand the words and keep the meaning to themselves as a century-old inside joke.

Contact Info Rocky Mountain National Park
1000 Highway 36
Estes Park, CO 80517-8397

General Park Information: (970) 586-1206
Visitor Information Recorded Message: (970) 586-1333
Backcountry Information (970) 586-1242
Campground Reservations (800) 365-2267

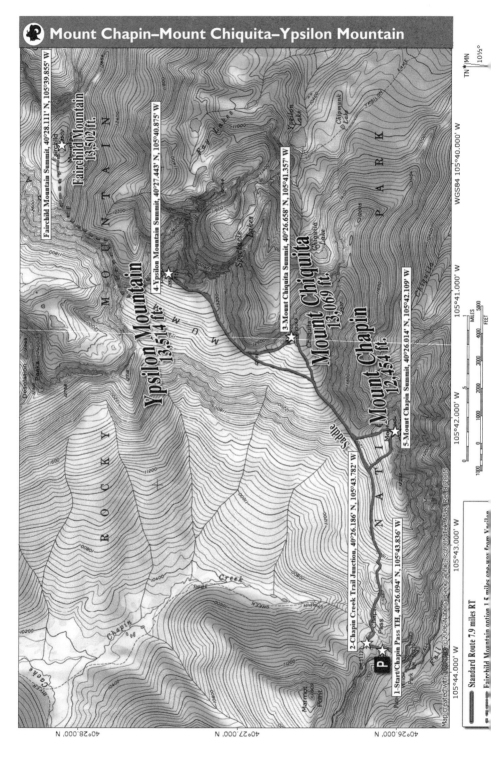

Mount Chapin–Mount Chiquita–Ypsilon Mountain

Fairchild Mountain Summit, 40°28.111' N, 105°39.855' W

Fairchild Mountain
13,502 ft.

4-Ypsilon Mountain Summit, 40°27.443' N, 105°40.875' W

3-Mount Chiquita Summit, 40°26.658' N, 105°41.357' W

Ypsilon Mountain
13,514 ft.

Mount Chiquita
13,069 ft.

Mount Chapin
12,454 ft.

5-Mount Chapin Summit, 40°26.014' N, 105°42.109' W

2-Chapin Creek Trail Junction, 40°26.186' N, 105°43.782' W

1-Start/Chapin Pass TH, 40°26.094' N, 105°43.836' W

Standard Route 7.9 miles RT

Fairchild Mountain option 1.5 miles one-way from Ypsilon

Map created with TOPO! © 2006 National Geographic; © 2005 Tele Atlas, Rel. 8/2005

WGS84 105°40.000' W

TN MN 10½°

11 Mount Chapin–Mount Chiquita– Ypsilon Mountain Traverse

These peaks are amongst the farthest north in Rocky Mountain National Park. Views from the high alpine tundra are top-notch on this peaceful, spacious hike.

Round Trip Distance	7.9 miles
Hiking Time	4–6 hours
Difficulty	4.5/10
Class	2
Start Elevation	11,148 ft., at Chapin Creek Trailhead
Peak Elevations	Mount Chapin: 12,454 ft.; Mount Chiquita: 13,069 ft.; Ypsilon Mountain: 13,514 ft.
Total Elevation Gain	3,373 ft.
Terrain	Good trail to easy alpine tundra
Best Time to Climb	June–September
Gear Advisor	Normal gear
Crowd Level	Moderate

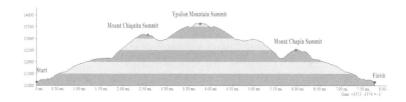

Location Mummy Range in Rocky Mountain National Park (RMNP), outside of Estes Park

Intro This threesome is very photogenic. Tourists have taken countless pictures of these mountains from the base of Old Fall River Road. Most of the hiking adventure takes place above timberline, offering expansive views of the Front Range, the Never Summer Range, and other Mummy Range peaks to the north. For those hoping to extend the day, there are several options to increase your peak count beyond this trio.

Why Climb It? The chance to bag three scenic peaks is tempting; to do so without heart-busting exertion seals the deal. Moderate alpine terrain brings you to these friendly mountains. The incredible perspective from the top of Ypsilon's southeast couloir down to Spectacle Lakes alone is worth the trip. Every step of the way is chock-full of scenery that elevates your senses. If three summits aren't enough, ambitious hikers can carry on to Fairchild Mountain. A walk along these mountains embodies the freedom of the hills.

Driving	Old Fall River Road is a very well-maintained dirt road and is passable by all vehicles.
How to Get There	From the Fall River entrance (US Highway 34), it is 2.1 miles to the right-hand turn (west) onto Old Fall River Road at Horseshoe Park. If you are coming from the Beaver Meadows entrance on US Highway 36, go 3.3 miles from the pay station and take the right (northwest) onto US 34. Go downhill 1.8 miles (passing a great photo opportunity of Mt. Chapin, Mt. Chiquita, and Ypsilon Mountain at a pulloff) and turn left onto Old Fall River Road. Follow the one-way dirt road (which is a novelty in itself) 6.8 miles to Chapin Pass Trailhead, on the right (north) side of the road in the midst of a section of switchbacks. Parking is limited in the area, so try to get in early. Remember when you are done to continue driving up on the one-way road, where you will exit at the Alpine visitor center.
Fees/Camping	It is $20 per car to enter Rocky Mountain National Park; annual passes are $35. Backcountry camping is available is designated areas only and requires a permit and $20 fee. There are several pay campgrounds in the park; call ahead to make reservations or to check availability.
Route Notes	My route hits the summit of Chapin on the return from Ypsilon and Chiquita; you are more than welcome to summit Chapin first, if you prefer. Both ways are on class 2 terrain.
Mile/Waypoint	**0.0 mi (1)** Start at the Chapin Pass Trailhead. Get on the trail, and head uphill to a small saddle.

0.1 mi (2) On the quickly reached saddle, turn right at the Chapin Creek Trail junction toward Chapin, Chiquita, and Ypsilon summits. There is a sign that will help point the way.

0.7 mi As you near Chapin, the trail fades a little and goes left of the peak. If you'd like to summit Chapin first, take the optional route to the summit and continue on to Chiquita.

1.8 mi The formal trail disappears as you reach the saddle between Chapin and Chiquita at 12,160 feet. Carry on northeast to Chiquita's summit on good alpine terrain that is a mixture of grass and rocks.

2.6 mi (3) Mount Chiquita's summit has a nice wind shelter and good views. Take a break here, and then continue northeast to Ypsilon.

3.8 mi (4) Ypsilon Mountain's summit looks similar to Chiquita's. As mentioned before, the views down to Spectacle Lakes are astounding. Vistas in every other direction are pretty good, too! For this route, return to the saddle between Chiquita and Chapin, bypassing Chiquita's summit (for the time-being).

5.7 mi Back at the saddle, start heading up an intermittent footpath to the summit of Chapin. This climb is only about 400 feet.

6.1 mi (5) Chapin's summit. This is my favorite summit of the three to sit and take in the scenery, which is why I suggest closing your hike with it.

From here, you can descend down the north slopes or take the optional walk down the west ridge back to the trail.

7.9 mi Finish. Remember to drive uphill on the one-way road to exit.

Options So this little sojourn was too easy for ya, huh, tough guy (or girl)? Why not try the traverse over to Fairchild Mountain? Its summit is 1.5 miles from Ypsilon's summit on class 2+/3 terrain. If that's not enough, you can continue on to Hagues Peak. A famous loop can be made by going from Hagues Peak to Mummy Mountain and down to Lawn Lake, where a second car should be parked. (You'll need to pick up additional quad maps if you'd like to give it a shot, as my humble little map doesn't cover these features.)

Quick Facts There are a few theories on which "Chapin" the mountain is named for. The most plausible is Frederick H. Chapin, another guy from Connecticut who came to Colorado to escape the flatlands and climb some *real* mountains (he was from Hartford). (I, too, hail from the Constitution State, having been born in Waterbury Hospital, elevation: 760 feet above sea level.) Chapin climbed in the state from 1886 to 1888 as a representative of the Appalachian Mountain Club. He also contributed to getting Hallett's Peak named after W.L. Hallett, who had acted as a tour guide for the plucky New Englander.

For some odd reason, Enos Mills (who was responsible for putting names on the map) was smitten by a character in the book *Chiquita, An American Novel: The Romance of a Ute Chief's Daughter.* The story hit a soft spot with old Enos, and the name he gave the mountain stuck.

Spectacle Lakes were named by Roger Toll in 1922 for their resemblance to eyeglasses, though they could just as well have been named for the spectacle they present.

Ypsilon is named after the snow couloirs in its east face that form the letter "Y" when filled with snow. Since Ypsilon sounds more sophisticated than "Y Mountain," that name was applied.

Fairchild Mountain is named after Lucius Fairchild (what a great name!), an accomplished diplomat and three-time governor of Wisconsin. He never climbed the peak, but his admirers did, and honored him thus.

One last note: Fall River Road was the first, steep road through the park; it was rendered to second-class duty when Trail Ridge Road was completed in 1932.

Contact Info Rocky Mountain National Park
1000 Highway 36
Estes Park, CO 80517-8397

General Park Information: (970) 586-1206
Visitor Information Recorded Message: (970) 586-1333
Backcountry Information (970) 586-1242
Campground Reservations (800) 365-2267

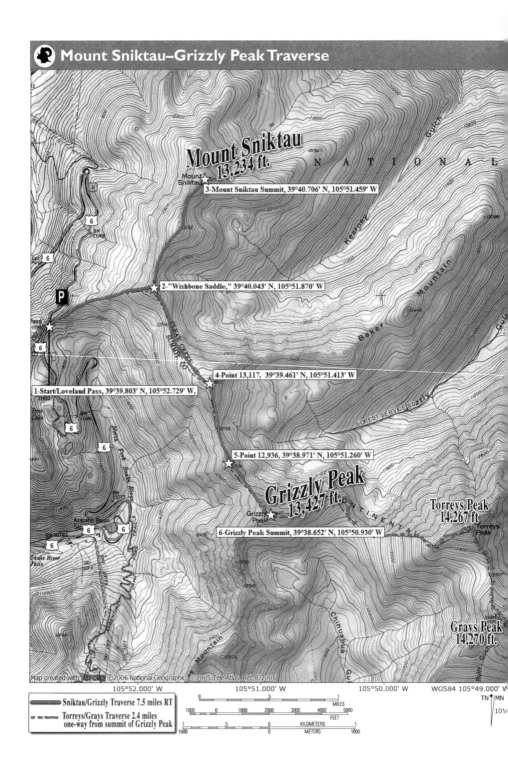

Mount Sniktau
13,234 ft.

3-Mount Sniktau Summit, 39°40.706' N, 105°51.459' W

2-"Wishbone Saddle," 39°40.043' N, 105°51.870' W

P

4-Point 13,117, 39°39.461' N, 105°51.413' W

1-Start/Loveland Pass, 39°39.803' N, 105°52.729' W,

5-Point 12,936, 39°38.971' N, 105°51.260' W

Grizzly Peak
13,427 ft.

Torreys Peak
14,267 ft.

6-Grizzly Peak Summit, 39°38.652' N, 105°50.930' W

Grays Peak
14,270 ft.

Map created with TOPO!® ©2006 National Geographic; ©2005 Tele Atlas, Rel. 8/2005

105°52.000' W   105°51.000' W   105°50.000' W   WGS84 105°49.000' W

━━━ Sniktau/Grizzly Traverse 7.5 miles RT
┅┅┅ Torreys/Grays Traverse 2.4 miles
      one-way from summit of Grizzly Peak

12 Mount Sniktau–Grizzly Peak Traverse

Stay above treeline as you traverse rolling alpine ridges, culminating with a spectacular ascent of Grizzly Peak. Wide, open spaces and views of familiar places await you!

Round Trip Distance	7.5 miles
Hiking Time	4–6 hours
Difficulty	5/10
Class	2
Start Elevation	11,930 ft., at Loveland Pass Summit
Peak Elevations	Mount Sniktau: 13,234 ft.; Grizzly Peak: 13,427 ft.
Total Elevation Gain	4,088 ft.
Terrain	Rolling alpine ridges with good footing
Best Time to Climb	May–October; a good winter hike as well
Gear Advisor	Normal gear
Crowd Level	Moderate

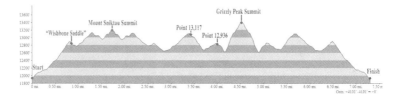

Location   Front Range in Arapahoe National Forest, just east of Loveland Pass

Intro   Mount Sniktau stands out when viewed from Interstate 70 near Loveland Pass; its lower slopes are home to a few runs at Loveland Basin Ski Area. Thanks to a high trailhead located at the summit of Loveland Pass, this entire hike is above the trees. Climbing from the pass to Sniktau is short and sweet; your rewards include amazing views of several mountain ranges and many familiar ski areas: Loveland, Arapahoe Basin, Keystone, and Copper Mountain. Turning south, the trek continues over a rolling ridge of unnamed summits, culminating with an 800-foot push to the top of Grizzly Peak (one of several Grizzly Peaks in the state).

Why Climb It?   Sniktau's easy access and familiar confines mean you'll have a quick drive from the Denver/Boulder/Golden area. An uphill push from the pass grants you access to this scenic ridge, which runs from the valley in I-70 to 14,267-foot Torreys Peak (and beyond). Because the entire hike is above the trees, you'll have grandiose 360-degree views the entire hike. After the moderate climb to Sniktau, roll south on the sky-high ridge to Grizzly Peak. It's a class 2 scramble up the northwest face of the Grizz. From the summit, Grays and Torreys peaks look *enormous.*

Driving Passenger cars can make it up Loveland Pass, which is paved and very well maintained year-round.

How to Get There   From I-70, take exit 216 (Loveland Pass/Loveland Ski Area exit) which is less than a half mile east of the Eisenhower/Johnson tunnel. Exit the highway, and then take a right to proceed up Loveland Pass (US Highway 6), which bypasses the Loveland Ski Area on your right; don't head left (east), or you'll simply end up at the lower part of Loveland. Continue up the steep, exposed pass 4.2 miles to the Loveland Pass summit; there is parking on the left. Be warned—it fills up quickly, especially in the winter.

Fees/Camping   There are no fees for hiking in this area. Camping is possible, but there are not many water sources. A good place to spend the night is at Herman Gulch, a few miles down I-70 east at exit 218 (there are no fees there either).

Route Notes   None.

Mile/Waypoint   **0.0 mi (1)** Start at the top of Loveland Pass. There is a large sign with the elevation; the trail uphill starts just behind it. There are no trail signs or markers, but the way up to the saddle is obvious. Follow the spine of the ridge northeast to "Wishbone Saddle," 900 vertical feet above.

0.8 mi (2) Wishbone Saddle. Catch your breath and grab a swig of water; the hardest part of your hike is behind you. Turn northeast and continue to follow the ridge.

1.3 mi You'll clear a 13,152-foot false summit en route to Mount Sniktau Summit. Between this point and Sniktau, there is often snow, especially on the east side. Continue to stay on the highpoint of the ridge and make the modest, 400-vertical-foot push up to Sniktau's summit.

1.8 mi (3) That was fast! You're already at the top of Sniktau. Did you bring your snowboard? You can drop directly down to the Loveland Ski Area from here. Wait, you're here to hike! Enjoy the awesome views up here: the Vasquez Mountains are to the north, the Gores to the west, the Front Range to the east, and in the southern distance are the Mosquito Range peaks. Far west, you may be able to see the Sawatch Peaks. Return to Wishbone Saddle.

2.7 mi (2) Back in the saddle again! This time, go south along the footpath that floats over the ridge to the base of Grizzly Peak.

3.5 mi (4) Point 13,117 is a subsummit. From here, you'll need to partake in fun class 2+ scrambling to stay directly on the ridge. Hikers wishing to bypass these outcrops can easily divert left (west). Continue to the base of Grizzly. Note that things get steeper and more rugged from here.

4.0 mi (5) Point 12,936. Grizzly's loose, rocky pyramid looms before you. Climb down to a low point in the ridge, at roughly 12,600 feet. From there, the 800-foot hike/scramble to the top follows a faint climber's trail. Be careful not to kick rocks down as you muscle up to the summit.

4.7 mi (6) Phewwww! Finally, Grizzly Peak's summit. That was quite a push, wasn't it? The incredible views make it all worthwhile, especially panoramic shots to the north of the ridge you just traversed. After you've seen what there is to see, return to the ridge and head north, back to Wishbone Saddle.

5.8 mi (2) Back in the saddle *again!* This time, turn west downhill and back to your vehicle.

7.5 mi Finish.

Options   This traverse bags a lot of peaks, but if you really want to push it, continue east from Grizzly Peak to the summit of Torreys Peak. There is a faint trail that follows a scrambly ridge east. It is possible to have an epic day by continuing over to Grays Peak and either making the arduous return the same way you came or looping down the Grays Peak Trail to Bakerville Trailhead (where you should have a second car parked). Torreys is 1.7 miles one way from the top of Grizzly; Grays is 2.4 miles from Grizzly. As an out-and-back, this is 12.4 miles round trip; as a one-way trek to Bakerville, it's about 11.5 miles.

Quick Facts   So what exactly is a "Sniktau"? An Indian term for "bear nose"? A missing letter of the Greek alphabet? As it turns out, it's neither. Rumor has it, the name was a pseudonym used by pioneer journalist E. Patterson, who "borrowed" his pen name (with a variant spelling) from fellow journalist W.F. Watkins. Look closely: "Watkins" backwards is "sniktaw." So the peak is named after the nom-de-plume of a snarky journalist—how'd they slip that one by the cartographers?

There are five Grizzly Peaks in Colorado; all five are 13ers. This Grizzly is the fourth highest of the pack.

Contact Info   Arapahoe National Forest
Clear Creek Ranger District
101 Chicago Creek Road
P.O. Box 3307
Idaho Springs, CO 80452
(303) 567-3000

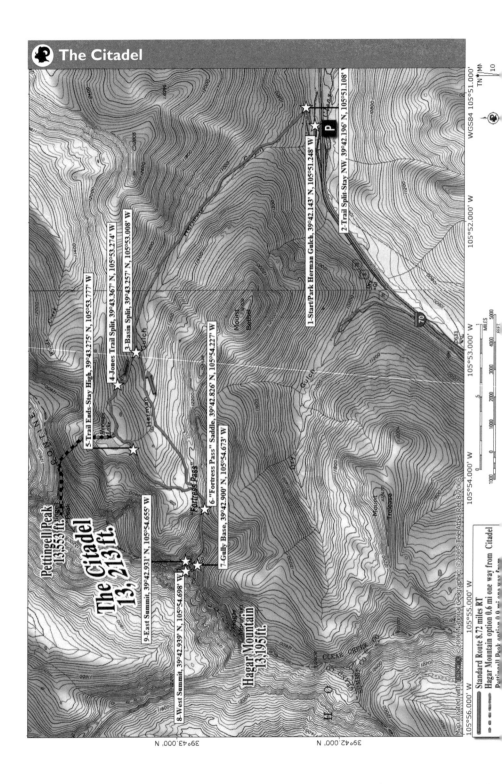

The Citadel

Petingell Peak
13,553 ft.

The Citadel
13,213 ft.

Hagar Mountain
13,195 ft.

1-Start/Park Herman Gulch, 39°42.143' N, 105°51.248' W

2-Trail Split-Stay NW, 39°42.196' N, 105°51.108' W

3-Basin Split, 39°43.257' N, 105°53.008' W

4-Jones Trail Split, 39°43.367' N, 105°53.274' W

5-Trail Ends-Stay High, 39°43.275' N, 105°53.777' W

6-"Fortress Pass" Saddle, 39°42.826' N, 105°54.227' W

7-Gully Base, 39°42.900' N, 105°54.673' W

8-West Summit, 39°42.939' N, 105°54.698' W

9-East Summit, 39°42.931' N, 105°54.655' W

"Fortress Pass"

Herman Gulch

Map created with TOPO! ©2006 National Geographic ©2005 TeleAtlas Rel 8/2005

Standard Route 8.72 miles RT
Hagar Mountain option 0.6 mi one way from Citadel
Petingell Peak option 0.9 mi one way from

13   **The Citadel**

The Citadel is a local favorite that you won't find on the map. Fun scrambling and easy trailhead access makes the Citadel a great dayhike—a hidden Front Range classic.

Round Trip Distance	8.72 miles
Hiking Time	5–7 hours
Difficulty	6/10
Class	3
Start Elevation	10,290 ft., at Herman Gulch
Peak Elevation	13,213 ft.
Total Elevation Gain	3,228 ft
Terrain	Mellow class 1 to Herman Lake; Fun, steep hike/ scramble to class 3 summit blocks
Best Time to Climb	Late June–September
Gear Advisor	Light hikers or trail runners; helmet
Crowd Level	High to Herman Lake/low from lake to summit

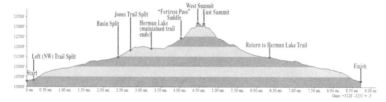

Location   Front Range in the Arapahoe National Forest near Loveland Pass

Intro   You don't want to miss this one. Tucked away just north of Interstate 70, "the Citadel" is the climber's name for a rock formation that is unnamed on official maps. Citadel's twin summits lie between Pettingell Peak to the north (13,553 feet, the highpoint of Grand County) and Hagar Mountain (13,195 feet) to the southwest. With very easy access and a surprisingly fun class 3 scramble, these worthy summits are great choices for the Denver/ Boulder/Golden crowd who want a great hike with a short drive.

Why Climb It?   You'll be surprised this climb is so close to the familiar stretch of I-70 just before Loveland Pass. An easy, class 1 prelude draws you away from the din of traffic and into a stunning alpine basin. Emerging out of treeline, Herman Gulch opens before you, a beautiful network of streams and small alpine lakes. Imposing views of the Citadel formation contrast with the smooth domes of neighboring mountains. As the trail ends, your trek continues. Cross the basin and head up the steep "Fortress Pass." Continue up a burly ridge to the back side of the Citadel's two summits. Reach the tops of both peaks with a good class 3 scramble.

Driving

The trailhead for the Citadel is passable for all vehicles and is easy to reach.

How to Get There

This one is easy. From either direction on I-70, take the Herman Gulch exit, 218, on the east side of the Eisenhower Tunnel near Loveland Pass. If you exit I-70 westbound, take a right at the end of the exit and then another quick right into the large parking area. If you exit I-70 eastbound, turn left off the exit and proceed to the parking lot. The trail begins at a large sign kiosk.

Fees/Camping

There are no fees to climb t he Citadel or camp in the area.

Route Notes

This is a very avalanche-prone area in winter/early spring.

Mile/Waypoint

0.0 mi (1) From the parking lot, start your journey on the Herman Gulch Trail (which coincides with a section of the Colorado Trail). The sign lists this as Trail #98. Herman Lake is your first goal.

0.18 mi (2) Early in the hike, the trail divides. Stay left (northwest) on the

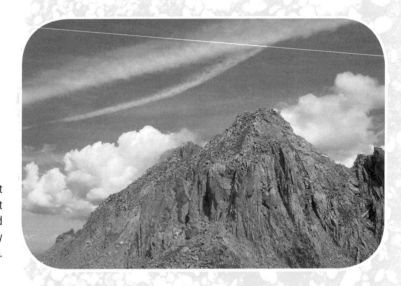

Both the east (forefront) and west summits are accessed by a convenient gully that splits the two.

Herman Gulch Trail at the split. From here, you have an easy-to-follow trail that leads all the way up to Herman Lake. Enjoy the gulch, and be ready for the Citadel's imposing, craggy visage to rise beyond the basin.

2.4 mi (3) Where the trail splits in the basin, stay on the main trail and continue uphill. This area is a good place to shortcut through the basin when there is snow; otherwise, stay on the trail. This split is also where you will rejoin the main trail on the way back if you follow the loop detailed in this route description.

2.75 mi (4) The Jones Pass South Trail splits off here; stay on course toward Herman Lake.

3.3 mi (5) Just past Herman Lake, the well-worn trail fades away. You'll need to traverse the basin southwest to "Fortress Pass," the saddle between the Citadel and Point 12,674. When the snow is cleared off, you'll see a distinct, switchbacking trail heading up this pass. Stay high in the basin during your traverse, as dropping to the lower section only adds elevation to your climb. Ascend the short, steep trail to the top of the saddle.

4.1 mi (6) From the saddle, head due west up the very steep ridge leading to the Citadel. When you reach the top of this ridge, the east summit of the Citadel will be before you. Do not directly ascend; rather, skirt left (south) on the back side and descend a short distance. You will pass several gray-ish/black gullies that are very tight; these class 3+/ 4 paths will lead you to the east summit, but I don't suggest you attempt them. Pass these gullies and continue 0.1 mile from the ridgetop down to a prominent, wider gully that has dirt and rock (and a small fan of talus) at the bottom.

4.5 mi (7) GPS users might want to note the coordinates of this waypoint, taken at the base of the gully. This class 3 scramble (finally, here it is!) is slightly loose; the rock is fairly solid, but it's easy to kick down smaller, loose rocks. This gully actually terminates directly between the two summits; from here it's a class 3 scramble up to either. My suggestion: veer left (west) about halfway up the gully, and scramble to the higher west summit.

4.7 mi (8) The west summit of the Citadel, 13,213 feet. Enjoy the views and scramble down to the top of the gully that splits the summits. From here, the scramble up to the east summit (13,203 feet) is a little trickier (perhaps class 3+); there is a great notch to wiggle up directly east of the gully's upper terminus. From here, it's a very short walk to the east summit. (Want a good picture? Take a photo from one summit of your friend on the other.)

4.8 mi (9) From the east summit, descend via the gully (waypoint 7) you came up (the eastern slopes lead to some sketchy class 3+/4 descents). Return to the ridge, descending back down to Fortress Pass (waypoint 6).

5.3 mi You can return the same way you came by ascending to Herman Lake, but crossing the basin as you descend is quicker. Follow the streams down (in the spring this may be quite muddy).

6.5 mi (3) As the basin blends in with the pine trees, cut off left (north) to intercept the Herman Gulch Trail. There are several faint paths leading from the basin to the main trail; any northward path through the pine trees will eventually connect with the main trail. Follow the trail back to the parking lot.

8.72 mi Finish.

Options Skilled scramblers looking for a good challenge can traverse 0.6 mile one way from the west summit of the Citadel southwest to the summit of Hagar Mountain. This ridge is class 3+ and may require some serious concentration in icy or wet conditions.

County highpointers can grind up the northeast slopes from Herman Lake to Pettingell's east ridge, and then follow it up to Grand County's highest point, the rounded summit of Pettingell Peak.

The gentle ridge leading over to Mount Bethel (12,705 feet) is another possible climb if you want to scramble over Fortress Pass saddle (waypoint 6) and continue east along the ridge. While Bethel doesn't look like much more than a nice hill from the saddle, automobiles emerging from the Eisenhower/Johnson tunnel on Loveland Pass will recognize the peak by its prominent snow fences, high upon the southwest face.

Quick Facts Despite being excluded from maps, the Citadel continues to be a local favorite for Colorado hikers. Climbers bestowed the Citadel's name as a compliment to its fortress-like presence in the Herman Gulch Basin.

Because of its easy accessibility, this area sees a lot of traffic in the winter. It is known for heavy avalanche activity. Skiers and hikers viewing the Citadel from Loveland Ski Area and Loveland Pass have also given it the innocuous title "Snoopy's Doghouse" because the snow on the twin summits resembles the snoozing beagle of cartoon fame.

Contact Info Arapahoe National Forest
Sulphur Ranger District
9 Tenmile Drive
P.O. Box 10
Granby, CO 80446
(970) 887-4100

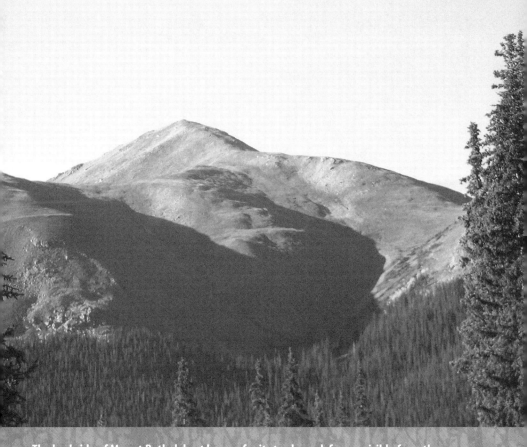

The backside of Mount Bethel, best known for its trademark fences visible from the eastern side of Eisenhower Tunnel

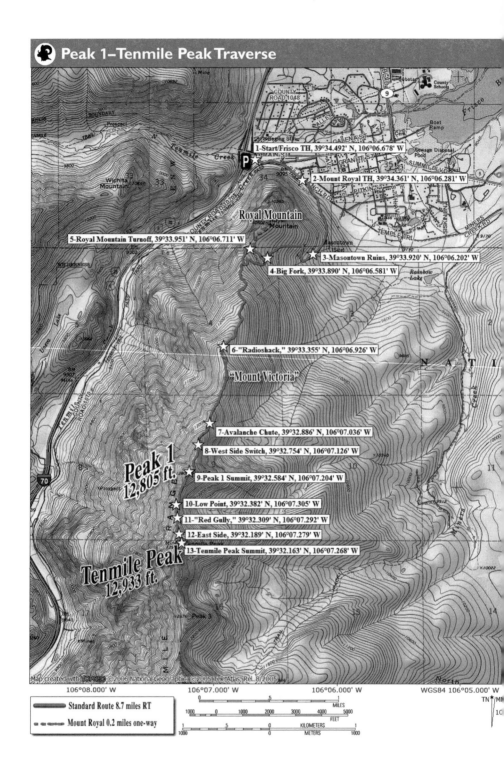

Peak 1–Tenmile Peak Traverse

1-Start/Frisco TH, 39°34.492' N, 106°06.678' W

2-Mount Royal TH, 39°34.361' N, 106°06.281' W

Royal Mountain

5-Royal Mountain Turnoff, 39°33.951' N, 106°06.711' W

3-Masontown Ruins, 39°33.920' N, 106°06.202' W

4-Big Fork, 39°33.890' N, 106°06.581' W

6-"Radioshack," 39°33.355' N, 106°06.926' W

"Mount Victoria"

7-Avalanche Chute, 39°32.886' N, 106°07.036' W

8-West Side Switch, 39°32.754' N, 106°07.126' W

Peak 1
12,805 ft.

9-Peak 1 Summit, 39°32.584' N, 106°07.204' W

10-Low Point, 39°32.382' N, 106°07.305' W

11-"Red Gully," 39°32.309' N, 106°07.292' W

12-East Side, 39°32.189' N, 106°07.279' W

13-Tenmile Peak Summit, 39°32.163' N, 106°07.268' W

Tenmile Peak
12,933 ft.

Map created with TOPO!® ©2006 National Geographic. ©2005 TeleAtlas, Rel. 8/2005

106°08.000' W   106°07.000' W   106°06.000' W   WGS84 106°05.000' W

──── Standard Route 8.7 miles RT

- ◆- ◆- ◆ Mount Royal 0.2 miles one-way

14 Peak 1–Tenmile Peak Traverse

Peak 1 and Tenmile Peak are often admired for their perfect conical shapes, as seen from Interstate 70. The hike over these two is a good challenge; pay attention for seashells on the ridge!

Round Trip Distance	8.7 miles
Hiking Time	6–8 hours
Difficulty	8/10
Class	3
Start Elevation	9,121 ft., at Frisco Trailhead
Peak Elevations	Peak 1: 12,805 ft.; Tenmile Peak: 12,933 ft.
Total Elevation Gain	4,353 ft.
Terrain	Good trail to rocky ridge traverse
Best Time to Climb	June–September
Gear Advisor	Normal gear
Crowd Level	Moderate to Peak 1; low to Tenmile Peak

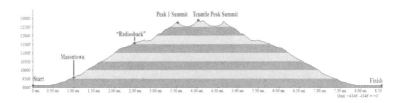

Location   Tenmile Range in Arapaho National Forest in the town of Frisco

Intro   The pointed summits of these two mountains stand sentry over the town of Frisco. Motorists can't help but be mesmerized by the picture-perfect profiles of the twosome—the view from I-70 westbound is stunning. Even though the trailhead starts in the town of Frisco, these mountains don't see as much traffic as you might think (especially Tenmile Peak). For those who have skied the number peaks in Breckenridge, this route covers the lowest-digit mountains of the Tenmile Range (Tenmile Peak is also known as Peak 2).

Why Climb It?   This is the easiest trailhead to reach of any hike in this book; the drive is relatively short from metro areas. I must have passed these mountains a hundred times, every time making a mental note to find out what they were and climb them. My curiosity served me well, as the hike and scramble on these two is a blast. The lower portion of the hike takes you through the ruins of an old mining town that was twice flattened by avalanches. Climbing above treeline offers great views of the city and reservoir below. You also get a sneak peek at hidden lakes and mountains that you can't spot from I-70. The class 3 ridge between the two keeps you on your toes! Much like the nearby Gore Range, the less-traveled parts of these mountains are dotted with fossils and seashells.

Driving Any vehicle can make it to the Frisco Trailhead; it is paved all the way.

How to Get There From I-70, take exit 201 to Frisco. If you are coming on I-70 westbound, take a left off the exit, pass under the highway bridges, go past the eastbound exit ramp and take a quick right into a big paved parking area that has restrooms. This area also serves as a launching point for cyclists on the bike path. If you are coming on I-70 eastbound, exit at 201, take a right off the exit and then a quick right into the parking area.

Fees/Camping There are no fees to hike Peak 1 and Tenmile Peak. The campsites around Dillon Reservoir are geared more toward the RV crowd and are a bit expensive. Overnight car camping is allowed in the parking lot.

Route Notes None.

Mile/Waypoint **0.0 mi (1)** Start. From the parking lot for the Frisco Trailhead, go left onto the concrete bike path and follow it southeast to Mount Royal Trail on your right.

0.4 mi (2) Turn right (west) onto the marked Mount Royal Trail. This trail sees a lot of local traffic, as it services the Mount Royal viewpoint. A wide trail continues up to the fabled town ruins of Masontown. Don't take any of the side trails that join along the way.

1.0 mi (3) On your right, you'll see a bit of garbage and a few brick foundations from Masontown. The better ruins are a little off-trail on the right side. Stay right when a junction trail comes in around Masontown on your left. It's easy to miss this "town" since there isn't much of it left standing. After the ruins, the trail goes "New England style"—straight up with no switchbacks.

1.5 mi (4) Wow, was that steep! At 1.5 miles, you come to a fairly large fork ("Big Fork") with well-worn trails both ways. In the summer of 2006, this junction did not have any signs. As the map shows, the right-hand path goes to a neat viewpoint of I-70 and continues over to Royal Mountain (5). Note there is a very faint wrap-around trail that rejoins the main path from here to the left of the viewpoint (I didn't discover this until I was on the way down). This faint trail begins in a sandy area and exits behind an old cabin and then connects with the main trail.

Going left (straight) at the big fork (4) is the main trail—straight uphill. A short 0.2 mile up from this point, you'll see the aforementioned cabin on your right. The main trail is obvious from here. It's quite steep up to the next waypoint, which is…

2.6 mi (6) … the "Radioshack," atop the rocky knoll known as "Mount" Victoria. A small radio transmission building and tower announce your exit out of treeline. Pass the shack and level off at a mild saddle between Victoria and Peak 1. The views to the east are really opening up at this juncture.

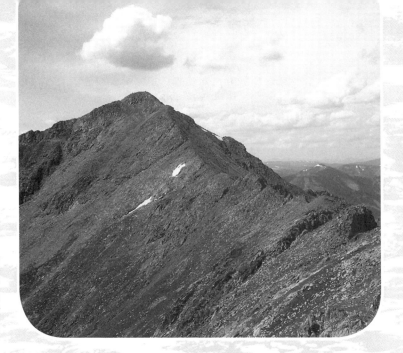

3.2 mi (7) At the saddle, look down at the swath of Aspen trees. This is the path dozens of avalanches have blazed—including the ones that flattened Masontown (twice!). A glance over the west side and down to I-70 reveals a much more rugged side of the mountain. Stay on the trail and continue south.

3.4 mi (8) Get ready to turn to the dark side. Much like "the Force" in Star Wars, this mountain has two sides. The east face is grassy and rounded; the west face is jagged and sharp. If watching movies has taught me anything (which it hasn't, really), it's that humans are always drawn to the dark side. In this case, the west side of the peak offers fun, class 2 scrambling to the upper reaches of the mountain. With all the effort you'll be putting forth, you'll find it hard to believe this isn't even a 13er.

3.7 mi (9) Peak 1's summit! The mileage to here isn't huge, but that was some tough stuff you just came up. There used to be a giant American flag atop the mountain, but it was gone when I last visited. There *was*, however, a mini-tower thing with two big flashlights taped to it.

From the top, keep going south toward the obvious ridge to Tenmile Peak. This is where the class 3 terrain begins. For the most part, you can stay on the ridge or just off to the east side until you reach the low point at waypoint 10.

3.9 mi (10) At 12,550 feet, you're at the low point of the range. There's a bamboo pole sticking out of the rock just past here, indicating where you should head next. Stay on the ridge or just below it on the east until you reach a sandy, red-colored gully just past the pole.

4.0 mi (11) This is "Red Gully." Cross this below the ridge (where it's safest) and quickly get back up on the ridge. This little diversion has a secret: I saw dozens of ancient seashells in the red rock. Please don't take any home, but do take some photos—or else people will think you were hallucinating. After climbing out of the gully, switch back over to the west side of the mountain, where the scrambling is better.

4.1 mi (12) One more switch! Want more? Get back on the east side and follow the easy, class 2 hill to Tenmile's summit.

4.3 mi (13) Tenmile Peak Summit! There's a neat, handmade monument on the spur to the east, perhaps a memorial for a beloved pet. This is a great summit for views. Take your photos, and return the way you came. The return on the ridge has one tricky move, back at Red Gully. Take your

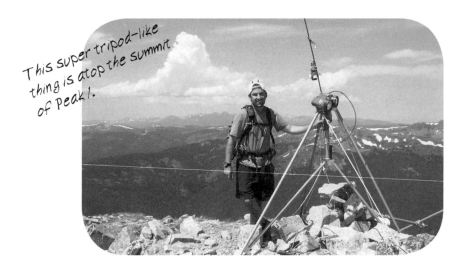

This super tripod-like thing is atop the summit of Peak 1!

time—the route-finding is a little tricky, but the scrambling is solid. Go back over Peak 1 and return the way you came.

6.8 mi One note on the descent: If you bypassed it the first time, you can take the side trail from the old cabin in the trees down to the Royal Mountain saddle viewpoint (waypoint 5). Go left on a faint trail (instead of a cairn, there's a bunch of old cans). Follow it down to the viewpoint and then down the wide trail to your right back to Big Fork.

8.7 mi Finish. As with many of these hikes, your mileage may vary slightly, depending on how direct the routes were that you took when off-trail.

Options The only option I've mapped out is the short trek over to Royal Mountain. This 10,502 viewpoint is worth the walk over and it's only 0.2 mile one way from waypoint 5.

There are some who get "numbers fever" and continue the traverse (class 3+) south to Peak 3 and over to Peak 4. Friends who have made the trek say the best route is to descend Peak 4 into town, and then take public transportation back to Frisco.

Quick Facts   Tenmile Peak takes on the name of the range it's in; it also goes by the alias "Peak 2" when it wants to fit in with the guys. The number peaks were labeled by a rather uninspired surveyor.

Masontown was the site of a profitable mill that serviced Victoria Mine. The town lifted its named from a place in Pennsylvania where the company's investors lived. At its peak, there were about 800 residents. The gold and silver from the mine were sent to the Denver mint until operations fizzled, around 1910. The town was demolished by an avalanche in 1912. Bootleggers capitalized on this misfortune and used the damaged town as a center for making moonshine—until they were flattened by an avalanche in 1926. The last structures that still resembled buildings were destroyed—not by ice, but by fire—when the place burned to the ground in 1968.

Contact Info   Arapahoe National Forest
Clear Creek Ranger District
101 Chicago Creek Road
P.O. Box 3307
Idaho Springs, CO 80452
(303) 567-3000

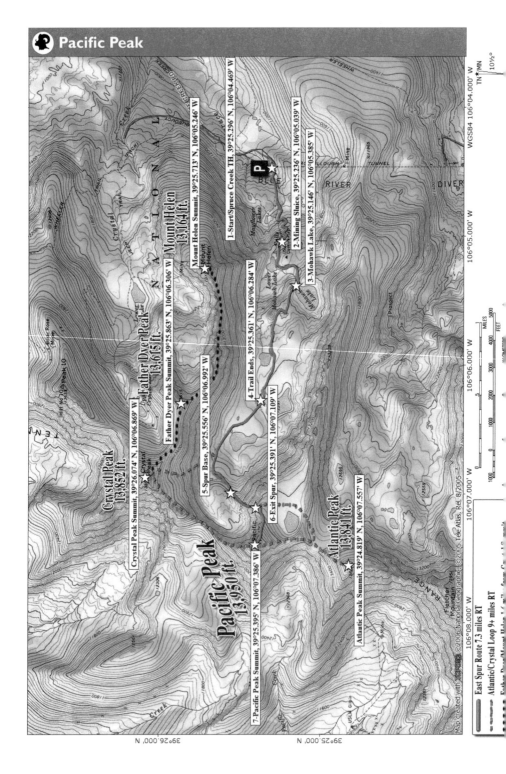

Mount Helen
13,164 ft.

Father Dyer Peak
13,615 ft.

Crystal Peak
13,852 ft.

Pacific Peak
13,950 ft.

Atlantic Peak
13,841 ft.

Mount Helen Summit, 39°25.713' N, 106°06.306' W

1-Start/Spruce Creek TH, 39°25.296' N, 106°04.469' W

2-Mining Sluice, 39°25.236' N, 106°05.039' W

3-Mohawk Lake, 39°25.146' N, 106°05.385' W

Father Dyer Peak Summit, 39°25.863' N, 106°06.306' W

4-Trail Ends, 39°25.361' N, 106°06.284' W

5-Spur Base, 39°25.556' N, 106°06.992' W

Crystal Peak Summit, 39°26.074' N, 106°06.869' W

6-Exit Spur, 39°25.391' N, 106°07.109' W

7-Pacific Peak Summit, 39°25.395' N, 106°07.386' W

Atlantic Peak Summit, 39°24.819' N, 106°07.557' W

East Spur Route 7.3 miles RT

Atlantic/Crystal Loop 9+ miles RT

WGS84 106°04.000' W

15 Pacific Peak

Pacific Peak has lots of appeal: mining history, beautiful lakes, and a great scramble. Link up to neighboring summits for extended time in this high-altitude playground.

Round Trip Distance	7.3 miles
Hiking Time	5–7 hours
Difficulty	7/10
Class	2+/3
Start Elevation	11,095 ft., at Spruce Creek Trailhead
Peak Elevation	13,950 ft.
Total Elevation Gain	2,795 ft.
Terrain	Good trail to rocky scramble to summit
Best Time to Climb	June–September
Gear Advisor	Sturdy boots
Crowd Level	Low

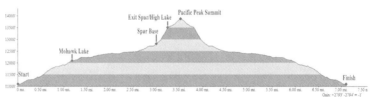

Location Tenmile Range in the Arapahoe National Forest outside of Breckenridge

Intro The Tenmile Range possesses riches and stark beauty in abundance. Not only are these mountains perched atop a wealth of minerals (the Colorado Mineral Belt has a strong presence), but these peaks avoided the heavy glaciations that smoothed out the nearby Sawatch, Mosquito, and Gore ranges. As a result, the Tenmiles have a jagged and raw appearance. Pacific Peak is in the middle of the range. Its prominent split summit can be seen from miles away.

Why Climb It? Breckenridge was once synonymous with mining, thanks to its hearty gold deposits. The old sluice and cabins at the start of this trail hearken back to the days of the great gold rush. Above the mines, Mohawk Lakes decorate a broad, colorful basin. It's a neat effect to come up to Mohawk Lake and have it appear at eye level, similar to the "infinity pools" popular at high-end resorts. A solid scramble leads to a very high unnamed alpine lake at 13,420 feet. Finish the climb to the top on a scenic ridge. There are several moderate options available for those who'd like to grab a few more summits.

Driving Driving on Spruce Creek Road pushes tough passenger cars to their limits; I was barely able to make the full length in my Accord. It has all the expected rocks and washboards, but it also has several rutted, waterbar-style speed bumps that are difficult for low-clearance vehicles. On the way down, I scraped many, many times, putting numerous dents in my exhaust system. (It wasn't quite as bad as the time I knocked the entire exhaust system off on nearby Kite Lake Road or the subsequent time I again unmoored my exhaust system on a dirt road near Peaceful Valley.) It's passable with a TPC, but you're risking damage from the inevitable bangs and bumps. Sport utility cars, SUVs, and 4x4s should have no trouble.

How to Get There   Drive south out of Breckenridge on Colorado Highway 9, about 2.5 miles from the edge of town. Just after the town limit sign for Blue River, turn right (west) onto Spruce Creek Road (Forest Service Road 800). There is a small street sign, and the turn comes up quickly. It is 3.0 miles up Spruce Creek Road to the trailhead. Spruce Creek Road begins as a well-maintained dirt road through a housing development; it continues up to a large parking area where several trails (good for mountain biking) intersect. Drive through the parking area and continue on the road, which does not get much rockier. Do not stray onto any of the side roads. After dropping into a low draw, you'll be on the final climb to the parking area, which is the roughest part of the road. The parking area shares space with a small water-treatment facility.

Fees/Camping   There are no fees to hike or camp in the area of Pacific Peak. There are a few car camping pulloffs on the way to the trailhead.

Route Notes   In September of 2006, volunteers rebuilt the lower portions of the Mohawk Lakes Trail to improve navigation through the mining ruins. By the time you read this, the work should be done, making the trip up to the lakes straightforward.

Mile/Waypoint   **0.0 mi (1)** Start from the Spruce Creek Trailhead and take the trail to Mohawk Lake/Continental Falls. This trail works its way up through an old mining operation, and you will bypass several cabins and a large sluice within the first mile. Because the mining area has some interesting relics, there are many subpaths that are easy to confuse with the main trail. If you get confused, follow the river up to the large sluice that is anchored with giant wires; the main trail passes by the very top of it.

0.7 mi (2) At the top of the sluice, the trail becomes much easier to follow. Stay on it as it goes by Lower Mohawk Lake and climbs up on the left side of Continental Falls. The cabin ruins along the way add a quaint ambiance to this lovely area.

1.2 mi (3) As you reach the basin, the eastern shore of Mohawk Lake will be at eye level. The trail continues up to some higher lakes but begins to fade out as you traverse across the meadow. Pacific Peak's distinct summit looms in the distance.

2.2 mi (4) At this point, north of the unnamed lake at 12,391 feet, the trail is but a whisper, fading away into the grass. Pass the two high lakes in the basin on their north sides. The southern sides of these lakes are a more direct path, but the boulders are big, unstable, and will slow you down considerably. Stay north on the grassy slopes and reach the base of the ridge spur (12,825 feet) that intersects with your larger goal, the east ridge.

3.0 mi (5) From the base of the spur, scramble up the slope, picking the line you feel is best. There are a few easy, class 3 moves, especially toward the top.

3.3 mi (6) Exit the spur, taking note of where you do so, in order that you will be able to recognize the line down when you descend. Check out the seemingly misplaced lake on a flat tract of land below Pacific's southeast face. Elevation here is roughly 13,500 feet. Follow the obvious east ridge westward to Pacific's summit.

3.6 mi (7) Pacific Peak's summit! From here, you have the option to go south to Atlantic Peak or north to Crystal Peak. Read the "Options" section for more information. Return the way you came.

7.3 mi Finish.

Options   It's a nice walk south to Atlantic Peak. This route is 0.7 mile one way from Pacific's summit on good, class 2 terrain. Note that Atlantic is not named on most maps—it is simply Unnamed Peak 13,841 feet.

The traverse north to Crystal Peak (13,852 feet) is longer and slightly more rugged, at 1.0 mile one way. You can then descend the rocky south slopes (class 2) of Crystal to get back into the lakes basin (rejoining the trail somewhere around waypoint 4), making this an excellent loop option.

A tour of all three peaks (Atlantic, Pacific, and Crystal) is roughly a 9-mile round trip. This mileage assumes you exit the top of the spur (waypoint 6) and walk past the high lake to Atlantic first, return over to Pacific, traverse to Crystal, and go down Crystal's south slopes. (I highly recommend this route if the weather is good.)

If you want to get yet *more* mountains, Father Dyer Peak (UN 13,615) can be reached via Crystal's east ridge. There is an interesting plaque on the mountain commemorating Father Dyer. From Father Dyer Peak, you can make a class 3 scramble out to Mount Helen (13,164 feet). Father Dyer is 0.6 mile from Crystal's summit, and Mount Helen is 1.0 mile farther to the east, 1.6 miles from Crystal's summit.

Quick Facts   Many men were made wealthy by the riches hidden in these mountains. Gold and silver in particular were found in abundance in this area. Amongst those who made their fortunes here was Methodist minister John L. Dyer. The "mining minister," Father Dyer met with moderate success at his Warrior's Mark Mine. He built a cabin at the site in 1881; a few years later, he sold the mine for $2,000. A small town sprung up in the area called Dyersville, which died out when the mining ceased.

Contact Info   Arapahoe National Forest
Clear Creek Ranger District
101 Chicago Creek Road
P.O. Box 3307
Idaho Springs, CO 80452
(303) 567-3000

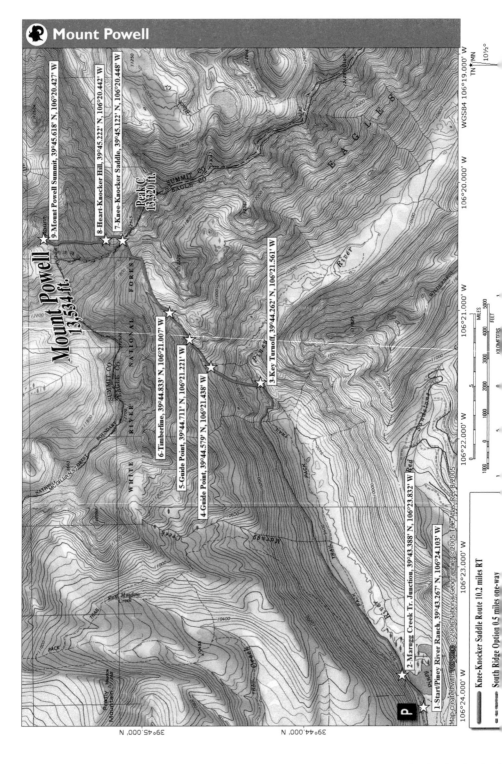

Mount Powell
13,534 ft.

Peak C
13,320 ft.

9-Mount Powell Summit, 39°45.618' N, 106°20.427' W

8-Heart-Knocker Hill, 39°45.222' N, 106°20.442' W

7-Knee-Knocker Saddle, 39°45.122' N, 106°20.448' W

6-Timberline, 39°44.833' N, 106°21.007' W

5-Guide Point, 39°44.711' N, 106°21.221' W

4-Guide Point, 39°44.579' N, 106°21.438' W

3-Key Turnoff, 39°44.262' N, 106°21.561' W

2-Maryeg Creek Tr. Junction, 39°43.388' N, 106°23.832' W

1-Start/Piney River Ranch, 39°43.267' N, 106°24.103' W

Knee-Knocker Saddle Route 10.2 miles RT

South Ridge Option 0.5 miles one-way

16   **Mount Powell**

Isolated in his daunting kingdom, the king of the Gore Range requests your company. Test your legs, lungs, and brains as you find your way to this regal peak.

Round Trip Distance	10.2 miles
Hiking Time	7–10 hours
Difficulty	9/10
Class	2
Start Elevation	9,368 ft., at Piney Lake Trailhead
Peak Elevation	13,534 ft.
Total Elevation Gain	4,930 ft.
Terrain	Tricky off-trail navigation to steep, challenging hill climbs
Best Time to Climb	June–September
Gear Advisor	Gaiters, trekking poles or ice axe, GPS
Crowd Level	Low

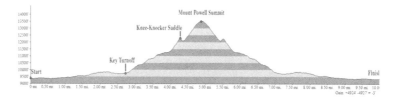

Location   Gore Range in the Eagles Nest Wilderness/White River National Forest outside of Vail

Intro   Mount Powell is the hidden patriarch of the Gore Range. It takes a bit of backcountry navigation savvy to locate the way up, but once you do, you're in for a heck of a fun day. After a nice approach on class 1 trails through the beautiful Piney Lake area, you will be off-trail for 2.1 miles of rugged terrain. Climb up a foliage-rich slope to a secret alpine basin at 10,800 feet. From here, the route becomes easier to see as you tackle Knee-Knocker Saddle and Heart-Knocker Hill. The summit is a special place with incredible views.

Why Climb It?   The Gore mountains stand out as some of the most beautiful and geologically significant peaks in Colorado. The Gores were pushed up by fault-blocks and further shaped by heavy glaciations. As a result, you have a hybrid range that has jagged peaks and glacial cirques, with terrain that reveals an occasional fossil to the keen-eyed hiker. Powell is the highest of these mountains, yet it has no standard route to its summit—which is part of its appeal. You make the summit in three pushes: a steep climb up a densely overgrown hillside, a steep climb up the basin to Knee-Knocker Saddle, and the final summit push up the steep Heart-Knocker Hill. The summit feels like an eagle's nest, with views of wilderness to the north and the Vail Ski Area to the south.

Driving

Passenger cars can make it up the dirt road to Piney River Ranch and the start of the trailhead. The road is bumpy at times, but it never gets too rocky or so washed out that you'll need a high-clearance vehicle. Trucks and high-clearance vehicles will fare better and will have no trouble reaching the trailhead.

How to Get There

From Interstate 70 westbound, take exit 176 into Vail. Take a right to enter the roundabout, and then take a left onto North Frontage Road (the sign reads N. FRONTAGE ROAD/WEST VAIL). Stay on this road 1.0 mile and take a right (north) turn onto Red Sandstone Road, which has a sign for Piney Lake. If you are coming from I-70 eastbound, take exit 173, follow the roundabout to Frontage Road and continue east for 1.7 miles to reach this same point, Red Sandstone Road.

Follow the paved Red Sandstone Road 0.7 mile uphill, where it turns to a well-maintained dirt road and becomes Forest Service Road 700. Reset your odometer. There will continue to be signs for Piney Lake and Piney River Ranch along the way. At mile 2.6, stay left on FS 700 at a split (at this juncture, you're officially off Red Sandstone Road). Stay on FS 700 as it climbs and drops through an unspoiled part of Vail. You will see several pulloffs for primitive camping along the way; if you plan on camping, wait a few miles for closer (and better) sites. At mile 6.6, stay right on FS 700 at the junction with FS 701. Go downhill; eventually you'll be driving next to a river. Be careful of the resident moose that live here. At mile 9.1, turn right where a small sign announces PINEY LAKE 2 MILES. Follow FS 700 to Piney River Ranch at mile 10.6. Park on the left at the end of the road and away from the lots closer to the buildings; the ranch here hosts many functions and needs the spaces for their guests. Please respect the private land around this area, as the ranch owners are the ones who make it possible to hike into the Gore Range.

Fees/Camping

There are no fees for hiking or camping in this area. There are great car camping sites along FS 700, starting around mile 8.9 (once you are near the river). From here to the parking area are several good places to pull off and set up a tent.

Route Notes

None.

Mile/Waypoint

0.0 mi (1) Start at Piney River Ranch and go west toward Piney Lake. Get on the Upper Piney Trail #1885 and enjoy a morning tour of this misty valley.

0.3 mi (2) At the west end of Piney Lake there is a junction with the Marugg Creek Trail #1899. Stay right on the Upper Piney Trail and follow it as it enters into dark woods, climbs up a hill, and descends back down.

2.8 mi (3) This is the key to your entire hike. Since GPS units are not perfectly precise, expect this turn to come between 2.79 and 2.91 miles on your receiver. You will have gone downhill and will be almost level with the river at roughly 9,750 feet. The barely there trail is usually marked by a few small cairns, which may or may not be there; the uphill trail starts where two skinny pine trees stand in the middle of the footpath. You will need to turn left (north) at this key turnoff and begin climbing. There is a very faint and overgrown trail that you can follow, but if you lose it, don't worry. This climb goes through some dense foliage with the occasional clearing; keep going up with a northeast trajectory.

3.1 mi (4) At this point, the trail is right next to a rocky waterfall/stream and actually crosses over it and continues up. Once you have found this stream, you can use it as a guide to lead you northeast to the basin. Waypoints 5 and 6 are on the map for GPS users, to help establish a route.

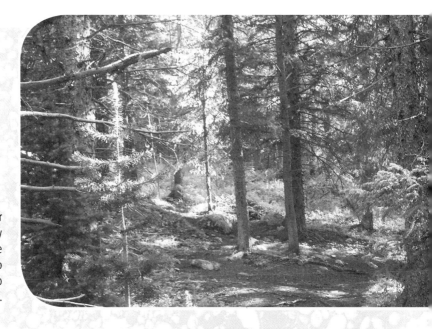

eep your eyes open for se "twin trees"—they signal your departure om the main trail onto he barely there path to Kneeknocker Saddle.

3.7 mi (6) Just above this waypoint, the basin opens up before you at 11,100 feet. It is rocky on the sides but has a nice grassy meadow in the middle. This area holds snow far into the summer. Magically, a hiking trail reappears to guide you to Knee-Knocker Saddle. Knee-Knocker Saddle is to the northeast, between the shoulder of Powell (you can't see the top from here) on the left and Peak C on the right. Climb more than 1,200 feet directly up to Knee-Knocker Saddle, staying on the rockier left side for better footing. The gully in the middle is loose and difficult to ascend, though it makes for good scree-surfing on the descent.

4.4 mi (7) At 12,300 feet, you're in Knee-Knocker Saddle and you'll finally have views of the summit. (A friend related this experience to *The Simpsons* episode in which Homer has to climb Mount Springfield. Each time he thinks he sees the top of the mountain, a comically larger one appears behind it, much to his chagrin. Same thing here!) There are permanent snowfields on the east side of this pass. To follow the class 2 route, drop down about 100 feet over the east side of the pass to the base of Heart-Knocker Hill to your left (north). Note that when the snowfield is filled in, you may have to descend on snow on the far side of the saddle, to the right, to make your way over to the base of the hill. The direct way to the hill may require you to use kicksteps to get down safely (or you can glissade a little, though the terrain may be a bit too steep for some people).

4.5 mi (8) You are now at the base of Heart-Knocker Hill, whose long, grassy, and rocky hill offers the best way up. What are you waiting for? It's only another 1,350-foot climb (in a half mile) to the top. Much like the previous climb, stay to the sides for better footing (in this case, the right side is best). When you get to a flat section at 13,470 feet, atop the gully, you'll need to scramble up a pile of boulders on your right, northeast to the highest point. The rocks are solid, but after all the work to get up here, you may be thinking you'll never see the summit.

5.1 miles (9) Phew! Finally, Mount Powell's summit! It sure is nice up here. Enjoy the views and let your heart rate slow down. Vail's ski areas are to the south, while there's more Gore goodness to the north.

To return, go back down the basin. (The descent will seem amazingly fast in contrast to your ascent.) The trail through the meadow of the basin is much easier to follow on the way down. You can always follow the stream down (or at least keep it in sight) to return to the main trail. Enjoy your hike out.

10.2 miles Finish.

Options From the top of Knee-Knocker Saddle, you can go right onto Powell's south ridge and ascend on class 2+/3 terrain that intercepts Heart-Knocker Hill about three quarters of the way up. It's a nice option for those comfortable with navigating ridges on which you'll need to make a few blind moves.

Quick Facts There are two mountains named after John W. Powell in Colorado; this one and Powell Peak in Rocky Mountain National Park. Powell actually climbed this mountain (with partner Ned Farrell) in the summer of 1868, shortly after his historic "first" ascent of Longs Peak.

To this day, many of the Gore Range peaks lack formal names (such as the letter peaks: C, N, G, etc.).

This is yet another mountain where I found seashells in the dirt.

Contact Info White River National Forest
Eagle Ranger District
125 W. Fifth Street
P.O. Box 720
Eagle, CO 81631
(970) 328-6388

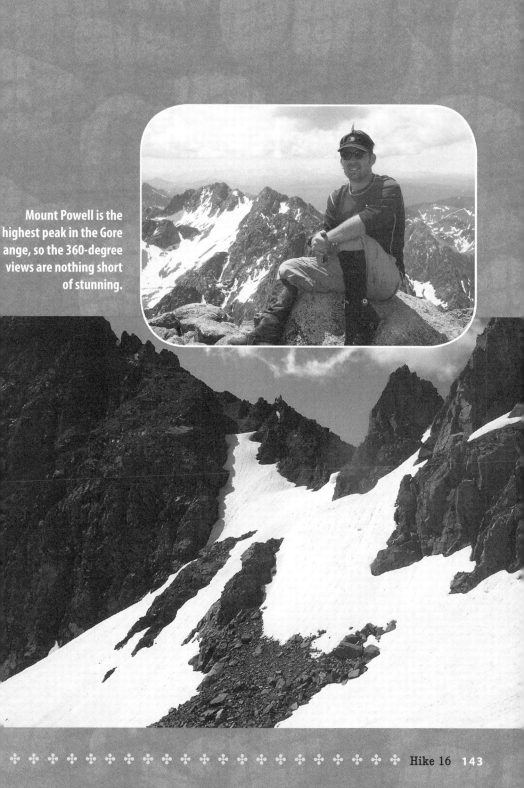

Mount Powell is the highest peak in the Gore ange, so the 360-degree views are nothing short of stunning.

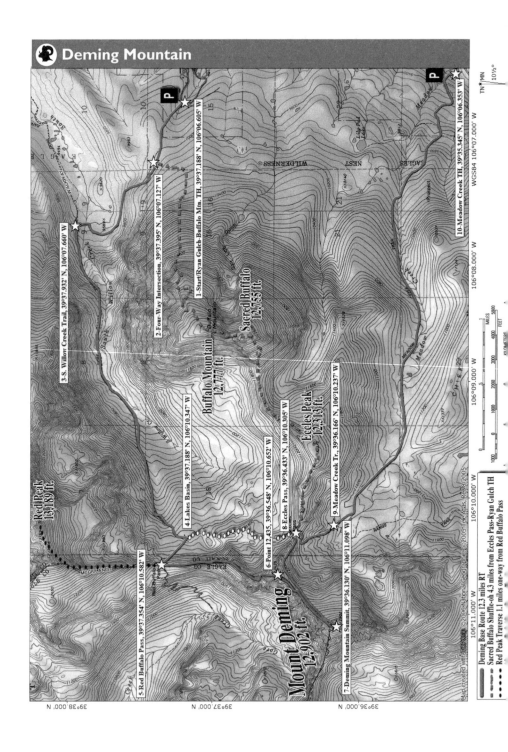

Red Peak
13,189 ft.

Mount Deming
12,902 ft.

Buffalo Mountain
12,777 ft.

Sacred Buffalo
12,755 ft.

Eccles Peak
12,313 ft.

1-Start/Ryan Gulch-Buffalo Mtn. TH, 39°37.188' N, 106°06.605' W

2-Four-Way Intersection, 39°37.395' N, 106°07.127' W

3-S. Willow Creek Trail, 39°37.932' N, 106°07.660' W

4-Lakes Basin, 39°37.188' N, 106°10.347' W

5-Red Buffalo Pass, 39°37.354' N, 106°10.582' W

6-Point 12,435, 39°36.548' N, 106°10.652' W

7-Deming Mountain Summit, 39°36.130' N, 106°11.098' W

8-Eccles Pass, 39°36.433' N, 106°10.305' W

9-Meadow Creek Tr., 39°36.166' N, 106°10.237' W

10-Meadow Creek TH, 39°35.345' N, 106°06.353' W

WGS84 106°07.000' W

106°08.000' W

106°09.000' W

106°10.000' W

106°11.000' W

39°38.000' N

39°37.000' N

39°36.000' N

Map created with TOPO!® ©2006 National Geographic ©2005 Tele Atlas, Rel. 08/2005

Deming Base Route 12.3 miles RT
Sacred Buffalo Shuffle-oh 4.3 miles from Eccles Pass-Ryan Gulch TH
Red Peak Traverse 1.1 miles one-way from Red Buffalo Pass

17 **Deming Mountain** *Good Overnight!*

Deming is a truly "Gore-geous" mountain! You have options galore on this overlooked Gore, including a fun class 2+/3 ridge, a class 2 walk up, and an epic loop!

Round Trip Distance	12–14 miles (read below)
Hiking Time	8–11 hours
Difficulty	7/10
Class	2/3
Start Elevation	9,760 ft., at Buffalo Mountain/Ryan Gulch Trailhead
Peak Elevation	12,902 ft.
Total Elevation Gain	3,775 ft. (one-way standard route)
Terrain	Good trail to rugged ridge or off-trail walk-up
Best Time to Climb	June–September
Gear Advisor	Normal gear
Crowd Level	Low

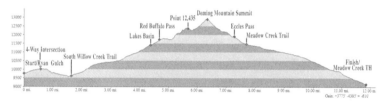

Location Gore Range in the Eagles Nest Wilderness/Arapahoe National Forest, outside of Frisco

Special Routes Deming Mountain has no standard route. The "Mile/Waypoint" description details a one-way, point-to-point route that requires two cars. This course encompasses the most optional routes, as there are many ways to hike the mountain. There are also two ways to reach the summit once you are near it: a good class 2 walk up or an exciting class 3 ridge scramble. Here's a summary rundown of the possibilities (please see map for actual route details).

Route 1: Full Tour (Base Route)
This route uses two trailheads to make an epic tour that nearly circumnavigates Buffalo Mountain. Starting at the Buffalo Mountain Trailhead, the route drops down to the South Willow Creek Trail and follows it west to Red Buffalo Pass. From here, the route follows Red Buffalo Ridge south on an exciting class 3 ridge scramble over to Deming. It then drops down to Eccles Pass and exits via the Meadow Creek Trail, ending at the Meadow Creek Trailhead. This route is about 12 miles total.

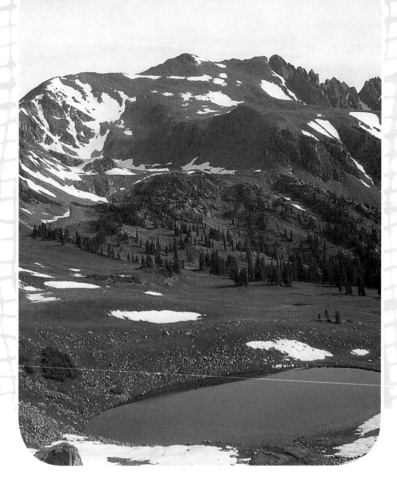

Looking back at Red Peak on the ridge scramble option to Deming

If you like this route but want to keep it class 2, avoid Red Buffalo Ridge/Red Buffalo Pass and hike to Eccles Pass, where you can traverse off-trail to the summit of Deming (this is the descent route in the Full Tour).

There are two solid variations to Route 1 that avoid using two trailheads and two cars.

Route 1, Option 1: Out and back starting from Buffalo Mountain Trailhead. This variation goes up to Deming as stated above, down to Eccles Pass and retraces your steps the way you came. Not a bad hike, but it makes for a very long day. Returning on the South Willow Creek Trail and back uphill to the parking lot is a bit tedious. It's also very long, about 14 miles. This option is advised if you like the wild, less-traveled path through South Willow Creek.

Route 1, Option 2: Out and back from Meadow Creek Trailhead. This is perhaps the most reasonable and efficient way to get up the mountain. It's about 12 miles round trip, but it's faster than the standard route, thanks to the approach on good trails. If you want to hike the ridge, you'll have to clear Eccles Pass and go north to Red Buffalo Pass, and then swing back down to Deming. If you are doing the class 2 route and want a quicker hike, this is the way to go.

Route 2: Sacred Buffalo Shuffle-oh

This route uses the trailhead of your choice, followed by a hike of Deming, then a return over Eccles Peak, a trip up and over "Sacred Buffalo" and Buffalo Mountain, ending at Buffalo Mountain/Ryan Gulch Trailhead. You gain a ton of elevation, somewhere close to 5,500 feet in the 13 to 14 miles of hiking. If you start from Buffalo Mountain Trailhead, you can make this an epic loop, requiring only one car.

As you can see, you can mix and match these options as you wish. I'll describe the base route and add my notes for Buffalo Mountain and Red Peak in the usual "Options" section.

Intro
Options abound! The class 3 ridge is a real challenge. From Red Buffalo Pass, it's 1.6 miles via ridges to Deming. All the hikes showcase the beauty of the Gore Range, an area overrun with wildflowers and teeming with wildlife.

Why Climb It?
Poor Deming doesn't see a lot of visitors. Go say hi. The approach in from either trailhead is very scenic, especially in the wild garden of the South Willow Creek Trail. Bear and moose are locals here and aren't terribly shy, so keep your eyes open and your bear bells jingling! The Gores are a beautiful range, and this hike, no matter which option you take, will showcase that magnificence. It should be noted that the basin north of Eccles Pass is an awesome place to camp. The extra time you gain by waking up in the mountains makes a complete dayhike of the four named peaks in the area—Deming, Eccles, Buffalo, and Red Peak—a more feasible task.

Driving
All vehicles can make it to either trailhead; they are both very close to I-70.

How to Get There
Ryan Gulch/Buffalo Mountain Trailhead: From Interstate 70, take exit 205 (Silverthorne) and head north on Colorado Highway 9. If coming off the westbound side, take a right off the exit and then take a left at the next light, onto Wildernest Road. This appears to be a frontage road, but it actually goes up through a condo development. Follow this road for 3.5 miles; after mile 1.0, it turns into Ryan Gulch Road (once you pass the Wildernest center). Parking is on the left-hand side of the road and the trail begins on the right-hand side, a short distance down the road you came up. Do *not* go up the road to the Lily Pad Lake Trailhead.

Meadow Creek Trailhead: Exit I-70 in Frisco at exit 203. Go around the roundabout to the north side and take a left (west) onto the dirt road, County Road 231, and continue for half a mile to the Meadow Creek Trailhead.

Fees/Camping
There are no fees to hike or camp in the area. If you do stay overnight, please keep one unfortunate reality in mind: the trailheads are easily accessed and are subject to a bit more crime than backcountry lots.

Route Notes
Following is the description for the base route, starting at Ryan Gulch/Buffalo Mountain and ending at Meadow Creek.

Mile/Waypoint
0.0 mi (1) Start at the Ryan Gulch/Buffalo Mountain Trailhead and make sure you get on the proper trail on the north side of the road, a little east

of the parking area. Your goal from here is to descend to the South Willow Creek Trail.

0.5 mi (2) There is a four-way intersection here. Go straight (north) and begin the downhill run to the basin bottom. The trail is worn and generally easy to follow, though tree fall has obscured portions and there's a short talus section that may make it difficult to spot. If you get off-trail, just keep descending to South Willow Creek.

1.6 mi (3) You've dropped down about 400 feet to the creekbed at 9,600 feet. Even though you are in a swamp, there are primitive camping areas here. The South Willow Creek Trail intersects here (and is signed) and goes for a long way west. Get on this trail and enjoy the walk through a wild area. The trail fades a bit in swampy areas but is otherwise easy to follow.

4.6 mi (4) Near the small lakes in the basin, turn north and go to Red Buffalo Pass. Or, if you're feeling good in the knees, go directly up one of the slopes and freelance scramble to the ridge from here. I'd say go to the pass: it's fun because it gives you the chance to experience the entire ridge as it evolves from a grassy slope to a broken, rocky traverse.

5.0 mi (5) Red Buffalo Pass. Go south and begin the ridge. The highpoint you see in the distance is not Deming; it is Point 12,435—which is your first goal, a mile from waypoint 5. Scrambling gets progressively harder as you go higher, culminating in some tricky class 3 moves just before Point 12,435. If you get stymied, try the pillars on the west side of the ridge—there are loose gullies you can use to skirt some of the harder parts. This is not a ridge for beginning scramblers, as the route-finding is deceptively difficult. In places, the rock is quite rotten and loose.

6.0 mi (6) Point, 12,435. Finally, you can see the gradual slopes leading to Deming. Follow the southwest contour of the ridge on class 2 terrain over to the summit. Just to ensure I'm not making up the name of this often unrecognized peak, check out the metal summit marker. What? It's not a USGS marker? Uh-oh!

6.6 mi (7) What were we here for again? Oh yeah, Deming Mountain! You're there! Hurray! Check out the heavenly view of the Cross Couloir on Mount of the Holy Cross from here. Descend eastward on the slanted slopes to the saddle of Eccles (rhymes with "freckles") Pass.

7.6 mi (8) Eccles Pass. From here, you're back on trail and the hard "work" is over. Drop south on the Gore Range Trail into another very lovely basin, much like the first, where the Meadow Creek Trail splits off to the left (east).

8.2 mi (9) Take the Meadow Creek Trail here and follow it east/southeast 4.1 miles to the parking area and your second car. You *did* remember to bring a second car, right?

12.3 mi (10) All done! Finish at the Meadow Creek Trailhead.

Options Besides the choices already mentioned, here are a few more: traverse to Red Peak (13,189 feet) along a good, class 2 ridge north of Red Buffalo Pass (waypoint 5). It is 1.1 miles from the pass to the summit, one way.

The Sacred Buffalo Shuffle-oh route starts at Eccles Pass (waypoint 8) and goes east to Buffalo Mountain along Buffalo's west ridge. Go to 12,313-foot Mount Eccles, 0.6 mile from the pass. Continue east along Buffalo's west ridge, which gets tougher as you get higher, in the style of Red Buffalo Ridge. After a long walk to the saddle between Eccles and Buffalo, climb up to "Sacred Buffalo," a subsummit of Buffalo, at 1.9 miles from the pass. Getting up and over Sacred Buffalo takes some class 3 moves; you can skirt to the southeast if you prefer. At 2.0 miles from the pass, you're on Buffalo Mountain's summit, at 12,777 feet. Descend via the Buffalo Mountain Trail back to Ryan Gulch, which is 2.3 miles away (4.3 miles total from the pass).

Quick Facts   Deming Mountain is named for an old homesteader, John J. Deming, who lived in the Frisco area with his family from 1890 until his death in 1924. It is interesting that the name does not appear on many maps, even though the Bureau of Reclamation has a marker proclaiming "Deming Mountain" on the summit. (The Bureau of Reclamation didn't "repossess" Deming because the USGS couldn't pay their bills; it's a subgroup of the USGS established in 1902 primarily to deal with environmental water concerns.)

Contact Info   Arapahoe National Forest
Clear Creek Ranger District
101 Chicago Creek Road
P.O. Box 3307
Idaho Springs, CO 80452
(303) 567-3000

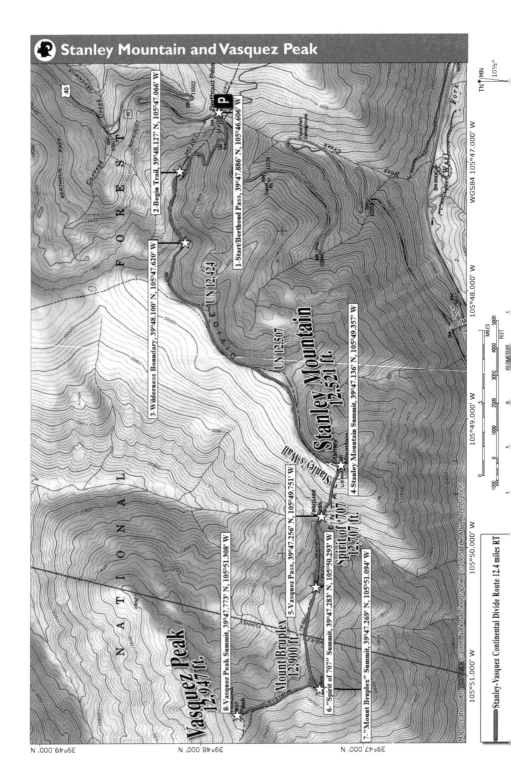

Vasquez Peak
12,947 ft.

8-Vasquez Peak Summit, 39°47.773' N, 105°51.308' W

Mount Bruplex
12,900 ft.

Stanley Mountain
12,521 ft.

4-Stanley Mountain Summit, 39°47.136 N, 105°49.357' W

Spirit of '707
12,707 ft.

5-Vasquez Pass, 39°47.256' N, 105°49.751' W

6-"Spirit of 707" Summit, 39°47.283' N, 105°50.293' W

7-"Mount Bruplex" Summit, 39°47.269' N, 105°51.094' W

Stanley's Wall

UN 12,507

UN 12,424

3-Wilderness Boundary, 39°48.100' N, 105°47.620' W

2-Begin Trail, 39°48.127' N, 105°47.066' W

1-Start/Berthoud Pass, 39°47.886' N, 105°46.606' W

F O R E S T

N A T I O N A L

WGS84 105°47.000' W

105°48.000' W

105°49.000' W

105°50.000' W

105°51.000' W

N 39°49.000' N

N 39°48.000' N

N 39°47.000' N

TN* MN 10½°

Stanley-Vasquez Continental Divide Route 12.4 miles RT

18 **Stanley Mountain and Vasquez Peak**
Plus bonus peaks "Spirit of 707"and "Mount Bruplex"

Peaks galore are yours for the bagging! Take a walk on the Continental Divide and discover the charm of the little-known Vasquez Mountains.

Round Trip Distance	12.4 miles
Hiking Time	6–9 hours
Difficulty	7.5/10
Class	2
Start Elevation	11,304 ft., at Berthoud Pass
Peak Elevations	Stanley Mountain: 12,521 ft.; Vasquez Peak: 12,947 ft.; Spirit of 707: 12,707 ft.; Mount Bruplex: 12,900 ft.
Total Elevation Gain	4,753 ft.
Terrain	Trails and good off-trail alpine tundra
Best Time to Climb	June–September; Year-round to Stanley Mtn. and back
Gear Advisor	Trekking poles
Crowd Level	Low

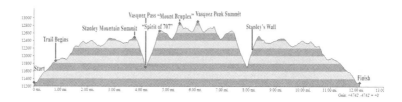

Location Vasquez Mountains in the Vasquez Peak Wilderness/Arapahoe National Forest near the top of Berthoud Pass

Intro The Vasquez Peak Wilderness is a relatively unknown area, despite its close proximity to Winter Park and its accessibility from the top of Berthoud Pass. This route begins with a sky-high walk along the Continental Divide to Stanley Peak, a hike that is possible year-round. Dropping down to Vasquez Pass gives you access to three rolling mountains, including the highpoint of the Vasquez Mountains, Vasquez Peak. The crazy elevation profile shows this hike is the true-to-life incarnation of that famous old-timer rant: you'll be hiking uphill both ways!

Why Climb It? The Vasquez Mountains make up a small range best known for their northern slopes, where most of the trails for Winter Park and Mary Jane ski areas are cut. This area is popular for backcountry skiers. The beginning of this hike was once within the boundaries of the now-defunct Berthoud Pass Ski Area.

Approximately 95% of this hike is above treeline, giving brilliant views of the Gore and Front ranges. The first half of the hike follows a mellow trail on high alpine plains to Stanley Mountain. The second half dips down, and gives you a chance to test your legs and lungs as you press on to three more mountains. On the west side of Vasquez Pass, the land feels very clean and pure and is punctuated with scarlet grasses and wildflowers. On the way back, get ready to push yourself up the giant grassy feature known as "Stanley's Wall."

Driving All vehicles can make it to the top of Berthoud Pass, which is paved and very well maintained. This parking area is open year-round and caters to backcountry skiers, snowboarders, and snowshoers in the winter.

How to Get There From I-70, take exit 232 (the Winter Park, Empire, Granby exit) and follow US Highway 40 approximately 15 miles to the top of Berthoud Pass. The flat summit of the pass has a large parking area on the right (east) side at the base of a ski hill; you'll see relics of the old Berthoud Pass Ski Area. Park here and cross the street to begin your hike.

Fees/Camping There are no fees to hike or camp in the area. There are a few pay campgrounds along Berthoud Pass on both the north and south sides; call the Forest Service number listed on page 153 for fee information.

Route Notes None.

Mile/Waypoint **0.0 mi (1)** Start at the parking area on the east side of Berthoud Pass. Cross the paved road and begin hiking on the dirt road on the west side. (There will be a gate and a sign for Continental Divide Scenic Trail; this is also Forest Service Road 786.) As you head up, make sure you stay on FS 786.

0.8 mi (2) The road ends and an obvious footpath continues left (northwest). This trail has a cairn at the start. Follow the path to a steep hill, which you'll ascend via several switchbacks.

1.5 mi (3) After climbing the switchbacks, you'll pass the Vasquez Wilderness boundary. You can see your trailing stretching far to the west—welcome to the Continental Divide!

1.9 mi The trail intersects with the old Mount Nystrom Trail, which overlaps the ambitious Continental Divide Trail. Stay left (southwest) and hike on the gently rolling hills of the divide, crossing over several small unnamed summits along the way. This is a very peaceful area with great views. Stanley Peak looks far off, but you'll be there sooner than you think.

3.8 mi (4) Stanley Mountain's summit! This is the end of your on-trail hiking (though the barely there Mount Nystrom Trail continues along the route in this description). Drop down Stanley's very steep western slope to the saddle of Vasquez Pass. This grassy hill has good footing but drops very quickly, earning it the nickname "Stanley's Wall." Trekking poles will help save your knees at this point.

4.2 mi (5) You're at a low point at Vasquez Pass, 11,700 feet. You may hear the din of machinery from Henderson Mine to the south. From here, a faint path pushes west up to the summit of "Spirit of 707 Peak." Make up all the elevation you lost, and then some, to reach the top.

4.8 mi (6) The top of Spirit of 707! From here things get much easier—and much prettier. Very few people venture to this section of the Vasquez Mountains. Continue west to "Mount Bruplex." A trace of the Mount Nystrom Trail may appear here and there as you hike along the alpine meadows.

5.5 mi (7) After a good class 2 hike/scramble, you're on the summit of "Mount Bruplex." The ridgeline between Bruplex and Vasquez is obvious as it heads north. The last brief section before Vasquez's summit has some rocky patches.

6.2 mi (8) You've finally reached the highpoint of the Vasquez Mountains, Vasquez Peak. Congratulations! On most days, you'll have the summit to yourself, so soak in the solitude and take lots of pictures.

Return the way you came, with the exception of skirting just below the top of Mount Bruplex. It may be tempting to shortcut from the knobby outcrop just north of Bruplex, but the footing is not very good. Continue back up and over 707, and then drop back down to Vasquez Pass.

8.1 mi (5) At this point in most hikes, you'd be done gaining elevation. Not so here—the climb back up to Stanley is a bugger! Again, trekking poles will be a big help. You're going from 11,700 feet to 12,490 feet in less than half a mile. Push, push, push your way back up "Stanley's Wall" to the summit, and you'll be home free. Enjoy the rest of the walk back to Berthoud Pass.

12.4 mi Finish.

Options If you count the unnamed summits on this hike, you'll be topping seven moderate peaks. What more do you want? The only option I recommend is hiking to Stanley Mountain in the winter. It's a good adventure on safe terrain. However, going down to Vasquez Pass would be very dangerous (this is prime avalanche terrain) and is not recommended when there is still snow.

Quick Facts Vasquez Peak takes its name from the brothers Vasquez. Louis is known for building a fort at Clear Creek in 1832; Antoine was member of Zebulon Pike's exploratory expedition. Stanley Mountain honors F.O. Stanley, creator of the Stanley Steamer. "Spirit of 707" (an unofficial name) celebrates the long forgotten events of the year A.D. 707, which included the death of Japanese Emperor Mommu and the Byzantines losing the Balearic Islands to the Moors (the world would never be the same). "Mount Bruplex" is unnamed on every map save this one, but every good mountain deserves a name. Bruplex happens to be the name of one of my cats.

Contact Info Arapahoe National Forest
Clear Creek Ranger District
101 Chicago Creek Road
P.O. Box 3307
Idaho Springs, CO 80452
(303) 567-2901

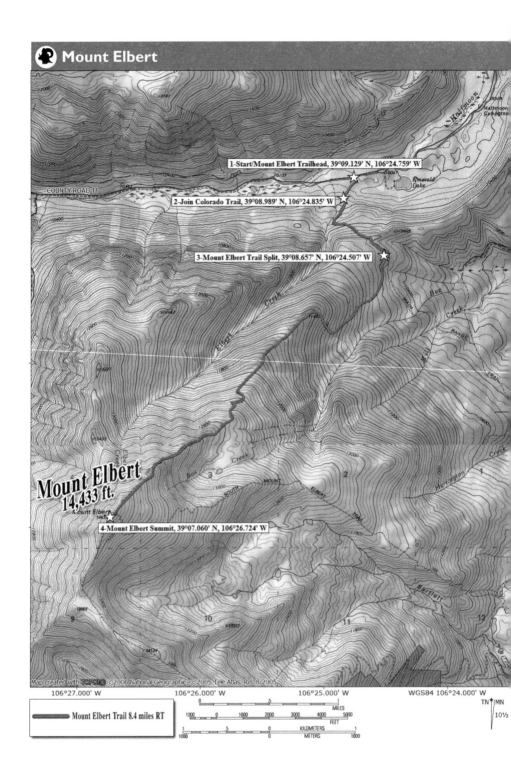

1-Start/Mount Elbert Trailhead, 39°09.129' N, 106°24.759' W

2-Join Colorado Trail, 39°08.989' N, 106°24.835' W

3-Mount Elbert Trail Split, 39°08.657' N, 106°24.507' W

Mount Elbert
14,433 ft.

4-Mount Elbert Summit, 39°07.060' N, 106°26.724' W

COUNTY ROAD 11

Map created with TOPO!® ©2006 National Geographic; ©2005 Tele Atlas, Rel. 8/2005

106°27.000' W   106°26.000' W   106°25.000' W   WGS84 106°24.000' W

Mount Elbert Trail 8.4 miles RT

MILES
FEET
KILOMETERS
METERS

TN / MN
10½

19 Mount Elbert

Welcome to Colorado's highest mountain! Elbert is a gentle giant whose lofty heights are also tops in all the Rocky Mountains. This king of 14ers is one of Colorado's best hikes.

Round Trip Distance	8.4 miles
Hiking Time	4½–6½ hours
Difficulty	5/10
Class	2
Start Elevation	10,066 ft., at Mount Elbert Trailhead/Elbert Creek Campground
Peak Elevation	14,433 ft.
Total Elevation Gain	4,643 ft.
Terrain	Well-maintained trail
Best Time to Climb	June–September
Gear Advisor	Light hikers
Crowd Level	Moderate; high on weekends

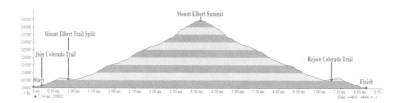

Location Sawatch Range in the Mount Massive Wilderness/San Isabel National Forest near Leadville

Intro Ask folks outside of Colorado what the highest mountain in the state is, and they'll probably guess Pikes Peak or Longs Peak. Humble Mount Elbert has little fanfare outside of the Centennial State, despite being the second highest mountain in the lower 48 states (and the 21st highest in the entire US, including Alaska). Only Mount Whitney (14,494 feet) in California is higher. Elbert's northeast ridge is a surprisingly moderate hike (roughly 8 to 9 miles round trip, and 5 to 7 hours of hiking) and is typical of the rounded, giant Sawatch mountains.

Why Climb It? The obvious draw to Mount Elbert is its height. The gentle northeast ridge that the Mount Elbert Trail follows is a true classic. The lower sections weave through a pristine pine forest and then switchback up to treeline, where Elbert's majesty is revealed. If treeline is reached in the early-morning dawn, the panoramic sunrise looking north to Leadville is stunning, especially when a low blanket of clouds hovers below. Hiking up past the notorious false summits leads to a flat apex with gorgeous 360-degree views. Elbert's moderate difficulty (altitude notwithstanding) makes it a good primer for more arduous hikes.

Driving   Elbert Creek and the Mount Elbert Trailhead can be reached by all vehicles. The dirt road is well maintained and easy to drive in normal conditions. Past the trailhead, the road gradually becomes rockier. A tough passenger car can make it far enough past the trailhead to park at some of the better primitive campsites.

How to Get There   From downtown Leadville, drive 3.5 miles south on US Highway 24 and turn right (west) onto Colorado Highway 300, which appears just after a service station on the right. Drive 0.7 mile, and then turn left (south) onto County Road 11. Turn right at 1.8 miles (when the road turns to dirt) and follow the signs to Halfmoon Creek Campground. Continue on this good dirt road 6.8 miles (bypassing the Halfmoon Creek Campground), until you reach the Mount Elbert Trailhead on your left; Elbert Creek Campground is across from the trailhead on your right. The Mount Elbert Trailhead is a large lot.

Fees/Camping   There are no fees to climb Mount Elbert. If you'd like to camp at Halfmoon Creek or Elbert Creek campgrounds (which have toilets and maintained sites), the fee is $11 per night, as of 2006. If you prefer to save a few bucks, there are several free primitive campsites past the Mount Elbert Trailhead (and beyond the Mount Massive Trailhead). These sites are between 0.25 and 0.5 mile from the end of the passenger-car-friendly road, though most cars can make it to the first sites.

Route Notes   None.

Mile/Waypoint   **0.0 mi (1)**   Start from the Mount Elbert Trailhead and take the Mount Elbert Trail. There's an informative sign at the beginning of the trail.

0.2 mi (2)   The Colorado Trail joins the Mount Elbert Trail, coming in from the right. Follow the signs for Mount Elbert and bear left (you'll feel silly if you take the wrong turn because it brings you directly back to the road). Get ready to start plugging uphill, passing a few cabin ruins during a level section.

0.9 mi (3)   The Mount Elbert Trail splits right (south), while the Colorado Trail goes straight and downhill. Turn right onto the signed Mount Elbert Trail and hike your way up toward treeline. After a straight, steep section, you'll continue to climb to 12,000 feet, where you will emerge from timberline.

2.4 mi   Exit treeline (12,000 feet). From here, you'll have a good look at the ridge up to Elbert's summit. Continue on the well-traveled trail.

3.1 mi   After a particularly steep section, top out on one of Elbert's false summits. There's one more (sort-of) false summit after this one, before you truly top out.

4.2 mi (4)   Mount Elbert Summit! You're now the highest thing in Colorado (unless you have a taller hiking companion!). Return the way you came up.

7.5 mi (3)   It's easy to zone out on the long descent; make sure not to miss the left turn on Mount Elbert Trail when it rejoins the Colorado Trail.

8.4 mi   Finish.

Options   With so many 14ers and high 13ers nearby, it's easy to pair Elbert up with another Sawatch climb. Some described in this book include: Mount Hope (Hike 21), Huron Peak (Hike 22), Mount Ouray (Hike 23), Mount Shavano and Tabeguache Peak (Hike 24). The most logical peak for a weekend excursion with Elbert is Mount Massive (14,421 feet), which is barely Colorado's second highest mountain (edging out Mount Harvard by a foot!). The Mount Massive Trailhead is less than a quarter mile west from the Mount Elbert Trailhead. Hiking Massive makes for a longer day, but it's still class 2 terrain, with a 13.6-mile round trip to bag its summit.

Quick Facts   Elbert's country-style name comes from former Colorado Governor Samuel Hitt Elbert, who served from 1873–74. Elbert, whose term was less than memorable, married the daughter of the next Governor, John Evans. Evans had a more notable term in office, but the 14er named in his honor (Mount Evans, 14,264 feet) had a lower elevation. This is another instance in which the mountain is not the measure of the man.

In the 1930s, there was a feud between Mount Elbert supporters and Mount Massive supporters; both argued their peak was the highest (the actual difference is a mere 12 feet). Massive fan club hikers (who apparently had quite a bit of free time) constructed large cairns on the summit of Massive to boost its height, only to have Elbert supporters tear them down. Ultimately, measurements determined that Elbert is the higher mountain, though it's safe to say Mount Massive has a more impressive name.

One final bit of interest: in 1949, a Jeep drove to the top of Elbert as part of survey to gauge the mountain's potential for development of a road or ski area. Several bicyclists have made ascents of the peak as well.

Contact Info   Hiking Mount Elbert is a good year-round adventure. During good snow conditions, one can make an enjoyable descent from the peak on skis or a snowboard. Contact the Forest Service for winter conditions, and remember to bring your avalanche beacon!

San Isabel National Forest
Leadville Ranger District
2015 North Poplar
Leadville, CO 80461
(719) 486-0749

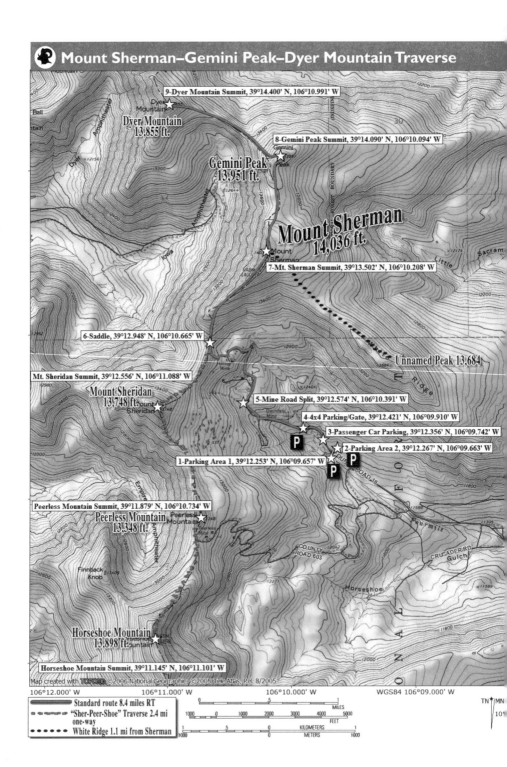

Mount Sherman–Gemini Peak–Dyer Mountain Traverse

9-Dyer Mountain Summit, 39°14.400' N, 106°10.991' W

Dyer Mountain
13,855 ft.

8-Gemini Peak Summit, 39°14.090' N, 106°10.094' W

Gemini Peak
13,951 ft.

Mount Sherman
14,036 ft.

7-Mt. Sherman Summit, 39°13.502' N, 106°10.208' W

6-Saddle, 39°12.948' N, 106°10.665' W

Unnamed Peak 13,684

Mt. Sheridan Summit, 39°12.556' N, 106°11.088' W

Mount Sheridan
13,748 ft.

5-Mine Road Split, 39°12.574' N, 106°10.391' W

4-4x4 Parking/Gate, 39°12.421' N, 106°09.910' W

3-Passenger Car Parking, 39°12.356' N, 106°09.742' W

2-Parking Area 2, 39°12.267' N, 106°09.663' W

1-Parking Area 1, 39°12.253' N, 106°09.657' W

Peerless Mountain Summit, 39°11.879' N, 106°10.734' W

Peerless Mountain
13,348 ft.

Finnback Knob

Horseshoe Mountain
13,898 ft.

Horseshoe Mountain Summit, 39°11.145' N, 106°11.101' W

Map created with TOPO!© ©2006 National Geographic; ©2005 Tele Atlas, Rel. 8/2005

106°12.000' W   106°11.000' W   106°10.000' W   WGS84 106°09.000' W

TN / MN

Standard route 8.4 miles RT
"Sher-Peer-Shoe" Traverse 2.4 mi one-way
White Ridge 1.1 mi from Sherman

MILES
FEET
KILOMETERS
METERS

20 Mount Sherman–Gemini Peak– Dyer Mountain Traverse

Get ready for great ghost mines, fun scrambles, and hallmark views of Colorado's highest mountains. These mountains are Mosquito Range classics, full of history.

Round Trip Distance	8.4 miles
Hiking Time	4½–6 hours
Difficulty	5/10
Class	2/2+
Start Elevation	11,885 ft., at County Road 18 Parking Area
Peak Elevations	Mount Sherman: 14,036 ft.; Gemini Peak: 13,951 ft.; Dyer Mountain: 13,855 ft.
Total Elevation Gain	3,742 ft.
Terrain	Good trail to Sherman, rocky traverse to Gemini and Dyer
Best Time to Climb	June–September
Gear Advisor	Normal gear
Crowd Level	Moderate

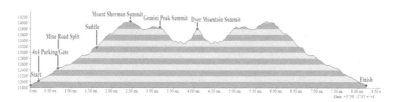

Location   Mosquito Range Pike National Forest/Bureau of Land Management (BLM) land outside of Fairplay

Intro   From most perspectives, Mount Sherman's flat summit appears unassuming, perhaps unexciting, as it stands on the horizon. It isn't until you close in on the peak that the allure of this mild 14er becomes apparent. Spooky mining ruins at the base of Sherman teem with history, including the enormous mill at the abandoned Leavick townsite. The gentle, rolling ridges between several peaks around Sherman make summit-bagging easy. From the central parking area, it's possible to collect six in a single day!

Why Climb It?   A trip to Sherman is likely to include more than summiting the 14er. The twisted mine ruins and old Leavick mill site are sure to stir the imaginations of those interested in Colorado's mining history, and the saddle between Sherman and Sheridan is the perfect place to view Colorado's two highest mountains, Mount Elbert and Mount Massive.

❖ Hike 20   **159**

Sherman is generally considered the easiest of the 14ers to climb, making it a good first 14er for the uninitiated. For more experienced hikers, the option to link several mountains is irresistible; the two additional peaks on the main route for this hike go north, while the optional three traverse south.

From the parking area, you can view the amazing glacial cirque on Horseshoe Mountain. The marking is natural, despite its resemblance to a Colorado strip mine.

Driving   Borrowing a cheeky term from the world of mountain biking, the dirt road to Sherman is littered with "baby heads"—dozens of rounded rocks on an otherwise smooth road. In normal conditions, passenger cars will be able to get within 0.2 mile of the closure gate—only a deeply washed-out rut prevents the last portion from being safely passed by low-clearance cars. The last section requires sport utility cars or more rugged vehicles. Note that there are sections of private land en route, so be respectful as you drive through.

How to Get There   One mile south of the intersection of US Highway 285 and Colorado Highway 9, just outside of Fairplay, turn west onto Park County Road 18. From here, it is roughly 11.5 miles on Park County Road 18 to the first of the parking areas, and 12 miles to the final parking area. The road is paved for a short distance; when you reach a four-way intersection, stay straight on PCR 18 as it turns to dirt. Remain on PCR 18 to the end of the road. Be ready for a barrage of small but steady bumps and washboards. You'll go in and out of private land, passing two campgrounds before reaching the enormous Leavick Mill at 10.5 miles. There is a large parking lot on the left here, but keep going farther—even passenger cars can make it up the road, and you'll spare yourself a longer walk than is necessary up to the trailhead. Good parking pulloffs begin 1.5 miles after the Leavick Mill on both sides of road. If you're in a passenger car, pick any of these; sport utility cars, SUVs, and trucks will have no problem making it to the parking area at the closure gate.

Fees/Camping   There are no fees to hike Sherman or the surrounding peaks, but please be aware most of the land is privately owned. There are two campgrounds en route to Sherman: Fourmile Campground (14 sites) and Horseshoe Campground (19 sites). Both sites are $10 per night, as of 2006, and have toilets and water sources.

Route Notes   On many maps, there are dozens of trails and subtrails that may confuse the aspiring hiker. It's important to note that the standard "trailhead" is not officially marked: it's simply a closed gate at the end of the Park County Road 18. I met several frustrated hikers who had been looking for a sign for Fourmile Creek Trailhead. While you *do* follow Fourmile Creek on the road up, don't frustrate yourself looking for trailhead signage—just get to the end of the road.

Mile/Waypoint   **0.0 mi (3)**   This route starts 0.2 mile east of the final 4x4 parking lot and closure gate. If you park here, walk up the road to the closure gate.

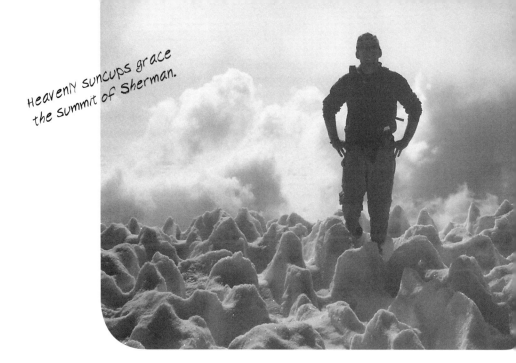

Heavenly suncups grace the summit of Sherman.

0.2 mi (4) At the gated end of the road, there are about 10 parking spots. You'll see the Dauntless and Hilltop mines from here. Go through the gate, and continue up the wide dirt road. Check out the mining relics along the way. A tower-supported aerial tramway once ran between the mine and the mill; there are still a few towers between the two (see "Quick Facts" on page 162). Stay straight (due west) on this road until mile 0.7.

0.7 mi (5) Turn right onto the dirt road that switchbacks up to the Hilltop Mine. The saddle between Sheridan and Sherman will be obvious, and you can reach it many ways; this way is the most scenic and easiest to follow. Hike up and past the Hilltop Mine and several abandoned cabins. (This area was actively mined from the late 1800s to the 1960s). Follow any of the several subtrails behind the cabins to a main trail on the west side of the ruins; eventually, one main trail appears and leads up a small hill to the saddle.

1.6 mi (6) As you gain the saddle, gorgeous views of Mount Massive and Mount Elbert appear on the horizon; you are looking out at the highest peaks in Colorado. Follow a well-worn trail northeast up the gentle, class 2 ridge. This is a pleasant hike with very good views.

2.5 mi (7) Mount Sherman's flat summit! You may be confused as to the actual highpoint; look for the summit log and USGS marker. In spring, Sherman is famous for its sun-cupped snowfield, which spikes up on the west side of the summit area. From here, continue north (there will no longer be a trail) to Gemini Peak. This traverse is gentle, dropping only 300 feet before climbing up to Gemini's mini-pyramid block.

3.3 mi (8) Gemini Peak's summit! You can scramble up on the slightly tricky west or south sides (probably class 2+), or find an easier path on the east face to reach the top. Some hikers are content with just these two peaks, which is totally reasonable. The route described here, however, continues on 0.9 mile to Dyer Mountain.

3.8 mi Head northwest 0.5 mile and then 600 feet down Gemini to the saddle between Gemini and Dyer. At 13,300 feet, you'll see huge wire-towers. (How the heck did they get those things up here?) Go under the wires, and make the class 2+ scramble up to Dyer Mountain Summit (this is like an extended version of the brief scrambling on Gemini).

4.1 mi (9) After a fun scramble, you have attained the summit of Dyer Mountain. Enjoy the views, and note the potential for continuing north for even more summits. Reverse your route back over Gemini and Sherman, returning down Sherman's ridge and back to the parking area.

8.4 mi Finish.

Options   You have plenty of options if you want to keep hiking after summiting Mount Sherman. At 1.1 miles southeast of Sherman (waypoint 7), you can venture out on White Ridge to Unnamed Peak 13,684, which affords some great views of the mining area.

From the saddle between Sherman and Sheridan (waypoint 6), you can start a 2.4-mile, class 2 traverse that crosses the summits of Mount Sheridan at mile 0.5, Peerless Mountain at mile 1.5, and Horseshoe Mountain at mile 2.4. This southern swing follows the obvious ridgeline that connects all three. Horseshoe Mountain is particularly impressive, with a huge glacial cirque on its east face.

Quick Facts   Mount Sherman was named by the Hayden survey party in 1872 for Civil War General William T. Sherman. Neighboring Mount Sheridan was named at the same time for Civil War General Philip Sheridan. Both were members of the Union Army. It seems just to me that the higher peak is named for Sherman, as Sheridan was involved in a great deal of violence against Native Americans during the US/Indian wars that followed the conclusion of the Civil War.

The mines in this area are evidence of the mineral wealth contained within these mountains. Silver was the draw for Felix Leavick, who bought the Hilltop Mine, following the "silver crash" of 1893. Along with business partner Brad DuBois, he restored the mining operations, modernizing the process with a railway and aerial tramway.

The prolific Leavick Mill was constructed in the spring of 1897. As in other boomtowns, Leavick's population was briefly sizeable enough to warrant a post office. The boom was shortlived, however, as residents began a mass exodus in 1899. Still, mining continued in the area until the 1960s, when most of the valuable veins of ore had been tapped.

Contact Info   Pike National Forest
South Park Ranger District
320 Highway 285
P.O. Box 219
Fairplay, CO 80440
(719) 836-2031

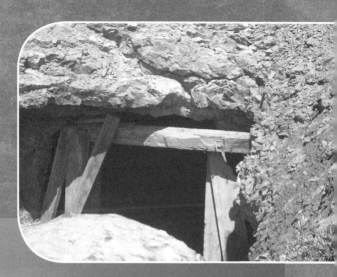

Mount Sherman is a wonderful blend of alpine scenery and mining history. The bonus traverse to Gemini Peak is a great additional summit to tag while you're up there.

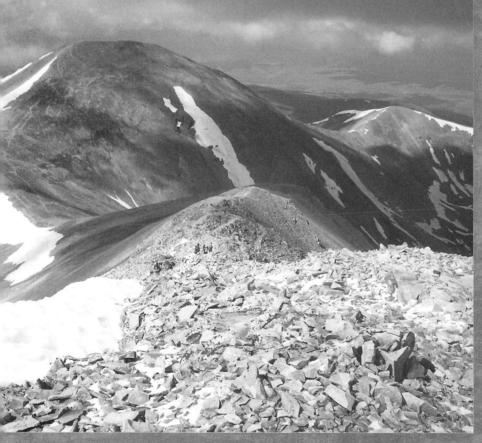

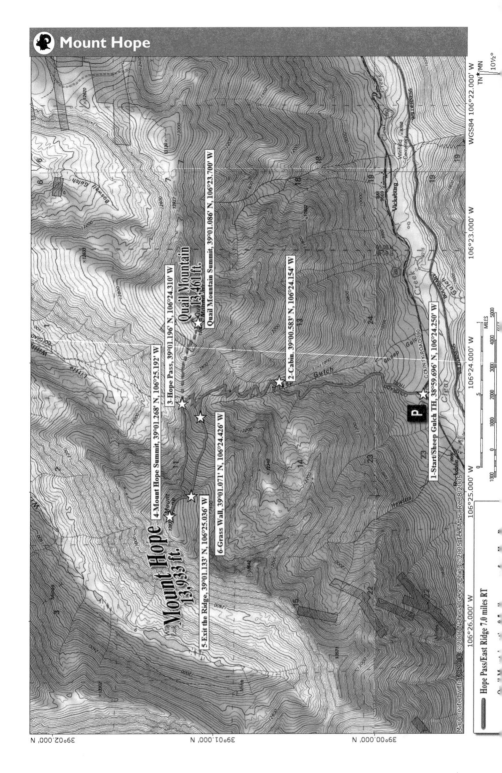

Mount Hope
13,933 ft.

Quail Mountain
13,461 ft.

4-Mount Hope Summit, 39°01.268' N, 106°25.192' W

3-Hope Pass, 39°01.196' N, 106°24.310' W

Quail Mountain Summit, 39°01.086' N, 106°23.700' W

5-Exit the Ridge, 39°01.133' N, 106°25.036' W

6-Grass Wall, 39°01.071' N, 106°24.426' W

2-Cabin, 39°00.583' N, 106°24.154' W

1-Start/Sheep Gulch TH, 38°59.696' N, 106°24.250' W

Hope Pass/East Ridge 7.0 miles RT

21 Mount Hope

Mount Hope's east ridge is a fun excursion on an overlooked mountain. Scramble on a solid ridge to a flat summit, which may surprise you with a gift of wildflowers!

Round Trip Distance	7.0 miles
Hiking Time	5–7 hours
Difficulty	7/10
Class	2+/3
Start Elevation	9,875 ft., at Sheep Gulch Trailhead
Peak Elevation	13,933 ft.
Total Elevation Gain	4,070 ft.
Terrain	Good trail to rocky but solid ridge walk
Best Time to Climb	June–September
Gear Advisor	Normal gear
Crowd Level	Low

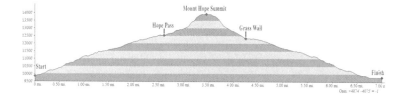

Location Sawatch Range in the Collegiate Peak Wilderness/San Isabel National Forest outside of Leadville

Intro Mount Hope is lost in the shuffle of the Sawatch giants, despite being a mere 67 feet lower than the prized 14ers. Maybe it's for the best, since the lack of traffic gives Hope a sense of solitude. The east ridge is a fine way to climb Hope; the scrambling has minimal exposure, which makes it a good first ridge scramble for the uninitiated. The approach to the ridge takes you through aspen forests and emerges from treeline, where stunning views to the south seem to invoke the Rocky Mountain spirit.

Why Climb It? The forest en route to Hope Pass is especially beautiful. Timberline dissipates slowly, with stray bunches of trees guiding you to Hope Pass. Scrambling on the ridge is mostly class 2+ with a few easy class 3 moves thrown in for fun. Daring scramblers can stay on the spine of the ridge and increase the number of class 3 moves. This summit has great views of La Plata Peak and Huron Peak; it is the highest place in which I've ever seen gardens of assorted wildflowers!

Driving	Any vehicle can make it to the trailhead. County Road 390 is a very well-maintained dirt road.
How to Get There	To reach Sheep Gulch Trailhead, start on US Highway 24 and turn west onto Chaffee County Road 390; this intersection is roughly 20 miles from Leadville and 15 miles from Buena Vista. Follow CR 390 for 9.4 miles, past Clear Creek Reservoir, to Sheep Gulch Trailhead, on your right. You can park here or along the road.
Fees/Camping	There are no fees to hike or camp in the area. Please note that the town of Winfield, just west of here, is privately owned, so if you're going to camp off the road, find a pulloff before or after that tiny and still functional town.
Route Notes	None.
Mile/Waypoint	**0.0 mi (1)** Start at the Sheep Gulch Trailhead and head north on the Hope Pass Trail, which is also the Colorado Trail. You'll hike by the old parking area as you enter the woods, and then gain an easy-to-follow singletrack trail up to Hope Pass. Enjoy the forest; it's one of my favorites!
	1.3 mi (2) On the way up, peek over to the right (east) into the woods. Can you find the cabin hiding in the trees? It must have been a laborious task to build it way up here.
	2.7 mi (3) At 12,550 feet you'll arrive at Hope Pass, between Quail Mountain and Mount Hope. The east ridge of Hope looms before you, in a series of hills. This entails very straightforward ridge scrambling with the occasional class 3 move. Some of the hike is best done down about 70 feet below

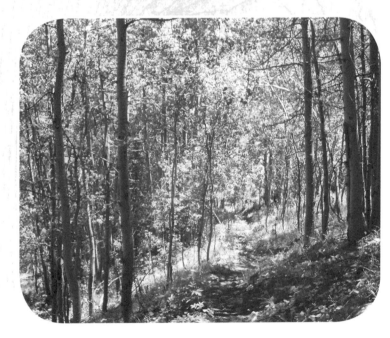

The approach to Mount Hope is a natural palace of aspen-lined corridors, making it one of the best autumn hikes in Colorado.

the ridge on the south side, where better footing will help you progress higher. The crux of the scramble is at 13,580 feet, where the rocky section to the final summit flats has a few easy class 3 moves that you have to link together. When you emerge on the summit flats, it's a short walk west on gentle terrain to the summit.

3.6 mi (4) Hope's optimistic summit! Views to the west of La Plata Peak are remarkable. To the north, check out Elbert and Massive; to the south, Huron and the Collegiate Peaks. You can go back down the east ridge if you like (a good option if you want to go climb Quail), but it will be slow going. The route described here is faster. Go south off the summit to the next waypoint.

3.8 mi (5) At 13,670 feet, find a good line down the steep wall, exit the ridge, and make your way into the basin. When there is soft snow, this is a good place to plunge-step with your heels (or glissade!). When there's no snow, it's rocky and a bit sketchy. The fact is, there's no easy way off Hope. The other options are descending the ridge you came up, or going down the south ridge—which will give you similar scrambling farther down and present you with a loose talus field to cross to regain the trail in the trees. Better to see where you are going! Stay north in the basin, and find a good high line back to the Hope Pass Trail. There's an easy talus field to cross here, and it is fairly stable.

4.5 mi (6) Just before connecting to the Hope Pass Trail, stay high (north) above the "grass wall." Doing so will give you better footing and reconnect you to the trail more quickly than trying to cut down on steep slopes. Once you are back on the trail, it's a quick hike back down to your vehicle.

7.0 mi Finish.

Options Mount Hope is a stalwart pile of rock that glaciers were forced to flow around. As a result, the only other peak connected to it is Quail Mountain (13,461 feet). From Hope's east ridge, Quail's scarred slopes resemble the bulbous chin of a tough old right whale. From Hope Pass, it's 0.5 mile one way on class 2 slopes to Quail's summit.

Quick Facts Mount Hope is unique in this area of the Sawatch, in that it doesn't have a long, gentle slope leading to its summit. The east ridge is arguably the easiest way to reach the top. The south ridge begins as the typical slope but gets broken off before making a smooth connection with the lowlands. This is evidence that the glaciers and rivers that carved the path now followed by Clear Creek were powerful enough to break apart the lower half of the ridge.

The Hopeful Couloir on the north face is a good spring snow climb. Expert skiers can enjoy a run down its thrilling 50-degree slopes.

Contact Info San Isabel National Forest
Leadville Ranger District
2015 N. Poplar
Leadville, CO 80461
(719) 486-0752

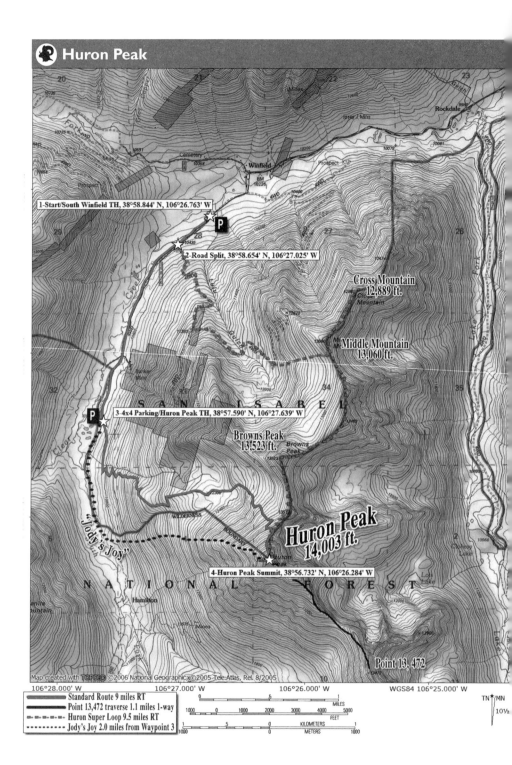

1-Start/South Winfield TH, 38°58.844' N, 106°26.763' W

2-Road Split, 38°58.654' N, 106°27.025' W

Cross Mountain
12,889 ft.

Middle Mountain
13,060 ft.

S A N   I S A B E L

3-4x4 Parking/Huron Peak TH, 38°57.590' N, 106°27.639' W

Browns Peak
13,523 ft.

Huron Peak
14,003 ft.

"Jody's Joy"

WILDERNESS

4-Huron Peak Summit, 38°56.732' N, 106°26.284' W

N A T I O N A L   F O R E S T

Point 13,472

Map created with TOPO! ©2006 National Geographic ©2005 Tele Atlas, Rel. 8/2005

106°28.000' W   106°27.000' W   106°26.000' W   WGS84 106°25.000' W

TN /MN

10½

Standard Route 9 miles RT
Point 13,472 traverse 1.1 miles 1-way
Huron Super Loop 9.5 miles RT
Jody's Joy 2.0 miles from Waypoint 3

MILES
FEET
KILOMETERS
METERS

22 Huron Peak

Huron is a classic climb on a pictue-perfect mountain! This 14er may be the most beautiful hike in the Sawatch Range, with excellent views from the summit pyramid.

Round Trip Distance	9.0 miles / 6.5 miles from 4x4 parking
Hiking Time	3–6 hours
Difficulty	4/10
Class	2
Start Elevation	10,286 ft., at South Winfield Trailhead
Peak Elevation	14,003 ft.
Total Elevation Gain	3,576 ft.
Terrain	Good trail, slightly rocky toward summit
Best Time to Climb	June–September
Gear Advisor	Trail runners
Crowd Level	Moderate; high on weekends

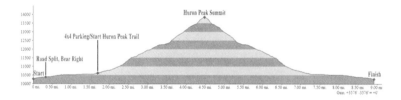

Location Sawatch Range in Collegiate Peaks Wilderness/San Isabel National Forest near Buena Vista and Leadville

Intro Look at that beautiful elevation profile! Huron is a very "clean" mountain with classic contours and a very well-maintained, class 2 trail. It's at the low side for 14ers, with the latest measurement putting its summit at 14,003 feet. Huron Peak has my favorite summit views of any Sawatch mountain, and the hike is a great intro to Colorado's higher peaks.

Why Climb It? Huron's locale in the southern Sawatch makes it the perfect perch for views of Colorado's highest peaks (Elbert, La Plata, etc.) to the north; the amazing views of Ice Mountain and the Three Apostles to the south ain't too shabby, either! The trail is very well maintained, making Huron a very good hike for non-hardcore hikers, dogs, and groups of mixed ability. A direct, on-trail ascent to the summit won't take long for fit climbers. Ambitious peak-baggers looking for more fun are welcome to head north of Huron and summit up to three more peaks, making for a longer day (which is nicely concluded as a loop). Alternately, scramblers can go for a "suicide push" up the steep but stable west ridge, a good off-trail option for those wanting to avoid crowds.

Driving Passenger cars can make it to the South Winfield Trailhead; the dirt road is a little bumpy but passable. Cars will have to park here. The 4x4 road beyond that is good, but it can be very rutted out; sport utility cars, SUVs, and 4x4s should be able to reach the 4x4 parking in normal conditions (I've seen several Outbacks and even a VW Eurovan at the 4x4 trailhead!).

How to Get There To reach the South Winfield Trailhead, start on US Highway 24 and turn west onto Chaffee County Road 390; this intersection is roughly 20 miles from Leadville and 15 miles from Buena Vista. CR 390 is a well-maintained dirt road; you'll be on it for just over 12 miles (you can follow the signs to Winfield). After passing the Clear Creek Reservoir on your left, you'll continue down the road until mile 11.8, where you'll see the (revived) ghost town of Winfield, a semirestored mining town with about 12 active summer cabins. It's worth a visit to Winfield's historic museums and cemetery after your hike. Follow the main road through Winfield (it curves left and then right) and continue 0.3 mile to the passenger car parking area. (The parking area is cleared out a bit; just past it, the road narrows and has a warning sign.) There are a few camping spots on the right side here. If you have a 4x4 vehicle, continue 1.7 miles to the end of the road and the Huron Peak Trail. There are tons of great camping sites between the South Winfield Trailhead and the end of the road. Make sure to stay on the main road (see "Mile/Waypoint" section for more info).

Fees/Camping There are no fees to hike Huron Peak or to camp in the wilderness along the access road. There are many great camping areas on the road between South Winfield Trailhead and the Huron Peak Trail.

Route Notes This is a straightforward hike with good views.

Mile/Waypoint 0.0 mi (1) Passenger cars park here. This is the South Winfield Trailhead. From here, it's a 1.7-mile hike/bike up easy terrain to the Huron Peak Trailhead (you gain only about 300 feet of elevation). Drive on, 4x4s!

0.3 mi (2) Stay straight on the main road. At this intersection, the road forks a bit; bear right (which is pretty much straight ahead). After that, the main road will be easy to follow as it passes a lush meadow on your right. Side roads mostly lead to camping areas.

1.7 mi (3) The Huron Peak Trailhead and 4x4 parking are at the closed Forest Service gate at the end of the road. Note that the Huron Peak Trail starts left of the sign and gate, not straight ahead (unless you are hoping for an off-trail scramble of the west ridge!). Once you are on the Huron Peak Trail, it's very easy to follow; there are no intersecting trails. Follow the switchbacks up above treeline, and then push up to the ridge between Browns Peak and Huron Peak. Stay right (south) and continue to follow the well-traveled trail to the summit of Huron Peak.

4.5 mi (4) Huron Peak's wonderful summit accommodates quite a few happy hikers. The prominent, powerful-looking mountain to the south is Ice

Mountain—you'll have a prime view of the Refrigerator Couloir on Ice, a wildly dangerous snow climb (due to heavy rockfall). The Three Apostles formation is just right (west) of Ice Mountain. Descend the way you came (or check out the "Options" section for more fun).

7.3 mi (3) Return to 4x4 parking lot.

9.0 mi Return to the South Winfield Trailhead.

Options To snag a few more peaks, head north from the summit of Huron Peak along the northern ridge (class 2) to Browns Peak (13,523 feet), 0.7 mile from Huron's top. Traverse northeast over Point 13,462, and proceed to Middle Mountain (13,060 feet), which is roughly 1.8 miles from Huron. A full 2.2 miles from Huron will bring you to Cross Mountain (12,889 feet). You can return to the access road by descending the western slopes between Browns and Middle mountains. There's a jeep trail you can eventually connect with that rejoins the main road (at the fork where you stayed right, 0.3 mile in, at waypoint 2).

From Huron Peak's summit (waypoint 4), you can follow the southeast ridge 1.1 miles down to Point 13,472.

Finally, for those looking for a fun scramble, try "Jody's Joy," a direct climb of the western ridge. Go straight at the forest gate (waypoint 3), instead of left onto the Huron Peak Trail. Follow this trail 0.8 mile to the wilderness boundary, and then turn left (west) and gain the western ridge. You can stay on the ridge or scramble up the gully just south of the ridge another 1.2 very steep miles (2.0 miles from the 4x4 parking area).

Quick Facts Huron Peak is indirectly named after the Huron Indians of Michigan; a mine near the peak was named Huron first, and the moniker was later transferred to the mountain. Since you'll be in the neighborhood, it's worth checking out the revamped ghost town of Winfield. Winfield was formally founded in 1881 after prospectors discovered copper and silver deposits nearby. (The town went through two names, Florence and Lucknow, before the name Winfield stuck.) With a maximum population of 1,500, circa 1890, some of the early residents of Winfield toughed it out until the last mines closed in 1912. Today, the area has a few restored summer cabins and two public museums. The Winfield cemetery is 0.25 mile up the road from the center of town. Vicksburg, a few miles north of Winfield, is another almost-ghost town. (There are a few functional residences in Vicksburg.)

Note that Huron is very close to Sheep Gulch Trailhead, which is the starting point for another hike in this book, Mount Hope (Hike 21). Doing both peaks in a weekend is a grand idea, especially in the early autumn.

Contact Info San Isabel National Forest
Leadville Ranger District
2015 North Poplar
Leadville, CO 80461
(719) 486-0749

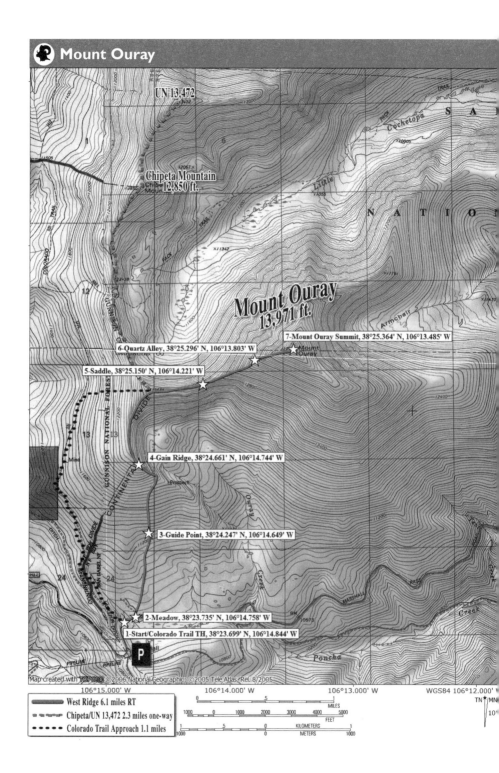

UN 13,472

Chipeta Mountain
12,850 ft.

Mount Ouray
13,971 ft.

6-Quartz Alley, 38°25.296' N, 106°13.803' W

7-Mount Ouray Summit, 38°25.364' N, 106°13.485' W

5-Saddle, 38°25.150' N, 106°14.221' W

4-Gain Ridge, 38°24.661' N, 106°14.744' W

3-Guide Point, 38°24.247' N, 106°14.649' W

2-Meadow, 38°23.735' N, 106°14.758' W

1-Start/Colorado Trail TH, 38°23.699' N, 106°14.844' W

Map created with TOPO! ©2006 National Geographic ©2005 Tele Atlas, Rel. 8/2005

106°15.000' W   106°14.000' W   106°13.000' W   WGS84 106°12.000' W

West Ridge 6.1 miles RT
Chipeta/UN 13,472 2.3 miles one-way
Colorado Trail Approach 1.1 miles

MILES
FEET
KILOMETERS
METERS

23 Mount Ouray

Ouray's west ridge is an adventure fit for a chief! Named after the great leader of the Utes, this southern Sawatch mountain is a great hike, with views to match.

Round Trip Distance	6.1 miles
Hiking Time	5–7 hours
Difficulty	6.5/10
Class	2
Start Elevation	10,813 ft., at Marshall Pass Trailhead
Peak Elevation	13,971 ft.
Total Elevation Gain	3,260 ft.
Terrain	Off-trail, easy-to-navigate terrain to long ridge walk
Best Time to Climb	July–September
Gear Advisor	Normal gear
Crowd Level	Low

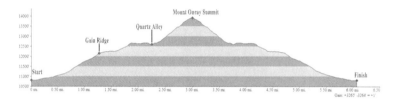

Location   Southern Sawatch Range in the San Isabel National Forest outside of Poncha Springs

Intro   Viewing it from the south just over Poncha Pass, Mount Ouray looks like a giant, gray, inflatable chair. The rounded contours and large cirque on the east face (another unholy "Devil's Armchair") are typical of Sawatch mountains. The long west ridge gives you a catwalk of nearly 2.0 miles each way, punctuated by views of two major ranges in Colorado: the Sawatch to the north and the Sangre De Cristos to the southeast. (Satan has had quite an influence on Colorado landmarks: Ouray has "Devil's Armchair," Lone Cone (Hike 50) is home of the "Devil's Chair," and you'll also find Devils Backbone, Devils Cow Camp (for naughty cows?), Devils Elbow, Devils Thumb, Devils Nose, Devils Punchbowl, Devils Kitchen, and Devils Head, to name a few.)

Ouray is one of the southernmost 13ers in the Sawatch Range—though it may actually be a 14er! Several people have noticed GPS readings over 14,000 feet on the top (I had a measurement of 14,005 feet with an error differential of +/- 7 feet.) Perhaps someday it will be admitted into the 14ers club, a fitting honor for Chief Ouray.

Why Climb It?	The off-trail approach through flowery meadows is a nice way to start the hike. Navigation is relatively easy, and once you are on the southern curl of the west ridge, you are treated to a long ridge walk to a scenic summit. The scrambling on the ridge is fun class 2 that is sustained the entire way. It's a straightforward Sawatch hike without the tedious switchbacks or gratuitous talus slog, making it a fine bookend to this hiker-friendly range.
Driving	Passenger cars can make it to the top of Marshall Pass. The road has a few rocky sections and some potholes but is otherwise well maintained.
How to Get There	From the junction of US Highway 50 and US Highway 285 in Poncha Springs, drive 5.1 miles south to the marked turnoff for Marshall Pass. If approaching from the south on US 285, it is roughly 2.4 miles from the top of Poncha Pass. Turn west onto the Marshall Pass Road (County Road 200), which is a dirt road. From here it is 14 miles to the top of the pass. The way up is very well marked. There is a right turn a little past mile 2.0 (it has a sign for Marshall Pass), and from there, the road is easy to follow. The trailhead is just east of Marshall Pass on the left side of the road. There is ample parking and a large sign kiosk for the Colorado Trail. **Note:** If you drive through the cool rock corridor to the top of the pass, you've gone about 0.1 mile too far.
Fees/Camping	There are no fees to hike or camp in this area. Campsites abound; there is a small primitive area behind the parking area as well as several similar sites off the summit of Marshall Pass.
Route Notes	This hike is quite straightforward; don't be intimidated by the fact that it does not use any trails.
Mile/Waypoint	**0.0 mi (1)** Start at the Colorado Trail Trailhead lot, just below the top of Marshall Pass. You will not be following trails on this route, though it is possible to take the Colorado Trail north roughly 1.0 mile and get off-trail east at the base of Ouray's west ridge. The off-trail route is more scenic and easy to follow. Walk east a hundred feet down the road to the open meadows on the north side of the road.

0.1 mi (2)   Head into the meadows and aim for the spur of Ouray's west ridge, which is above treeline. This is easy terrain to navigate; it's mostly open meadows. Get a compass bearing here to the ridge and follow it. There are a few patches of pine trees along the way. In a mile, you'll emerge from the intermittent timberline.

0.7 mi (3)   This is a guide point for those using GPS.

1.0 mi   As you clear the trees, the way to the ridge is obvious. The best footing is found by taking the spur ridge to reach the west ridge.

1.3 mi (4)   Gain the spur ridge and follow it as it curves into the west ridge. There are a few ups and downs here. The views of the peak are spectacular from this vantage point.

1.9 mi   At 12,670 feet you are now "officially" on the west ridge. Enjoy the hiking and easy scramble as you head toward the summit.

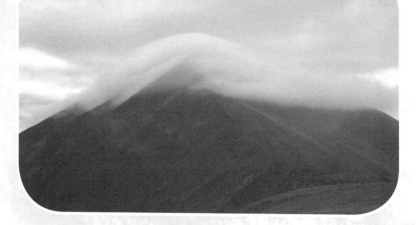

stical fog envelops the mmit of Mount Ouray.

2.3 mi (5) A windy saddle at 12,600 feet is the low point of the ridge. Keep heading up.

2.7 mi (6) A band of white quartz is high on the mountain, at 13,350 feet. This quartz alley is the "crux" of the climb, though you can easily bypass it on the left (west) side. Scrambling up is fun, but the surface is slick when wet. Top the quartz band and continue to the summit.

3.1 mi (7) Mount Ouray's summit! Check your altimeter; you may be on an unrecognized 14er. Return the way you came. The trek through the trees is nothing to worry about. If you get disoriented, just keep heading south and you'll intersect the Marshall Pass Road.

6.2 mi Finish.

Options Chipeta Mountain (12,850 feet) is an easy walk from the end of Ouray's west ridge (between waypoints 4 and 5). It is 1.5 miles one way to the north. From here, it is 0.8 mile to a large unnamed peak (UN 13,472). The easy class 2 out-and-back to these two mountains is 4.6 miles round trip, starting from Ouray's west ridge.

Quick Facts Chief Ouray (pronounced YOO-ray) was a leader of the Tabeguache Utes who tried to negotiate peace between his people and the white men. White leaders appreciated his intellect and willingness to compromise (he met two presidents in his lifetime); Utes respected his leadership and drive. Unfortunately, all his good intentions were in vain—his people were exiled to a Utah reservation in 1880, the year of his death.

Chipeta Mountain honors Ouray's wife, who was exiled to Bitter Creek, Utah, along with the rest of the Utes. She passed away in 1924 and was brought back to Colorado to be buried next to her husband.

Mount Ouray's status as a high 13er or a low14er has yet to be resolved. Some sources claim the peak is 29 feet higher than its official height. While it seems apparent the peak is slightly higher, it may still fall short of being a 14er. Let the controversy rage on!

Contact Info San Isabel National Forest
Salida Ranger District
325 Rainbow
Salida, CO 81201
(719) 539-3591

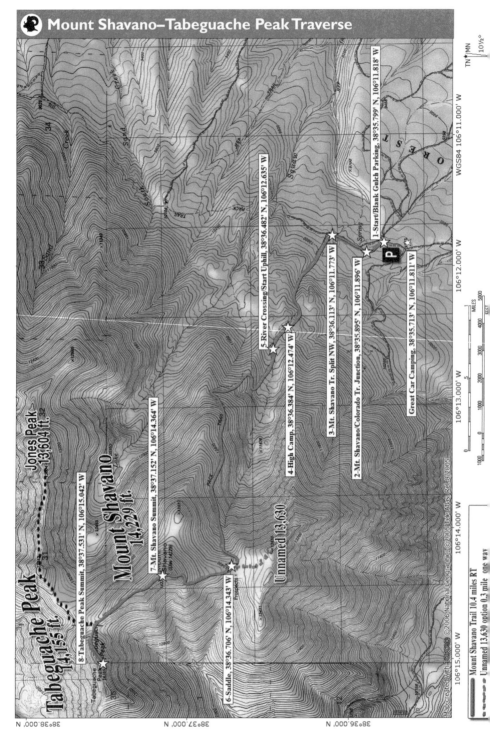

Mount Shavano–Tabeguache Peak Traverse

Tabeguache Peak 14,155 ft.

Jones Peak 13,604 ft.

Mount Shavano 14,229 ft.

Unnamed 13,630

8-Tabeguache Peak Summit, 38°37.531' N, 106°15.042' W

7-Mt. Shavano Summit, 38°37.152' N, 106°14.364' W

6-Saddle, 38°36.706' N, 106°14.343' W

5-River Crossing/Start Uphill, 38°36.482' N, 106°12.635' W

4-High Camp, 38°36.384' N, 106°12.474' W

3-Mt. Shavano Tr. Split NW, 38°36.113' N, 106°11.773' W

2-Mt. Shavano/Colorado Tr. Junction, 38°35.895' N, 106°11.896' W

1-Start/Blank Gulch Parking, 38°35.799' N, 106°11.818' W

Great Car Camping, 38°35.713' N, 106°11.811' W

Mount Shavano Trail 10.4 miles RT

Unnamed 13,630 option 0.3 mile one way

24 Mount Shavano–Tabeguache Peak Traverse

If it's a great day for a summit hike, why not do two! Even if you can't pronounce their names, these mountains offer a fine, Sawatch-style traverse with plenty to see along the way.

Round Trip Distance	10.4 miles
Hiking Time	5–8 hours
Difficulty	6.5/10
Class	2
Start Elevation	9,740 ft., at Blank Gulch Trailhead
Peak Elevations	Mount Shavano: 14,229 ft.; Tabeguache Peak: 14,155 ft.
Total Elevation Gain	5,162 ft.
Terrain	Good trail that gets a bit rocky; rocky but stable ridge walk
Best Time to Climb	Mid-May–September
Gear Advisor	Good boots for rocky terrain
Crowd Level	Moderate

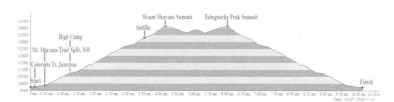

Location Sawatch Range in the Collegiate Peaks Wilderness/San Isabel National Forest outside of Poncha Springs

Intro These two mountains honor the memory of Chief Shavano and his tribe, the Tabeguache Utes (more on this in the "Quick Facts" section). The chance to top two 14ers in one day is a major draw; the fun and non-technical traverse between the summits is another. Because they are set in the southern Sawatch, the views east are particularly striking. Bucolic Buena Vista looks like a giant, dreamy farm from the heights. The "Angel of Shavano" snowfield graces the east face, famously spreading her wings across a deep indentation in the mountain.

Why Climb It? These two mountains are a blast to climb in one day, thanks to the great ridge that conjoins the summits. The Blank Gulch approach exits treeline into an impressive bowl that leads to a high saddle between Shavano and Unnamed Peak 13,630. Ascend Shavano via a good scramble and traipse roughly 1.0 mile to nearby Tabeguache Peak. Shavano is a very prominent peak, especially when viewed from US Highway 285 just north of Poncha Springs.

Driving   Passenger cars can make it to the trailhead, but they may get banged up a little; tough passenger cars are perfect for these road conditions. The road is rocky and has some extended washboards, but there isn't anything that will blast pieces off your car. Obviously, more rugged vehicles will have no problem reaching the trailhead.

How to Get There   From US Highway 285, turn west onto Chaffee County Road 140. This turn is about 20 miles south of the US 285/US 24 junction, just outside of Buena Vista, or 1.0 mile north of the US 285/US 50 junction in Poncha Springs. The road is paved. Follow it 1.7 miles and turn right (north) onto County Road 250 (there will be signs for Shavano and Tabeguache along the way). After a little pavement, the road becomes dirt. At mile 5.7, stay left on CR

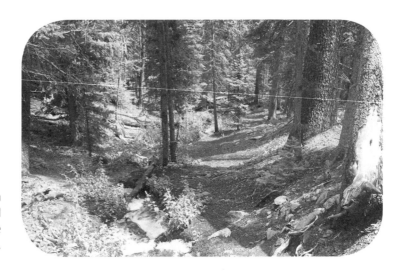

The rocky approach to Shavano is typical of Sawatch Range mountains.

252 (again, it will be signed). A pipe/bridge over Placer Creek follows a steep downhill at mile 6.5. Stay straight on CR 252, making sure not to take any lefts or rights. Signs will continue to point the way. Pass a gap in a fence and reach Blank Gulch Trailhead at mile 9.0. There is plenty of parking here. If you go left (west) through the parking lot and drive down the road a few hundred feet (still passable by all cars), there is a very large clearing that makes a great place to camp.

Note: You can also get on Chaffe CR 250 by turning north off US Highway 50 just west of Poncha Springs (this is a good option for folks coming from the Gunnison area). After about a half mile, you'll come to the four-way intersection with CR 140; you continue straight ahead (north) and follow the directions above.

Fees/Camping	There are no fees for hiking Shavano and Tabeguache. There is great camping just west of the Blank Gulch Trailhead parking lot, as described in the directions.
Route Notes	After reaching the "High Camp" waypoint, the trail gets slightly tricky to follow. Runoff gullies will mislead you; the easiest way to stay on target is to remain close to the stream until mile 1.4, where you will turn right (northwest) onto a wide trail that leads to some mild switchbacks. From there, the trail becomes more obvious and easy to follow to the summit.
Mile/Waypoint	**0.0 mi (1)** Start at the Blank Gulch parking area. There is an information kiosk and signs for the Mount Shavano and Colorado trails. Head out on the Mount Shavano Trail.
	0.1 mi (2) The starting connector trail intersects with the Colorado Trail. Turn right (north) and proceed; the Colorado Trail and the Mount Shavano Trail will overlap for a short distance.
	0.4 mi (3) The Mount Shavano Trail splits left (northwest) from the Colorado Trail, which continues northeast. Even though this turn is marked, it's easy to miss. You'll know you got it right when you start climbing up a steep slope covered in a sheet of baseball-sized rocks.
	1.3 mi (4) After 0.9 mile of tough climbing, the trail levels off a little and gets less rocky. If you are backpacking, this is a nice place to set up your tents (high camp) for the night. The next 0.2 mile can be a little tricky to follow, but stay close to the trail that is close to the stream.
	1.5 mi (5) A simple river crossing will have you on the right (north) side of the stream. The trail heads northwest up another rocky hill and then follows a section of rocky switchbacks that lead you up to treeline.
	2.5 mi Clear treeline at 12,200 feet. The trail continues through a few small shrubs and then opens up into the huge bowl and heads to the saddle south of Shavano. The trail is still easy to follow; if there is snow, just aim for the saddle via the easiest route.
	3.6 mi (6) After burning up your legs and lungs, you'll be at the broad saddle between Shavano to the north, and Unnamed Peak 13,630 to the south. If you take a snack break here, look around for signs of prospectors' mines scattered across the plateau. Continue north on the trail as it goes directly for the summit pyramid of Shavano. Toward the very top, you'll have some easy class 2 scrambling to reach the summit proper.
	4.2 mi (7) Mount Shavano's summit! Climb up on the highest block and let out a mighty yodel! Tabeguache Peak is not far off at this point; you'll see it clearly to the northwest. Scamper downhill along Shavano's northeast to another high saddle between the two 14ers. It is 0.6 mile to the 13,690-foot saddle, an elevation difference of roughly 540 feet.
	4.8 mi The Shavano/Tabeguache saddle. You'll gain Tabeguache's northeast ridge, which has a vague trail on rocks to the top. Navigation is easy: just keep heading up the short, steep talus slope to the summit.

5.2 mi (8) Make up your lost elevation and reach Tabeguache Peak's summit. The views back to Mount Shavano are most impressive. Return the way you came, back to Blank Gulch.

10.4 mi Finish back at Blank Gulch.

Options   Because these two peaks are huge, hiking them doesn't leave a lot of room for worthwhile side trips. A trek over to the Unnamed Peak 13,630 gives you a few fresh southern views. If you're really feeling ambitious, you can traverse the ridge northeast of the saddle between Shavano and Tabeguache to Jones Peak, a modest 13,604-foot outcrop that has an unnamed 13,712-foot point en route to its summit. This traverse is 1.3 miles one way from the saddle.

If you'd like to try a good, easy snow route, the Angel of Shavano is a great first-timer. Crampons are necessary if it has been very cold, but the angle is mild enough for most ascents to be done in boots (the route is in prime condition in May and early June). You start at the Blank Gulch Trailhead and simply follow the stream up the basin instead of diverting right to the main trail cut into the east ridge. The Angel is a good climb and has a wicked fun glissade (or ski or snowboard run) on the way down.

Quick Facts   First off, the correct pronunciations of the peaks are "SHAV-uh-no" (with an emphasis like "bungalow") and "TAB-uh-wahsh." Not Shimano and Tabber Guchie, nor Shamu and Tubberclutch, or any other odd pronunciation. Taberguache was the white man's spelling of the word the Southern Ute Indians used for the Northern Utes.

Shavano is a phonetic spelling of the name of a Ute chieftain known as Che-Wa-No. Che-Wa-No was a highly respected, intelligent, and wise leader who received his rank from the greatest Ute of all, Chief Ouray. He did his best to promote peace between Indians and whites, acting as a mediator to resolve several major conflicts. He was even taken to Washington and honored by white men for resolving an uprising led by Chief Kaneache. Despite his noble intentions and peaceful demeanor, he was exiled to Utah in 1881, along with his people.

Mount Ouray, a very high 13er, is climbed less often than Mount Shavano, Chief Ouray's higher rank notwithstanding. Both Ouray and Che-Wa-No were peaceful and strong leaders who were overpowered by the white man's ambitions to control the land.

The famous Angel of Shavano has been compared to the Cross Couloir on the Mount of the Holy Cross for its religious significance, though native people referred to it as the Indian Princess.

Contact Info   San Isabel National Forest
Leadville District
2015 North Poplar
Leadville, CO 80461
(719) 486-0749

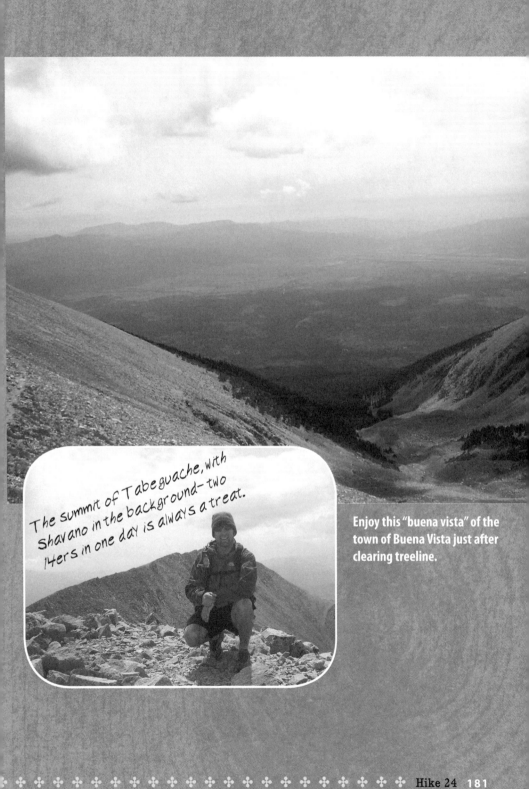

The summit of Tabeguache, with Shavano in the background— two 14ers in one day is always a treat.

Enjoy this "buena vista" of the town of Buena Vista just after clearing treeline.

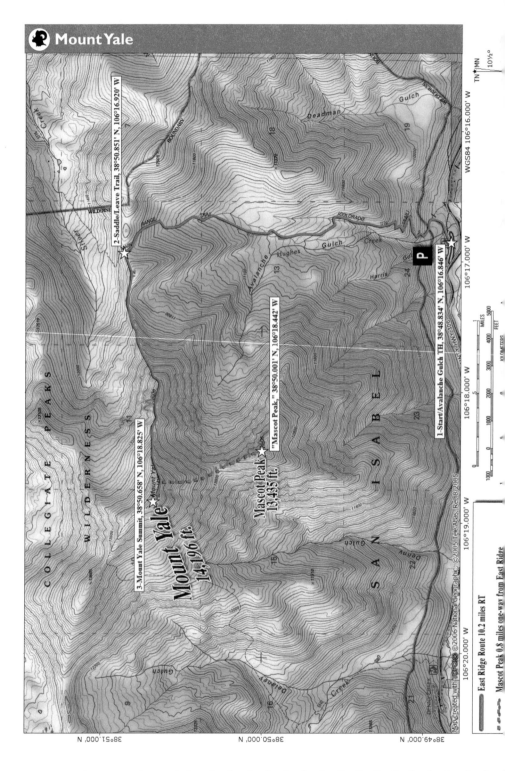

Mount Yale

2-Saddle/Leave Trail, 38°50.851' N, 106°16.920' W

1-Start/Avalanche Gulch TH, 38°48.834' N, 106°16.846' W

"Mascot Peak," 38°50.001' N, 106°18.442' W

3-Mount Yale Summit, 38°50.658' N, 106°18.825' W

Mascot Peak
13,435 ft.

Mount Yale
14,196 ft.

COLLEGIATE PEAKS

WILDERNESS

SAN ISABEL

East Ridge Route 10.2 miles RT

Mascot Peak 0.8 miles one-way from East Ridge

25 Mount Yale

Yale's 2-mile east ridge is an exciting scramble that prolongs the fun of hiking on a narrow ridge. Exposure is minimal but the route is thrilling nonetheless.

Round Trip Distance	10.2 miles
Hiking Time	6–8 hours
Difficulty	7/10
Class	2+
Start Elevation	9,389 ft., at Avalanche Gulch Trailhead
Peak Elevation	14,196 ft.
Total Elevation Gain	4,950 ft.
Terrain	Good trail to rocky ridge walk
Best Time to Climb	July–September
Gear Advisor	Normal gear
Crowd Level	Low

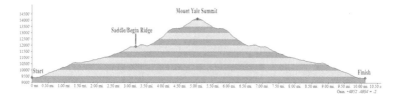

Location Sawatch Range in the Collegiate Peaks Wilderness/San Isabel National Forest outside of Buena Vista

Intro One can only ponder the way our maps would look if this mountain was named after a *different* Connecticut college. We could have been hiking Mount Mattatuck Community College! No matter what you call it, Yale is a prominent 14er cast from the classic, rounded Sawatch mold. The east ridge is not the standard route on Yale, perhaps due to the slightly technical nature of the ascent. At 2.0 miles one way, it's one of the longest ridge walks in Colorado.

Why Climb It? The drawn-out east ridge has good, easy scrambling. It's a fine first ridge walk for those who have only done on-trail hiking. This slight variation on the Sawatch theme means you won't be grinding up miles of talus. The east ridge is broad and gives the excitement of a narrow walkway without the dangerous exposure. Views from Yale are great, as it is smack in the middle of the Sawatch Range, standing apart from the other Collegiate Peaks.

Driving Avalanche Gulch Trailhead is off a paved road and any vehicle can make the trailhead.

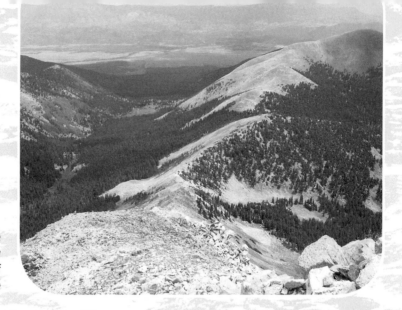

A look back to the saddle from halfway up the east ridge of Mount Yale

How to Get There   From downtown Buena Vista on US Highway 24, turn west onto County Road 306 (Cottonwood Pass Road). Follow the road 9.2 miles and turn right (north) into the Avalanche Gulch Trailhead parking lot, which is quite large. The turnoff is just west of Rainbow Lake.

Fees/Camping   There are no fees to hike Yale, but note that camping is not allowed at the spacious Avalanche Gulch Trailhead. The large and beautiful Collegiate Peaks Campground is 1.7 miles farther west on CR 306. There are 56 sites available, and the cost is $10 per night. There are some good backcountry campsites 1.4 miles in along this trail.

Route Notes   If you got a late start or weather seems to be moving in quickly, you may want to reconsider getting out on the ridge. You'll be walking 4.0 miles (round trip) on exposed terrain with very little shelter. It's not technical, but you won't be moving as fast as you would on a trail. Start a little extra early on this peak; I've seen some of the most violent and fast-forming storms in Colorado in this area of the Collegiate Peaks.

Mile/Waypoint   **0.0 mi (1)**   Start at the Avalanche Gulch Trailhead. Get on the Colorado Trail and go north toward the saddle of Yale and Point 12,505. From lower elevations, you won't be able to see Yale's summit; the large, rocky peak to your left (west) is Unnamed Peak 13,435, on Yale's south shoulder. Some call this mountain "Mascot Peak."

0.2 mi   A small connector trail joins from the right; stay left on the Colorado Trail. This should be obvious, and it is just before the trail starts switchbacking up an open hillside. From here, the well-worn Colorado Trail is very easy to follow as it winds through the woods. Enjoy the warm-up.

3.2 mi (2)   Your time in the woods comes to an end as you reach the saddle at 11,900 feet. There are a few trees, but the views are mostly open, especially to the north. Here you will leave the trail, turning left (west) onto the east ridge. There are intermittent trails you can follow. Use them as you see fit.

From this point, the hiking is very straightforward. You'll see Mount Yale directly in front of you. The ridge is long and without any major obstacles. A few rock outcrops can be scrambled or skirted and none of the easier routes exceeds class 2+. Navigation is easy—just stay on the highpoint of the ridge and head west. At points 13,420 and 13,900 there are some larger outcrops that may be considered "false summits" (though you'll have views of Yale's true summit the entire time). At 13,600 feet, you'll actually go downhill slightly before the final push to Yale's lofty summit.

5.2 mi (3) Yale's summit! To the north, you'll see many of the Collegiate Peaks, notably Mount Columbia, Mount Harvard, and the Missouri group. To the south, Mount Princeton, Mount Antero, and Tabeguache Peak will stand out. Try to reach the top of this peak no later than 10 A.M. (it's about a four-hour ascent).

On your descent, be aware that it takes quite awhile to get back down the ridge. Return the way you came.

Options You can drop off Yale's east ridge just below the final "summit hill" and take the south ridge 0.8 mile over to 13,435 "Mascot Peak." While it's feasible to descend Mascot's southeast ridge, going through the woods is rocky, rough, and not much fun. You may be inclined to do so if your navigation skills are adequate (or if the thought of reclimbing 600 feet to the east ridge is not your cup of tea).

Quick Facts Mount Yale was named by Professor Josiah D. Whitney, head of the Harvard Mining School. Did he lose a bet? Why would he name it after Harvard's Ivy League rival? As it turns out, Whitney graduated from Yale and thus honored his alma mater after a surveying trip in 1869. Of course, he named the higher 14,420-foot peak to the north Mount Harvard. Take that, old chap!

Contact Info San Isabel National Forest
Leadville Ranger District
2015 N. Poplar
Leadville, CO 80461
(719) 486-0752

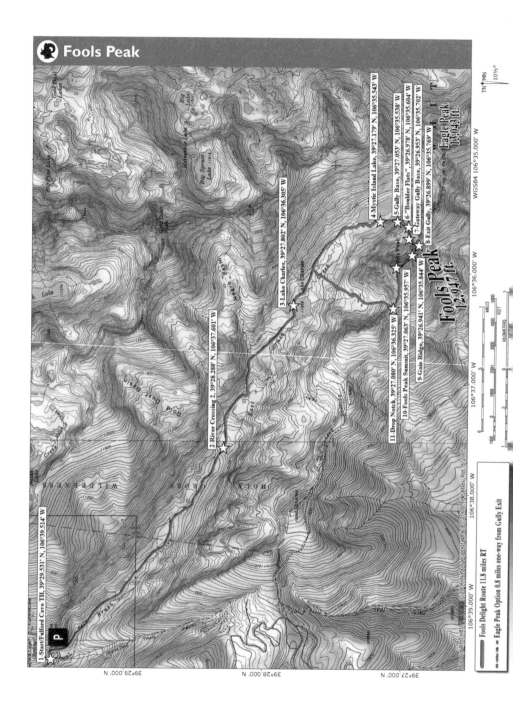

Fools Peak
12,947 ft.

Eagle Peak
13,043 ft.

1-Start/Fulford Cave TH, 39°29.531' N, 106°39.514' W

2-River Crossing 2, 39°28.288' N, 106°37.601' W

3-Lake Charles, 39°27.802' N, 106°36.305' W

4-Mystic Island Lake, 39°27.179' N, 106°35.543' W

5-Gully Base, 39°27.053' N, 106°35.538' W

6-"Boulder Flats", 39°26.978' N, 106°35.604' W

7-Gateway Gully Base, 39°26.953' N, 106°35.702' W

8-Exit Gully, 39°26.899' N, 106°35.769' W

9-Gain Ridge, 39°26.941' N, 106°35.844' W

10-Fools Peak Summit, 39°27.063' N, 106°35.957' W

11-Drop Notch, 39°27.080' N, 106°36.325' W

Fools Delight Route 11.8 miles RT

Eagle Peak Option 0.8 miles one-way from Gully Exit

26 **Fools Peak** *Good Overnight!*

You'd be foolish to miss this spectacular peak! A unique gully scramble tops out on a ridge that features exceptional class 3 terrain. A great climb with very good camping.

Round Trip Distance	11.8 miles
Hiking Time	7–10 hours
Difficulty	8/10
Class	3
Start Elevation	9,430 ft., at Charles Lake/Fulford Cave Trailhead
Peak Elevation	12,947 ft.
Total Elevation Gain	3,470 ft.
Terrain	Good trail to interesting, mixed terrain gully; rocky descent
Best Time to Climb	July–September
Gear Advisor	Gaiters, helmet, solid boots
Crowd Level	Low to lakes; hermit on peak

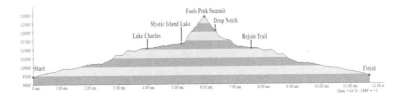

Location Sawatch Range in the Holy Cross Wilderness/White River National Forest outside of Eagle

Intro Mystic Island Lake and Lake Charles are grand destinations for overnight camping. Situated in a brilliant basin, surround by high-rising mountains, this rugged area is unlike any other in the Sawatch Range. Fools Peak is a visually stunning mountain, especially when viewed from the small lakes just east of Lake Charles. If you're ready for an off-trail adventure to one of Colorado's best-kept secrets, this is the hike for you.

Why Climb It? I could rave on and on about the beauty of the lakes below Fools; only the Lion Lakes at Mount Alice rival them for pure splendor. Even though this is a very feasible dayhike, I highly recommend camping. Not only does an overnight give you an early jump on the mountain, it gives you glorious views of the deep, dark night sky. On clear evenings, stars sparkle in the black canopy, often smeared with the faint glow of the Milky Way. The pure ambiance is complemented by a great class 3 gully that scrambles up watery cliffs and steep boulders. A final gully deposits you Fools' southwest ridge, a short sections that features some of the best class 3 scrambling around. A rocky descent lets you loop back down to the lakes.

Driving Passenger cars can make it to the Fulford Cave Trailhead on a well-maintained dirt road. Please note that you are heading toward Fulford Cave, not the ghost town of Fulford.

How to Get There From I-70, take exit 147 to Eagle. Exit south toward the town of Eagle. At the roundabout, take the first right. As of the summer of 2006, there was a lot of construction; the following are the directions as of that time. (Note that when the work is done, you can follow the brown Sylvan Lake forest access road through town.) From the right at the roundabout, turn left onto Broadway, then left onto Fifth Street, then right onto Capital. The distances between these turns are only 0.1 to 0.2 mile each, so keep an eye out for signs. Going south on Capital will bring you to a stop sign. Turn left onto Brush Creek Road (note that going straight instead brings you to a nice park—a good place to hang out after the hike). At 0.7 mile after the left at the stop sign, turn right to continue on Brush Creek Road, which is now labeled Forest Road 400. Follow this paved road 9.0 miles to the junction of Brush Creek Road and Forest Road 415 (this split turns to dirt).

Take a left and continue on this road 7.4 miles, following the signs for Fulford Cave Campground/Fulford Cave. Stay on the obvious main road (there are a few 4x4 road turnoffs along the way). At mile 6.3, you'll see a sign that reads FULFORD CAVE CAMPGROUND 1 MILE and FULFORD 4 MILES. Do not take the road up to the ghost town of Fulford; stay on the main road to its terminus at 7.4 miles. There is a small campground, toilets, and some sign kiosks at the trailhead (as well as a stinky, swampy pond). Don't camp here unless you have to—the bugs are atrocious!

Fees/Camping There are no fees to hike here, though the Holy Cross Wilderness requires you to acquire a permit, which is free. The camping is $7 per night at Fulford Cave Campground; there are only six sites. Only camp here if you have to—the backcountry camping is free. The best campsites are between Charles and Mystic Island lakes and on the south side of Mystic Island Lake.

Route Notes This scramble requires good route-finding in the gully; it's not a good choice for inexperienced scramblers. Since this is a loop, you can feel confident that any tricky sections you ascend won't have to be downclimbed.

Mile/Waypoint **0.0 mi (1)** Start at the Fulford Cave Trailhead and head east on the Lake Charles Trail (#1899). Do not take the Ironedge Trail (at the very beginning of the hike), which goes west and downhill. The Lake Charles Trail starts uphill and climbs steadily before following East Brush Creek.

Once you are on the trail, it is well-worn and easy to follow. There are two river crossings that are accomplished by means of downed trees and rocks in the water—nothing too serious.

2.5 mi (2) At the second river crossing, you'll begin gaining elevation. There are a lot of windblown trees down, so you'll need to take detours where they block the trail. As you get higher, you'll see spectacular black rock walls on both sides of the trail. These are your clues that you are nearing the first of the lower lakes.

4.2 mi (3) The trail emerges into a large meadow; you'll come to a few small lakes before reaching Lake Charles. The hill above Lake Charles is a good place to camp. Not only are the views good, but you will end the loop portion of the hike in this area. Trails get sort of spotty between here and Mystic Island Lake, but the way up is obvious: just follow the creek.

5.2 mi (4) The trail officially ends at Mystic Island Lake. Continue along the west side of the lake (there's good camping here, too). You'll see several gullies on the right; finding the correct one to continue up can be tricky.

5.3 mi (5) The proper gully to ascend is here at waypoint 5, at an elevation of 11,480 feet. There is a dirt patch that looks like a possible trail at its base; it is the first notch after a large gray rock with black water "stains" and lichen.

It's only 0.15 mile to your next goal, "Boulder Flats," but you'll be gaining 450 vertical feet on tricky terrain. This is the hardest scrambling of the hike. The best line stays to the right of the gully, near the solid rock that makes up the "right wall." You'll alternate between rocky outcrops and grassy ledges; there are also some miniwaterfalls running down the safest routes. Good scramblers will have no problem finding a good route. Keep climbing! Even when it looks like you may "top out," there are always good options—and remember, you don't have to descend what you climb up.

5.5 mi (6) This semiflat ledge I like to call "Boulder Flats." (It would be a very neat place to pitch a tent.) The hardest climbing is behind you, and

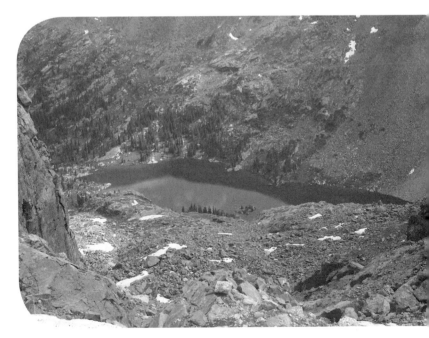

Mystic Island Lake from
the gully up Fools Peak

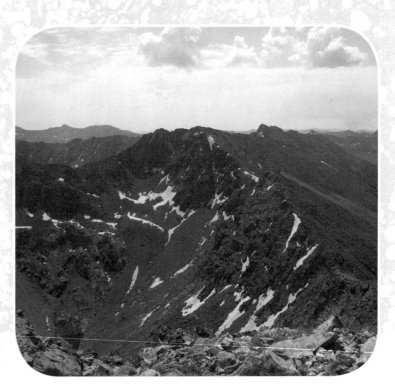

Eagle Peak is one of the more remote 13ers.

from here, you can see the good line to the ridge. The dirt-filled Gateway Gully beckons. Hop on the boulders to its base.

5.6 mi (7) This is the base of the gully (a waypoint for those using GPS). The better footing is on the right-hand side. Follow it up to the ridge.

5.7 mi (8) Exit the gully. The optional traverse to Eagle Peak goes to the left (east) from here. If you plan to get it, camp out and get an early start. The way to Fools is to the right (west). There is a steep rock outcrop guarding the ridge, so you'll need to skirt around the south side of the mountain. Go around the outcrop and take the first "lane" up to the ridge you feel comfortable scrambling. Boulders are set in the grassy slope and the scrambling is good. Climbing should not exceed class 3; if you feel the route is too tricky, go slightly farther west before ascending north onto the ridge.

5.8 mi (9) Gain the ridge. All the fun scrambling has led to this last hike to the summit, which tops out in dramatic fashion. You'll feel like you're on top of the world in just a few more steps!

6.0 mi (10) White rock surrounds you on the summit of Fools Peak. The yodeling is quite good up here! The 360-degree views are awesome. Peer over the north edge and wave to hikers down at Mystic Island Lake—they may be shocked to see you up here. Once you've had your fun, continue down the west ridge. Proving it is in fact a Sawatch peak, the slope down to Drop Notch is paved with boulders of all sizes. It's class 2, but step lightly. At the low point of the west ridge, you'll exit north to a high, swampy area.

6.4 mi (11) Get off the ridge and scramble down the steep, talus-filled slopes of Drop Notch. Aim for the ponds at the base of the gully. The rock here is loose and a bit annoying, but it is not exposed. When you finally reach the spongy grass around the lakes, your knees will thank you. Bushwack north to intercept the trail—the foliage isn't dense, but there are a few areas where you might "cliff out" on small cliffs. I found staying slightly right (east) gave me the best line. You'll have good sight lines to Charles Lake, so just keep going north and you'll eventually hit the trail.

7.4 mi Rejoin the trail and return the way you came. Well done!

11.8 mi Finish.

Options The hike to 13,043-foot Eagle Peak is a class 2 traverse covering 0.8 mile from the top of Gateway Gully. If you hike over to it, return back over Fools and follow the standard route down.

Though it's not covered in this book due to its technical nature, a May or June ascent of the April Day Couloir on the north face of the mountain is a great snow climb once the avalanche danger has cleared.

Spelunkers should take a trip up to Fulford Cave, a large labyrinth of stalagmites and stalactites. Please call rangers for more information on exploring this unique cave.

Quick Facts The rangers and historians I consulted were unable to tell me the origin of the name Fools Peak. It was likely named for some joker who probably got into a heap of trouble on the mountain. Mystic Island Lake is so named for the small, enchanting island on the southern side of the chilly lake.

Fulford Cave and the ghost town of Fulford honor the memory Arthur H. Fulford, an affable prospector who perished in an avalanche in 1892.

Contact Info White River National Forest
Eagle District
125 W. Fifth Street
P.O. Box 720
Eagle, CO 81631
(970) 328-6388

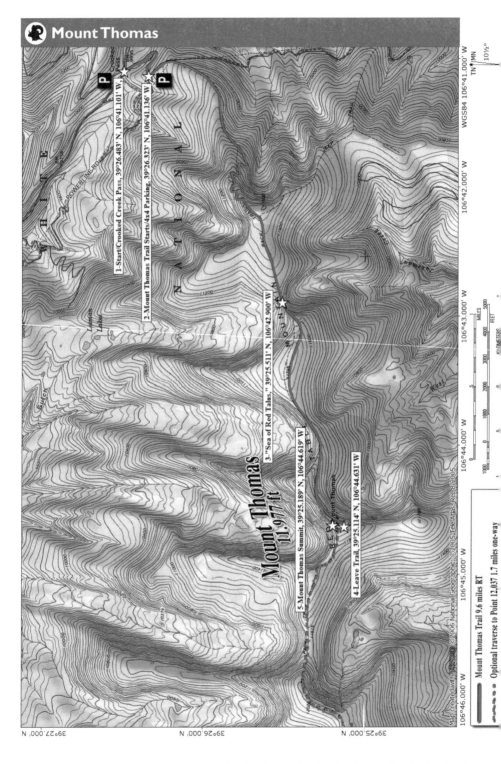

Mount Thomas
11,977 ft

1-Start/Crooked Creek Pass, 39°26.483' N, 106°41.101' W

2-Mount Thomas Trail Starts/4x4 Parking, 39°26.323' N, 106°41.136' W

3-"Sea of Red Talus," 39°25.511' N, 106°42.900' W

4-Leave Trail, 39°25.114' N, 106°44.631' W

5-Mount Thomas Summit, 39°25.189' N, 106°44.619' W

——— Mount Thomas Trail 9.6 miles RT

– – – Optional traverse to Point 12,037 1.7 miles one-way

27 Mount Thomas

Mount Thomas is a relatively easy hike but one filled with many surprises. This wildflower haven features unique geology with great talus rivers and spicy red rocks.

Round Trip Distance	9.6 miles
Hiking Time	4½–6 hours
Difficulty	2/10
Class	1
Start Elevation	10,007 ft., at Crooked Creek Pass
Peak Elevation	11,977 ft.
Total Elevation Gain	2,850 ft.
Terrain	Easy trail on unique terrain and amidst gorgeous scenery
Best Time to Climb	May–October
Gear Advisor	Normal gear
Crowd Level	Low

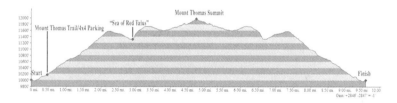

Location Red Table Mountain in the White River National Forest near Eagle and Sylvan Lake

Intro Mount Thomas has a different flavor than other hikes in this book; it's a mellow, peaceful hike with an emphasis on the beauty and unique geology of Red Table Mountain. From a distance, the crimson cliffs resemble the foundation of a giant, unfinished mountain. Because it lacks the glamour and notoriety of other wilderness areas, the chances of seeing pure Colorado alpine scenery are greatly increased. Climbing Mount Thomas affords views into five different wilderness areas, not to mention exceptional views of Pyramid Peak, Mount Sopris (Hike 35), Fools Peak (a class 3 climb, Hike 26), and panoramic vistas of the towns of Aspen and Snowmass Village.

Why Climb It? If the Garden of Eden was to be relocated to an alpine setting, Mount Thomas would be an obvious choice. Wildflowers grow in ponds of swirling colors, complemented by legions of vibrant butterflies patrolling for pollen. After a deceptively modern start under crackling power lines, it soon becomes apparent mankind has left a softer bootprint in these immaculate alpine meadows. Wildlife has taken refuge in the vanilla- and pine-scented forest; mountain lions, black bears, badgers, elk, porcupine, marmots, and even the rare lynx are all acquainted with Red Table Mountain. Half of this hike is above treeline, and the 360-degree views are amongst the best in the state. At times, the beauty of this area is overwhelming; it will recharge your spirit in the same way that clear, fresh mountain air refreshes your body.

Driving Passenger cars can make it to the top of Crooked Creek Pass, a well-maintained dirt road. The walk from the top of the pass to the formal trailhead is short and pleasant. If you have a jeep or rugged 4x4, you can try to drive the 0.4 mile on a violently rutted and washed-out road to a small parking area. SUVs would probably not make it or would get banged up in the process. When I hiked the peak, I was able to walk up the road faster than a jeep was able to drive up.

How to Get There From I-70, take exit 147 to Eagle. Exit south toward the town of Eagle. At the roundabout, take the first right. As of the summer of 2006, there was a lot of construction; the following are the directions as of that time. (Note that when the work is done, you can follow the brown Sylvan Lake forest access road through town.) From the right at the roundabout, turn left onto Broadway, then left onto Fifth Street, then right onto Capital. The distances between these turns are only 0.1 to 0.2 mile each, so keep an eye out for signs. Going south on Capital will bring you to a stop sign. Turn left onto Brush Creek Road (note that going straight instead brings you to

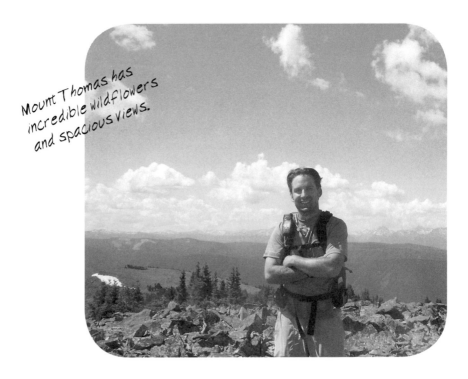

Mount Thomas has incredible wildflowers and spacious views.

a nice park—a good place to hang out after the hike!). At 0.7 mile after the left at the stop sign, turn right to continue on Brush Creek Road, which is now labeled Forest Road 400. Follow this paved road 9.0 miles. Where the road forks (and turns to dirt), bear right and continue to follow the signs to Sylvan Lake. From the intersection, it is 4.4 miles to Sylvan Lake. Go past the lake and continue up the road toward Crooked Creek Pass. After you pass through an opened gate, this road gets a little narrow but is still in very good condition. Continue 5.3 miles (you'll cross a cattle gate) to the top of Crooked Creek Pass, where there's a sign that reads EAGLE 20/THOMASVILLE 12. You can park here on the right. Your hike will begin by going right on the dirt road that drops down off the top of the pass. (Do *not* start on the trail marked RED TABLE MOUNTAIN 8). Those driving 4x4s can try the road to the trailhead if they feel so inclined.

   Note: Even passenger cars can drive a short distance down this road and park in a bumpy lot on the left at the bottom of the hill. There are some nice, big pine trees here to keep your vehicle in the shade while you hike.

Fees/Camping   There are no fees to hike or camp in the Mount Thomas area. There are some primitive camping sites at the top of Crooked Creek Pass and several fee sites below at Sylvan Lake.

Route Notes   None.

Mile/Waypoint   **0.0 mi (1)** Start at the top of Crooked Creek Pass. After the cattle gate, start by walking (or driving if you have a 4x4) right (south) down a shady 4x4 road. Stay on this road to the Mount Thomas Trailhead. Note that there is one split in the road; stay left (you'll see a sign for Forest Service Road 431), and hike up the steep hill. As you continue up the road, you'll see and hear crackling power line towers above you.

   0.5 mi (2) Look for a worn parking lot off to the right, near the top of a hill. You'll be hiking directly under the power lines just before reaching the right turnoff (it can fit about three jeeps!). Cross under the power lines and to your surprise, you'll see a nice sign for the Mount Thomas Trail (#1870). The hardest part of your hike is over! Once you're on this trail, you can turn on cruise control and take in the sights, smells, and sounds of untainted nature.

   0.7 mi The trail is easy to follow and diverts from the intrusive powerlines. Head southwest and continue a steady climb. I don't want to ruin any surprises, but get ready for some stunning wildflower meadows! You'll climb in and out of aspen and pine trees, with views opening up the higher you get. There isn't much signage, but the trail is very well worn. Continue west on this fine trail.

   2.6 mi Though this hike never truly breaks treeline, you'll come to an open mountaintop area where the trees will be spaced out in sporadic pockets. The views just keep getting better!

   2.9 mi (3) Continue on the trail as it crosses the "sea of red talus," a giant slide of red boulders that looks like a stone river cascading down the mountainside. Stay the course on the trail (which you'll note is slightly south of the mapped trail, as it doesn't quite follow the ridgetops—though you are welcome to do so if you wish).

4.7 mi (4) At mile 4.7, you'll be just below the summit of Mount Thomas. Get off the trail for a short distance to make your way up.

4.8 mi (5) Mount Thomas Summit! Enjoy the incredible views, especially of the continuing chain of peaks on Red Table Mountain, to the west. Check out the "Options" section for a bonus trek over to the highest peak on Red Table Mountain. Regardless of which option you take, simply follow the trail back to your car.

9.7 mi Finish.

Options As you can see from the top of Mount Thomas, the pack trail continues west over to the highpoint of Red Table Mountain, the unnamed point at 12,037 feet. The traverse from Thomas's summit covers 1.7 miles, one way. It's a nice peak, but you won't be seeing too much more than you do from Thomas (though you get a nice view of Mount Thomas from Point 12,037).

Quick Facts Red Table Mountain has remained unspoiled by humans throughout history. Outside of a few grazing pastures and short-lived sawmills, the area has remained relatively untouched. Geologically, Thomas is made of the same metamorphic sedimentary mudstone that makes up the Maroon Bells. This hardened mud gives both Red Table Mountain and the Maroon Bells their ruddy hue. Mount Thomas is one of the areas that was on the bottom of the ancient inland sea that covered Colorado some 70 million years ago.

Contact Info White River National Forest
Eagle Ranger District
125 W. 5th Street
P.O. Box 720
Eagle, CO 81631
(970) 328-6388

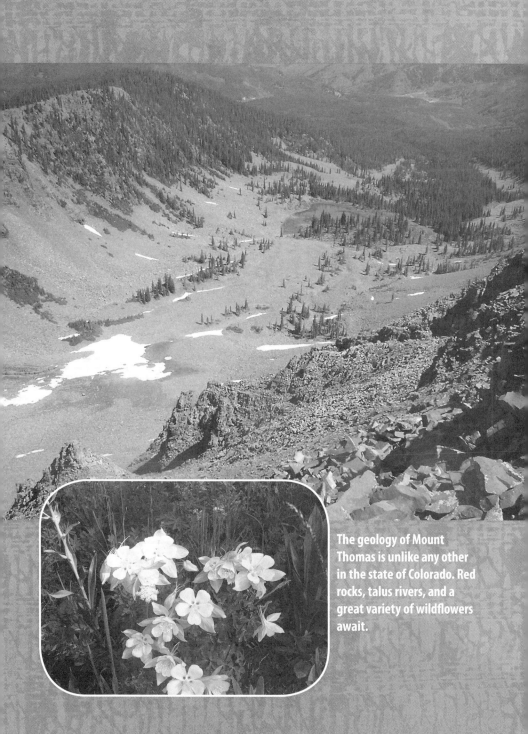

The geology of Mount Thomas is unlike any other in the state of Colorado. Red rocks, talus rivers, and a great variety of wildflowers await.

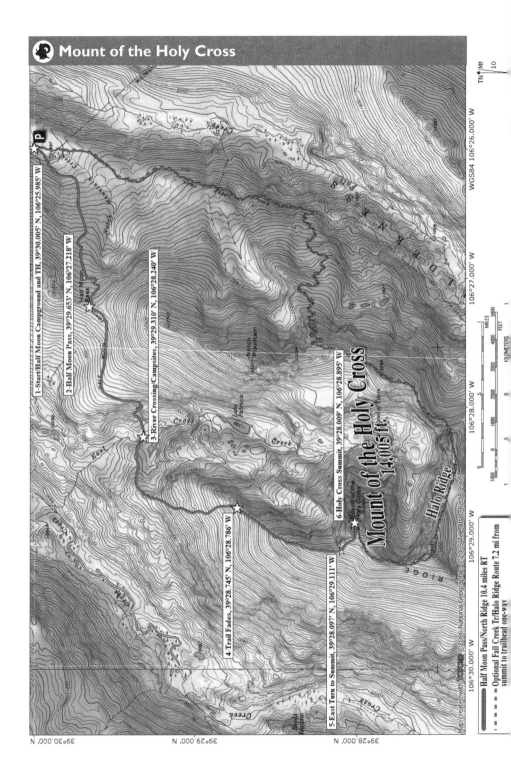

Mount of the Holy Cross
14,005 ft.

1-Start/Half Moon Campground and TH, 39°30.005' N, 106°25.985' W

2-Half Moon Pass, 39°29.653' N, 106°27.218' W

3-River Crossing/Campsites, 39°29.310' N, 106°28.240' W

4-Trail Fades, 39°28.745' N, 106°28.786' W

5-East Turn to Summit, 39°28.097' N, 106°29.111' W

6-Holy Cross Summit, 39°28.009' N, 106°28.895' W

WGS84 106°26.000' W

TN MN
10

Half Moon Pass/North Ridge 10.4 miles RT

Optional Fall Creek Tr/Halo Ridge Route 7.2 mi from summit to trailhead one-way

Halo Ridge

28 **Mount of the Holy Cross**

Good Overnight!

Holy Cross, Batman! This sturdy 14er is a favorite for hikers of all denominations, thanks to some heavenly routes that utilize the mountain's long, stable ridgelines.

Round Trip Distance	10.4 miles
Hiking Time	7½–10 hours
Difficulty	7.5/10
Class	2
Start Elevation	10,315 ft., at Half Moon Campground and Trailhead
Peak Elevation	14,005 ft.
Total Elevation Gain	5,627 ft.
Terrain	Good trail leads to big, stable boulders to summit
Best Time to Climb	June–September
Gear Advisor	Normal gear
Crowd Level	Moderate

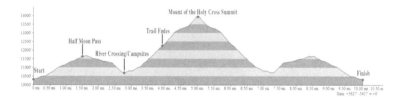

Location   Sawatch Range in the Holy Cross Wilderness/White River National Forest near the town of Minturn

Intro   Mount of the Holy Cross is named for the enormous, crumbling cross of couloirs and crevasses that dominate its east face. The cruciform has drawn hundreds of pious pilgrims of many faiths; those who believe in the power of a good hike won't be disappointed. Once considered a national monument, Holy Cross was demoted to a plain ol' mountain in 1954. In classic Sawatch style, Holy Cross has several drawn-out ridges that are perfect for class 2 ascents. Alpinists can take a shot at the fabled Cross Couloir or the more subtle Angelica Couloir on the northeast face.

Why Climb It?   Does Holy Cross have divine healing powers, as professed by dozens of visitors? It could be, though any visions you receive might be due to a lack of oxygen. As with other Sawatch peaks, the standard routes to the summit are solid, gradual ascents. One difference is the summit massif, which is mildly steep and will require some easy scrambling. While the Cross Couloir is an impressive site, the enormous north face is equally as beautiful. The hiking is very good on Holy Cross, and you'll have many opportunities to peer down the steep northeast features from the safety of the north ridge. Those looking for an epic day can tour the mountain via the optional 13-plus-mile loop.

Driving   Passenger cars can make it to the trailhead, though they will encounter some bumps and bangs; if you have a tough passenger car (TPC), no problem! Tigiwon Road is a rutted dirt road. I made the trailhead unscathed with my Accord. Cars will have to drive slowly to avoid legions of potholes; the entire road looks like it has sustained a mortar attack. Sport utility cars, SUVs, and 4x4s will have no problem. Tigiwon Road is open seasonally and is closed once the snow piles up.

How to Get There   Take exit 171 (Minturn) off I-70; this exit is approximately 5.0 miles west of downtown Vail. Go south on US Highway 24 (east) for 2.0 miles to the charming town of Minturn. Roughly 3.0 miles after the end of town, turn right onto Tigiwon Road (Forest Service Road 707; there's a National Forest Access sign). Tigiwon is a dirt road that goes under a trestle before climbing into the woods. It is a slow-going 8.5 miles to the Half Moon Campground and Trailhead. Along the way, you'll pass the Tigiwon Community House at mile 6.0, and Tigiwon Campground at mile 6.2. Reach the trailhead at mile 8.5.

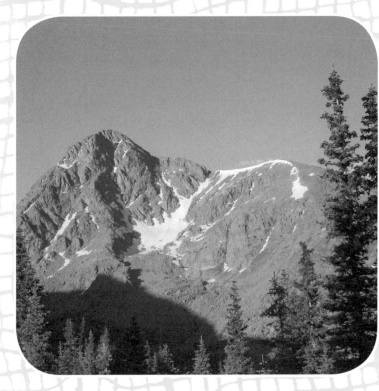

The standard route doesn't afford a look at the famous Cross Couloirs, but it's still a great hike.

Fees/Camping   There is no fee to dayhike the peak or to backcountry camp, though you need to fill out a free user permit. There are great backcountry spots to pitch a tent near the River Crossing waypoint; if you don't mind a short hike, there are also good areas near Patricia Lake. If you'd like to camp at Half Moon Campground, be warned: the few spaces fill up quickly, though you can always retreat to Tigiwon Campground 2.5 miles down the road. As of 2006, sites were $8 a night.

Route Notes   Many hikers are intimidated by the elevation gain presented by this hike. While you need to be in good shape to climb Holy Cross, the climb isn't as strenuous as the raw measurements make it seem (unless you do the entire Halo Ridge Loop). On the standard route, you climb to Half Moon Pass and then descend roughly 1,000 feet to the riverbed below. There are dozens of great, free campsites here for backpackers (and it's only 2.8 miles in).

The out-and-back mileage on the standard route is 10.4 miles, which makes this a better dayhike than some people suppose—though the dread of hiking 1,000 feet back up to Half Moon Pass after descending the summit is intimidating. I had the good fortune to double-check the distance with a park ranger using an advanced Trimble GPS system, as the distances published in various other guides were different than those I had recorded

Note: The standard route does not offer a view of the Cross Couloir; you can see it by making the full Halo Ridge Loop or by hiking up the Fall Creek Trail to the south saddle of Notch Mountain.

One more thing: many people have become disoriented above treeline on Holy Cross. Bringing a compass and GPS will increase your margin of safety.

Mile/Waypoint   **0.0 mi (1)** Start your hike out of the Half Moon Campground and Trailhead. Note that there are two major trails here: the Half Moon Trail, which is the start of the standard route and goes uphill; the other is the Fall Creek Trail, which descends initially and leads to Notch Mountain and the Halo Ridge route. For the route detailed here, take the well-traveled Half Moon Trail.

1.5 mi (2)   In a brief 1.5 miles, you'll have climbed 1,350 feet to the top of Half Moon Pass. From the top, you'll see a phalanx of mountains in the distance. Which one is Holy Cross? Continue down the trail a few hundred yards, past the obstructive shoulder of Unnamed Peak 12,743. Look to your left and prepare to have your jaw drop. Follow the switchbacking trail downhill to the riverbed.

2.8 mi (3)   At the bottom of the hill, there's an easy river crossing. Make sure to stay on the correct trail after the crossing; the Holy Cross Trail goes west and uphill. Avoid the trail that follows the river south to Lake Patricia. There are dozens of great campsites along this stretch of trail; the last good sites are about 0.25 mile west of the river.

3.5 mi   Hike uphill through a rocky forest and pop out of treeline at 11,600 feet. A confusing series of cairns denoting a few different routes will appear. I prefer to stay close to the spine of the ridge, though it is steeper and lacks knee-preserving switchbacks. The terrain gets steep and rocky for a while.

4.0 mi (4) For all intents and purposes, the main trail has disappeared by mile 4.0. Continue south on the ridge; as long as visibility is good, the way up will be obvious.

4.5 mi Finally, a reprieve from the steep climbing! The ridgeline gets less sharply inclined and more defined. A trail reappears on the spine of the ridge, leading to the base of the final summit pyramid.

4.9 mi (5) This is the base of the final summit pyramid. Glance down to the left to see one of the exits of the Angelica Couloir. The push to the summit has the same multicairned confusion as you encountered on the lower section of the mountain. Pick a good line and head east to the top.

5.2 mi (6) Mount of the Holy Cross Summit. Return the way you came up; this is often easier said than done. The perspective on the descent can be momentarily confusing. Take your time and regain the north ridge. Once you pass the Angelica Couloir, it gets easier.

6.3 mi (4) About here, regain the original trail and follow it back into treeline. If visibility is bad, remember you can head east-northeast to reach the river basin and follow it north to the trail. From the river crossing, slog back up to Half Moon Pass.

8.8 (2) Revisit Half Moon Pass. Good news: it's all downhill from here!

10.4 mi Finish.

Options As noted on the map, ambitious folks can make a monster loop of this hike by continuing on from the summit of Holy Cross (waypoint 6), and following Halo Ridge, a class 2+ traverse that circles the Bowl of Tears Lake and rejoins a well-worn trail at a shelter house on the south saddle of Notch Mountain. This vantage point is ideal for photos of the Cross Couloir. From the saddle, a trail zigzags down to a juncture with the Fall Creek Trail; follow it north to return to the Half Moon Trailhead. You can also reverse the route by starting at the Fall Creek Trail instead of Half Moon Pass Trail, which is a less strenuous option since the north ridge descent is easy to follow and you can go on autopilot once you find the trail in treeline.

   The Halo Ridge option is 7.2 miles from the summit of Holy Cross to Half Moon Trailhead (a full loop is between 12.5 and 13.3 miles, depending on how well you navigate and how many switchbacks you take).

Quick Facts Mount of the Holy Cross was a hidden treasure for many years. Many doubted it even existed, until it was officially surveyed in 1873. William H. Jackson took the first famous photo of the cross that captured the imagination of the public. In 1874, Thomas Moran (famous for his Yellowstone paintings) made an ethereal painting of the cross hanging in mist, which added to the mountain's mystique. Images of the peak inspired Henry Wadsworth Longfellow (who never saw Holy Cross in person) to write "The Cross of Snow," a depressing poem that uses the obscure word "benedight" (which means "blessed").

   From the 1920s on, religious pilgrimages made up a large portion of the tourism in the area. Mount of the Holy Cross was made a national monument in 1950, only to lose its status in 1954, due to a lack of visitors. For a

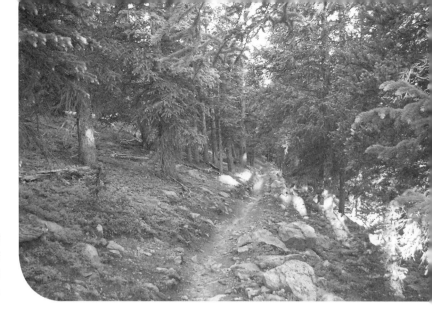

long time, Holy Cross was very difficult to reach. It did not receive "official" 14er status until 1964. It wasn't until the establishment of a good road that traffic finally increased (for better or for worse). Observant historians have noticed that the right side of the cross's horizontal bar is rapidly eroding, which may eventually cause the name of the peak to be changed to "Mount of the Holy T-Square."

One more fact: Tigiwon Community House has served as the launching point for religious retreats since 1927. "Tigiwon" is the phonetic English interpretation of the Ute word for "friend."

Contact Info   White River National Forest
Holy Cross Ranger District
24747 US Highway 24
Minturn, CO 81645
(970) 827-5715

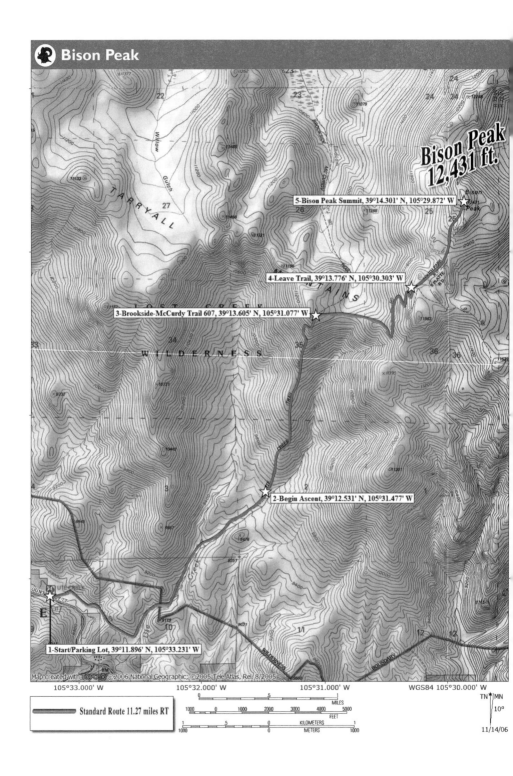

Bison Peak
12,431 ft.

5-Bison Peak Summit, 39°14.301' N, 105°29.872' W

4-Leave Trail, 39°13.776' N, 105°30.303' W

3-Brookside-McCurdy Trail 607, 39°13.605' N, 105°31.077' W

2-Begin Ascent, 39°12.531' N, 105°31.477' W

1-Start/Parking Lot, 39°11.896' N, 105°33.231' W

Map created with TOPO!® ©2006 National Geographic; ©2005 Tele Atlas, Rel. 8/2005

105°33.000' W   105°32.000' W   105°31.000' W   WGS84 105°30.000' W

Standard Route 11.27 miles RT

MILES
FEET
KILOMETERS
METERS

TN MN
10°

11/14/06

29 **Bison Peak**

Welcome to another planet! Bison Peak's incredible rock formations must been seen to be believed. This all natural super-Stonehenge is a unique Colorado experience.

Round Trip Distance	11.27 miles
Hiking Time	6–8 hours
Difficulty	3/10
Class	1
Start Elevation	8,719 ft., at Ute Creek Trailhead
Peak Elevation	12,431 ft.
Total Elevation Gain	4,315 ft.
Terrain	Well-maintained trail/grassy meadows
Best Time to Climb	May–October; this is a year-round option, due to low grade
Gear Advisor	Trail runners, trekking poles
Crowd Level	Low

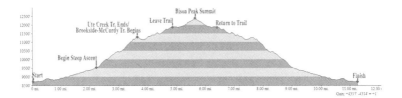

Location Tarryall Mountains in the Lost Creek Wilderness/Pike National Forest outside the town of Jefferson

Intro Bison Peak is unlike any other mountain in Colorado. Don't be intimidated by the mileage and elevation gain. This entire hike is class 1 on a well-maintained trail. After a pleasant walk through the woods, pop out of treeline into another world. Bison's enormous stone monoliths grace the summit in wild and wonderful formations. Rounded rocks sit impossibly atop one another and there are dozens of fun climbs, caves, and scrambles to enjoy.

Why Climb It? Magical rock formations atop the peak are incredible to behold. The hike in is long but peaceful; anyone in decent shape will be able to handle the class 1 trail. Beside the impressive rock gardens, Bison's place as the highpoint of the Tarryall Mountains offers beautiful panoramas of Pike National Forest and several Mosquito Range peaks. The isolation and grandeur of this peak bring to mind images of the fabled Elysian Fields of Greek mythology. Blur your vision, and watch the monoliths turn into a herd of giant bison!

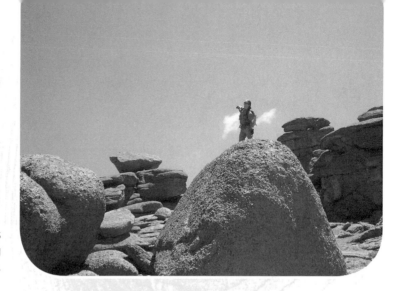

You can play for hours in Bison's amazing boulder gardens.

Driving The Ute Creek Trailhead is reached on paved roads, passable by all vehicles.

How to Get There From US Highway 285, find your way to the tiny town of Jefferson. If you are coming from the Denver area, you'll have to go over Kenosha Pass. From Jefferson, turn southeast onto Park County Road 77, also known as Tarryall Road. An easy way to find PCR 77: the junction is at Jefferson's general store and gas station. Continue on patchy paved road. At mile 17.0, you'll pass the Tarryall Resevoir on your right. At the end of the reservoir, it's approximately 3.4 miles to the Ute Creek Trailhead on the left side of the road (you'll pass some old barn buildings on the left). This parking area has a Lost Creek Wilderness sign, and a bridge spanning Tarryall Creek is visible from the road and parking lot.

Fees/Camping There are no fees to hike Bison Peak. As of 2006, there are no fees to camp in the Lost Creek Wilderness. (Call phone numbers in "Contact Info" section for more up-to-date information).

Route Notes None.

Mile/Waypoint **0.0 mi (1)** Start your hike from the Ute Creek Trailhead parking lot. Head north, cross the bridge, and begin hiking on Ute Creek Trail #629. You will cross into the Lost Creek Wilderness. This trail is well maintained and easy to follow—assuming there is no snow on the ground. You'll be cruising through beautiful stands of Aspen and evergreens as you ascend.

2.2 mi (2) After a nice warm-up, the trail begins to climb in earnest. As you ascend, you'll begin to see the southern rock formations through the trees. It's easy to mistake Point 11,963 for Bison Peak at this point.

3.7 mi (3) The Ute Creek Trail ends and the Brookside-McCurdy Trail #607 begins. This trail heads north and east; you'll want to turn right (east) and climb up to treeline.

4.9 mi (4) After you've climbed some switchbacks to this highpoint, more formations will be visible to the north. Leave the trail (which fades out a bit in the upper meadows) and proceed northeast to Bison's summit. Follow the high, flat ridge until the truly amazing formations appear. You'll descend a short 150 feet, and then climb up to the largest rock formation, where Bison's summit awaits. Don't worry: the summit is an easy scramble and doesn't require any technical or scary moves.

5.6 mi (5) Bison's summit is marked with a USGS marker and summit register (there are actually a few USGS markers up there!). There are a few, weathered wooden structures and some other debris around, including dozens of long metal nails driven into the stone. Return the same way you came, regaining the Brookside-McCurdy Trail where you left it.

11.27 mi Finish.

Options   Exploring the rock formations and scrambling on them can keep you busy for hours. A southwest traverse over the open meadows leads to McCurdy Mountain (12,165 feet). Even though it may look close, it's 2.2 miles one way from Bison to McCurdy, so be prepared to add more than 4.0 miles to an already long hike (which in turn makes for a really long day) if you decide to check it out.

Quick Facts   The Lost Creek Wilderness (designated in 1980) is an amazing place of gravity-defying rocks, mostly rounded granite blocks piled in assorted fashions. No other wilderness area boasts such unique terrain, especially in alpine tundra areas above treeline. Bison Peak was named for the similarity the huge monoliths on its summit bear to the tawny brown ungulates.

Contact Info   Pike and San Isabel National Forests
South Park Ranger District
320 Highway 285
Fairplay, CO 80440
(719) 836-2031

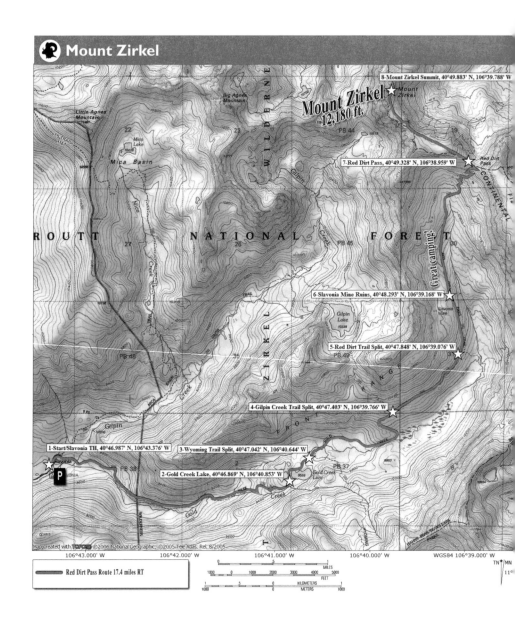

8-Mount Zirkel Summit, 40°49.883' N, 106°39.788' W

Mount Zirkel 12,180 ft.

7-Red Dirt Pass, 40°49.328' N, 106°38.959' W

6-Slavonia Mine Ruins, 40°48.293' N, 106°39.168' W

5-Red Dirt Trail Split, 40°47.848' N, 106°39.076' W

4-Gilpin Creek Trail Split, 40°47.403' N, 106°39.766' W

1-Start/Slavonia TH, 40°46.987' N, 106°43.376' W

3-Wyoming Trail Split, 40°47.042' N, 106°40.644' W

2-Gold Creek Lake, 40°46.869' N, 106°40.853' W

Red Dirt Pass Route 17.4 miles RT

30 **Mount Zirkel** *Good Overnight!*

A northern setting and a low-elevation peak makes Mount Zirkel a haven for color: wildflowers, grasses, red dirt, and snowy summits all decorate this pristine sanctuary.

Round Trip Distance	17.4 miles
Hiking Time	8–12 hours
Difficulty	7/10
Class	2
Start Elevation	8,388 ft., at Slavonia Trailhead
Peak Elevation	12,180 ft.
Total Elevation Gain	4000 ft.
Terrain	Good trail to good off-trail alpine plateau
Best Time to Climb	June–September
Gear Advisor	Gaiters, trekking poles, sandals for river crossing
Crowd Level	Low

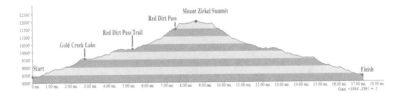

Location Park Range in the Mount Zirkel Wilderness/Routt National Forest outside of Steamboat Springs

Intro Mount Zirkel is the showpiece of the Mount Zirkel Wilderness. The mountains here hold more water than other areas, giving rise to great splashes of color. Hike early in spring to see white snow, green grass, and blue sky. Summer brings wildflowers, and autumn changes aspen leaves bright yellow. There is a calming and refreshing atmosphere in this peaceful and immaculate realm. The abundance of water, wide open spaces, and nontechnical terrain make this the perfect hike for your canine pals!

Why Climb It? You can climb Zirkel in a day; despite the long mileage, strong hikers will move quickly on the trail up to Red Dirt Pass. Better still, take your time and spend a night out in the alpine basin. The trail up to Zirkel is rich and teeming with flora and fauna. Diverging from the pass, you'll climb up to a secret plateau carpeted by thousands of wildflowers. An easy scramble leads up to an amazing summit. When I last did this hike and topped out, I wasn't alone. Two deer were lounging on the rocks, enjoying themselves on the lofty apex.

Driving	The road to Slavonia Trailhead is a very well-maintained dirt road. All vehicles will be able to make it to the trailhead.
How to Get There	From Steamboat Springs, start out on US Highway 40, west of town, and turn north onto County Road 129 toward Hahns Peak/Clark. Follow the road 17 miles to the town of Clark; from here, drive another 0.8 mile to the right (east) turnoff on Forest Service Road 400/County Road 64 (Seedhouse Road). Follow this road 11.8 miles to the eastern terminus at the Slavonia Trailhead; the first 5.9 miles are paved, and then it becomes a dirt road.
Fees/Camping	There are no fees to hike in the area or to backcountry camp. There are several primitive campsites along FS 400 and two pay campgrounds with facilities: Seedhouse and Hinman. Both places are $12 per night. There is fantastic camping along the trail, starting at mile 5.8, the Slavonia Mine ruins.
Route Notes	None.
Mile/Waypoint	**0.0 mi (1)** Start at Slavonia Trailhead and head west on the Gold Creek Trail. This is a good class 1 trail that is easy to follow. Take it to Gold Creek Lake.
	2.7 mi (2) Arrive at the lovely Gold Creek Lake. Stay on the north side of the lake; there's a river crossing here that may run high in the spring. Cross it and return to the trail, heading westward.
	3.0 mi (3) The Wyoming Trail splits off here, on the right. Stay on the Gold Creek Trail toward Red Dirt Pass.
	4.4 mi (4) The Gilpin Creek Trail splits off here, to the left. Again, stay straight on the Gold Creek Trail, which is turning into the Red Dirt Pass Trail.
	5.2 mi (5) There is an anemic trail sign here that designates a split in the trail. Stay left on the Red Dirt Trail that heads north, higher into the basin. The wrong-way Ute Pass Trail heads left and downhill. Do not take it!
	5.8 mi (6) As the basin opens up, there is great camping. The Slavonia Mine is just left (west) of the trail, and has some interesting ruins to explore. Near the mine is a small pond with some funky water in it; I would advise that you don't drink it, for obvious reasons. Note that there is a small, grassy, wet section where the trail disappears. Just keep heading north, and you can pick it back up when it reappears. You'll also get your first look at Red Dirt Pass from here. Drop down into the basin, cross a low-flowing river, and take the switchbacks up to the top of Red Dirt Pass.
	7.5 mi (7) Red Dirt Pass. At 11,500 feet, you've reached the top of the saddle. Leave the trail and head up the grassy/rocky slope to your left (northwest). Climb this slope to 11,870 feet, where a broad plateau will reveal your first glimpse of the craggy summit of Mount Zirkel. Walk across the beautiful meadow and make a class 2 scramble on solid rock to Zirkel's prized summit. Note that when you first see it, you may not be able to tell which "lump" is the top. Luckily, the summit isn't the peak on the far

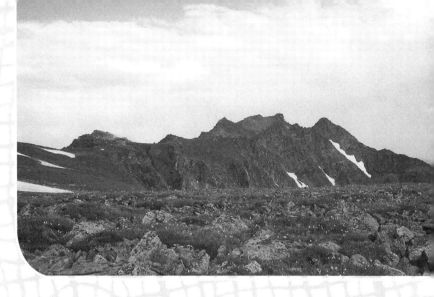

The final approach to
Zirkel's summit

right—it's the blocky piece left of that point, on the other side of the U-shaped saddle.

8.3 mi (8) Mount Zirkel's summit. You have exceptional views from the top, especially of Big Agnes Peak to the west. The optional traverse over to Zirkel's lower north summit is an exposed, class 3 thrill. Be careful, the rock is a little rotten on the way over. Once you have had your fill, drop back down to Red Dirt Pass and return the way you came.

17.4 mi Finish.

Options From Red Dirt Pass (waypoint 7), you could go right (east) instead of west, to check out the rolling mesa of the appropriately named Flattop Mountain. Amazingly, the huge, photogenic mountain you see to the northeast—from the top of Red Dirt Pass—is unnamed; maps list it as Unnamed Peak 11,931. It makes a good second peak to climb if you are camping in the area.

Quick Facts Mount Zirkel is named for Ferdinand Zirkel, a German petrologist who was a big help to survey parties, despite having a name that sounds like it belongs to a Muppet. I wonder what kind of woman Big Agnes was? Is it a compliment or an insult to have such a mountain named after you if you're a woman? My guess is that she wasn't a delicate flower of femininity but could probably cook some mean flapjacks and pull the family plow if the ox needed a day off.

Slavonia Mine had solid yields of zinc in its prime. If you had to work a mine, this was a beautiful place to do it. There is a bit more information on Slavonia at the trailhead.

Contact Info Routt National Forest
HahnsPeak/Bears Ears Ranger District
925 Weiss Drive
Steamboat Springs, CO 80487-9315
(970) 879-1870

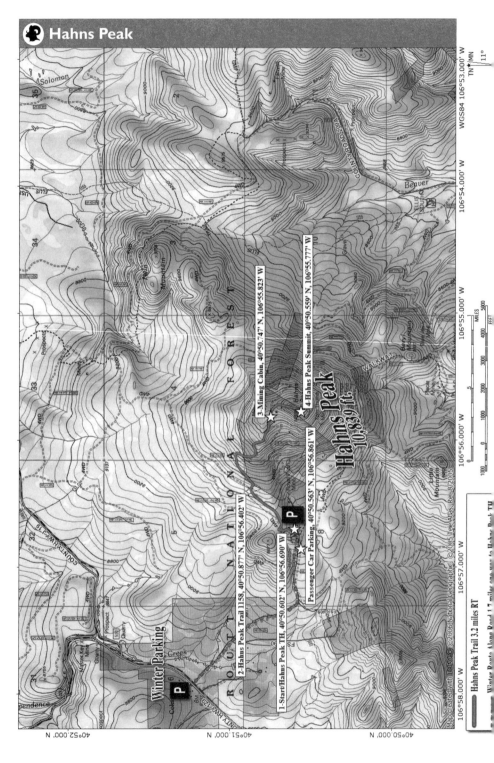

Hahns Peak
10,839 ft.

3-Mining Cabin, 40°50.747' N, 106°55.823' W

4-Hahns Peak Summit, 40°50.559' N, 106°55.777' W

Passenger Car Parking, 40°50.563' N, 106°56.861' W

2-Hahns Peak Trail 1158, 40°50.877' N, 106°56.402' W

1-Start/Hahns Peak TH, 40°50.602' N, 106°56.690' W

Winter Parking

ROUTT   NATIONAL   FOREST

Hahns Peak Trail 3.2 miles RT

Winter Route: Along Road 1.7 miles one way to Hahns Peak TH

WGS84 106°53.000' W

TN MN
11°

31 Hahns Peak

Miles of bright aspen trees and crystal clear lakes unfold before you from Hahns Peak's summit. This easy hike is the perfect complement to any trip to the Steamboat area.

Round Trip Distance	3.2 miles
Hiking Time	2–4 hours
Difficulty	1/10
Class	1; 2 for the last ½ mile
Start Elevation	9,407 ft., at Hahns Peak Trailhead
Peak Elevation	10,839 ft.
Total Elevation Gain	1,316 ft.
Terrain	Well-maintained trail with a slightly rocky hike to the top
Best Time to Climb	Year-round
Gear Advisor	Normal seasonal gear
Crowd Level	Moderate

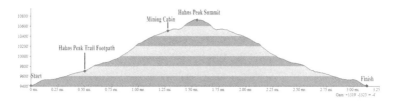

Location Elkhead Mountains in the Routt National Forest outside of Steamboat Springs

Intro Hahns Peak overlooks the aspen forests of Steamboat like a benevolent guardian. From the Steamboat Lake area, the perfectly conical mountain appears much higher than 10,839 feet; this may be due, in part, to the mountain's low timberline. The northern locale of the mountain presents a lush and gentle landscape. In the autumn, expansive acres of aspen turn bright yellow, and the crisp scent of fallen leaves may leave you feeling sentimental for another time and place.

Why Climb It? Hahns Peak is by far the easiest hike in this book. Taken just by the numbers, this mountain may seem too mellow to mention. So why put such a simple trek alongside such brawny adventures as Lead Mountain (Hike 5), Storm King Peak (Hike 45), and Mount Powell (Hike 16)? My rationale for including Hahns is simple. First of all, it's a fun hike that offers the best views I've seen of the beautiful Steamboat Springs and Steamboat Lake areas. The old mining ruins are intriguing, and the fire tower on the summit is a nice touch. But my main incentive to include Hahns is that it's a great complementary adventure to any visit to Steamboat Springs.

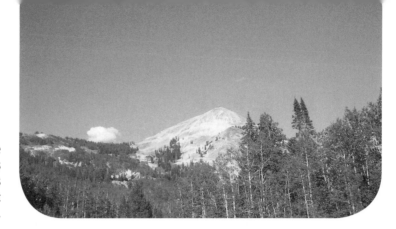

The old fire lookout affords incredible views of the Steamboat Springs area.

Chances are you would be coming to Steamboat Springs to mountain bike, ski, camp, or just be in the outdoors. Hahns takes only a half day to climb, meaning you can mix it in with other activities. In the winter, climbing Hahns from the paved road only adds another 3.0 miles, round trip, to the adventure. Its low angle makes it relatively safe to climb in snow. Hahns brings to focus the distinct beauty of the Steamboat area year-round.

Driving The road is a bit rocky and rough, but tough passenger cars can make it to the Hahns Peak Trailhead. There is a good bail-out point for cars 0.2 mile from the trailhead. Since this is a short hike, it may be a good idea to stop there if you don't want to bang up your car. High-clearance 4x4s and jeeps have the option to drive beyond the trailhead to a very small parking area at the start of the foot trail, but I recommend that you don't. There is only one spot to park, and the walk up the road is actually quite nice.

How to Get There From US Highway 40 in Steamboat Springs, drive to the north end of town. Turn right (north) onto County Road 129, which has a sign for the town of Clark, the airport, and Hahns Peak. Stay on this scenic road for 29.0 miles, passing the towns of Clark and Hahns Peak. You'll also pass Steamboat Lake and State Park, which will be on your left. At mile 29.0, you'll need to turn right onto Forest Service Road 490 (this is directly across from the Columbine General Store). If you're hiking in the winter, you'll have to park at the store and hoof it or ski in. Follow FS 490 for 1.4 miles on a progressively rockier road; at this point, the road splits. If you like, you can park your passenger car here—the roughest part of the road is the next short section. Stay left on FS 418 (there will be signs for Hahns Peak Trail #1158 to guide you) for slightly less than 0.2 mile and arrive at the large, well-marked trailhead. From here, the trail follows a true 4x4 road west and north 0.5 mile to the Hahns Peak Trail. As mentioned above, you can crash your 4x4 up the road, but the parking is limited at the footpath (plus it's very easy to miss if you're not paying attention). My advice is to park in the main lot.

Note: There has been a lot of construction on private land on the first mile of FS 490. There may be turnoffs for driveways and other new dirt roads; stay on FS 490 until the junction with FS 418. Don't camp on the land before the trailhead.

Fees/Camping	There's no fee to hike or camp in the Hahns Peak area, which is in the Routt National Forest. Please be aware of the private land. There are several pay campsites at Steamboat Lake and nearby Pearl Lake State Park.
Route Notes	None.
Mile/Waypoint	**0.0 mi (1)** Start at the Hahns Peak Trailhead parking lot. Head north on the 4x4 road (at the very beginning, avoid the downhill road to the left, after the fences). This is a surprisingly nice hike in the trees, with views opening up to the west as you get higher.
	0.5 mi (2) Turn right (east) onto the marked Hahns Peak Trail #1158. If you've taken your 4x4 up this road, you'll need to park in the small spot on the left-hand side of the road. This is a well-traveled, class 1 trail. Follow it up through the woods.
	1.3 mi (3) As you clear out of timberline (a relatively low 10,330 feet), there's an old mining cabin on your right. Shortly thereafter, you'll come to a crisscross of old mining roads that overtake your humble footpath. Getting up to Hahns Peak from here won't be hard: the fire tower is in clear sight, and there is a trampled path in the rocks that goes east and then cuts south to the summit. The rock on this final push is like a giant pile of broken ceramic plates, making audible "clangs" as you ascend.
	1.6 mi (4) That was quick! You've reached the lookout station on the summit. In the autumn, the views are particularly good. To make sure you are on the right trail when descending, hike down the rock pile, and make sure you pass the old mining cabin. Return the way you came.
Options	The options for this hike are a bit different than others in this book. First off, I'd like to suggest this as a winter trip. You'll have to park at the Columbine General Store off County Road 129, and it's a great adventure. If you are hiking in the summer, complement your trip with some great mountain biking on Emerald Mountain or a paddle on Steamboat Lake. This is also a good place to bring friends who aren't rabid hikers but still enjoy a good day out. It may be a short and easy summit, but it's too good not to mention!
Quick Facts	Hahns Peak is named after prospector Joseph Henn (or Henne); the English version of this German name takes the phonetic spelling "Hahn." Ol' Joseph did pretty well getting himself on the map, having both a mountain and a town named in his honor. As with the names of many other Colorado mountains, Hahns Peak lacks an apostrophe, in accordance with the USGS rule of eliminating them from all geographical names.
Contact Info	Routt National Forest Hahns Peak/Bear Ears Road Ranger District 925 Weiss Road Steamboat Springs, CO 80487 (970) 879-1870

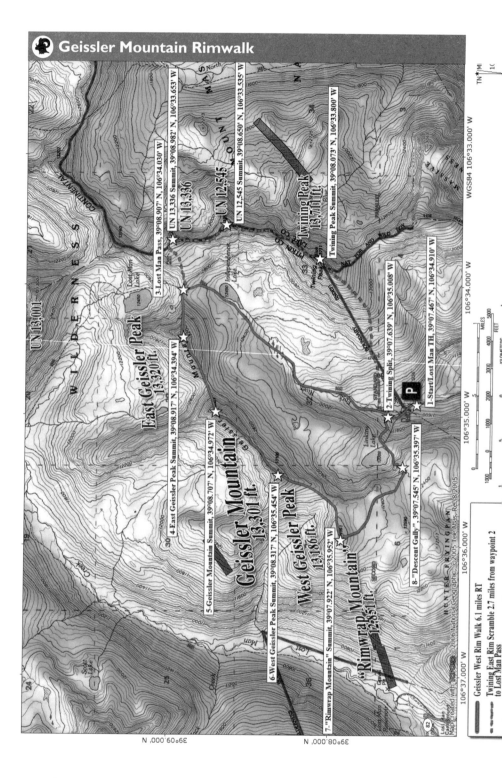

Geissler Mountain Rimwalk

UN 12,545

UN 12,545 Summit, 39°08.982' N, 106°33.653' W

Twining Peak 13,711 ft.

Twining Peak Summit, 39°08.073' N, 106°33.800' W

WGS84 106°33.000' W

UN 13,336

UN 13,336 Summit, 39°08.982' N, 106°34.030 W

3-Lost Man Pass, 39°08.907' N, 106°34.030' W

UN 13,001

2-Twining Split, 39°07.639' N, 106°35.008' W

1-Start/Lost Man TH, 39°07.467' N, 106°34.910' W

East Geissler Peak 13,320 ft.

4-East Geissler Peak Summit, 39°08.917' N, 106°34.394' W

Geissler Mountain 13,301 ft.

5-Geissler Mountain Summit, 39°08.707' N, 106°34.972' W

West Geissler Peak 13,180 ft.

6-West Geissler Peak Summit, 39°08.317' N, 106°35.454' W

"Rimwrap Mountain" 12,851 ft.

7-"Rimwrap Mountain" Summit, 39°07.922' N, 106°35.952' W

8-"Descent Gully", 39°07.545' N, 106°35.397' W

106°35.000' W

106°34.000' W

106°37.000' W

106°36.000' W

Map created with TOPO! ©2006 National Geographic; ©2005 Tele Atlas, Rel. 8/2005

Geissler West Rim Walk 6.1 miles RT

Twining East Rim Scramble 2.7 miles from waypoint 2 to Lost Man Pass

39°09.000' N

39°08.000' N

32 Geissler Mountain Rimwalk

Geissler Mountain is actually a collection of peaks that frame a beautiful, rugged alpine basin. The standard route collects four summits in a single day, while the optional route bags seven.

Round Trip Distance	6.1 miles
Hiking Time	4–6 hours
Difficulty	5/10
Class	2
Start Elevation	11,535 ft., at Lost Man Pass Trailhead
Peak Elevation	13,301 ft.
Total Elevation Gain	2,615 ft.
Terrain	Good trail to semirocky ridge traverse
Best Time to Climb	June–September
Gear Advisor	Normal gear; helmet for the optional loop on Twining
Crowd Level	Moderate

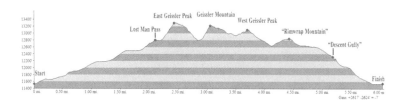

Location   Sawatch Range in the Hunter-Fryingpan Wilderness/White River National Forest just past the top of Independence Pass

Intro   Even though the Geissler Mountains are easily accessed, not many people know about them. Located just off Independence Pass, the multiple summits on the western rim of Independence Lake Basin make a great dayhike that gets to the good stuff right away. The access trail begins a mere 0.3 mile from the middle of the basin. For those who like scrambling and want to tour the whole rim, a thrilling 3+ traverse of Twining Peak and a pair of burly unnamed mountains await.

Why Climb It?   If you've ever driven over Independence Pass, you've no doubt looked up at the big peaks in the area and wondered what their names are and how to reach them. The Geissler Mountain may well be among those that have piqued your curiosity. The mountain of many peaks is very easy to access, and you have a ton of options once you are in the area. The Geissler summits (four in all) present a fun, class 2 ridge traverse that opens up incredible views from Aspen to Leadville. For those who love scrambling and want a longer, more challenging day, the Twining-Geissler Loop hits the whole rim—an exciting and novel experience!

Driving	Any vehicle can make it to the trailhead, the road is paved the entire way. Note that Independence Pass is closed from mid-autumn to mid-spring.
How to Get There	The Lost Man Trailhead is 1.9 miles from the summit of Independence Pass on the Aspen (west) side of the pass. If you are coming from the east, from the junction of US Highway 24 and Colorado Highway 82 (Independence Pass) drive 25.6 miles west on CO 82, up and over the pass, and down 1.9 miles to the trailhead parking area. It is on the north side of the road, off a tight, switchbacking turn. There are signs and a small information kiosk.
Fees/Camping	There is no fee to hike or camp in the area; nearby Lost Man Campground (a few miles west of this trailhead on CO 82) provides drive-in camping spots for $13 per night.
Route Notes	None.
Mile/Waypoint	**0.0 mi (1)** Start at the Lost Man Trailhead. Get on the trail and head north. In almost no time, you're in the basin! How's that for service?

0.2 mi (2)   This waypoint is here to show the split (east/northeast) for the Twining-Geissler Loop. Stay on the Lost Man Trail as it passes the inky Independence Lake and continues up to Lost Man Pass.

2.1 mi (3)   Two miles of easy hiking have brought you to Lost Man Pass, at 12,800 feet. Geissler and its attendant summits are to your left (west), and the western rim walk is easy to see. If you'd like to grab a couple more peaks without doing the optional route, you can go east here and check out Unnamed Peak 13,336 and Unnamed Peak 12,545. The standard route, however, goes west, up the ridge to East Geissler Peak. The rock here is a little loose, but the route never gets more difficult than class 2. Views from here show this is a very unique basin, with black and gray rock covering everything in sight.

2.5 mi (4)   East Geissler Peak is the first of your summits, at 13,320 feet. Take in the great views, and then continue southwest along the ridge to a saddle, and up to the middle summit.

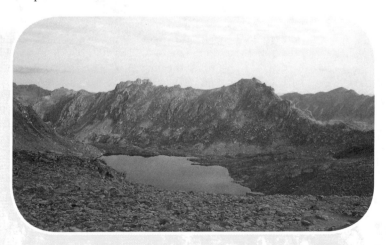

The Hunter-Fryingpan Wilderness is easily accessed from Independence Pass.

3.1 mi (5) The center peak is the official Geissler Mountain Summit, despite being lower than the east peak. This 13,301-foot peak has good views of Twining Peak and the eastern rim. Drop down again and head over to your third summit, West Geissler Peak.

3.8 mi (6) West Geissler Peak! This summit is more craggy and rugged than the previous two. At 13,186 feet, it's the wee Geissler of the family. (As of 2006, there was a broomstick poking out of the highest point. Add this to the ravens I saw circling around, and the eerie gothic color scheme, and I might as well have been standing on Halloween Peak!) Continue on southwest to your next summit.

4.5 mi (7) "Rimwrap Mountain" wraps up the rimwalk at 12,851 feet. From West Geissler, it looks impressive, but from down below it doesn't even resemble a mountain. From here, walk on the broad plateau southeast to the top of a trail that drops down to Linkins Lake.

5.3 mi (8) The "Descent Gully" is more of a slope. There is a faint trail here, but you can get down the slope whatever way is easiest. Once you get on the level with Linkins Lake, there is a cairned trail that goes back to the parking area.

6.1 mi Finish.

Options

The optional Twining-Geissler full rim hike is an exciting scramble. Bring your helmet for this one—you'll be on loose rock that gets up to class 3+ (maybe even class 4) in difficulty. You shouldn't need ropes in normal conditions, but there are some committing moves. At waypoint 2, go up the slope to Twining Peak; this is an easy class 2 hump up to 13,711 feet. Twining is the highest mountain in the rim. From here, you'll have a challenging ridge traverse over and around a few tricky rock pillars. You'll need good route-finding skills and a boost of courage to stay on the ridge. You'll eventually get to UN 12,545, a rugged peak that is officially unnamed despite its prominent profile. From here, continue north toward UN 13,336 on some more challenging terrain. There continues to be loose rock and some tough, short sections that require class 3 maneuvers. Once you reach the summit of UN 13,336, the hard stuff is over. Drop down to Lost Man Pass (waypoint 3), and pick up the Geissler Loop on the west rim from here.

Quick Facts

The Hunter-Fryingpan Wilderness is so named because the area serves as the headwaters of the Hunter and Fryingpan Rivers. It is somewhat unique, in that the area is easy to access yet sees little traffic. It was designated in 1978 and expanded in 1993, making it a relatively new wilderness region.

The mountain you see directly in front of you (north) when you get into Lost Man Pass is Unnamed Peak 13,001, the lowest officially ranked Colorado 13er (number 637 of 637).

Contact Info

White River National Forest
Aspen Ranger District
806 W. Hallam
Aspen, CO 81611
(970) 925-3445

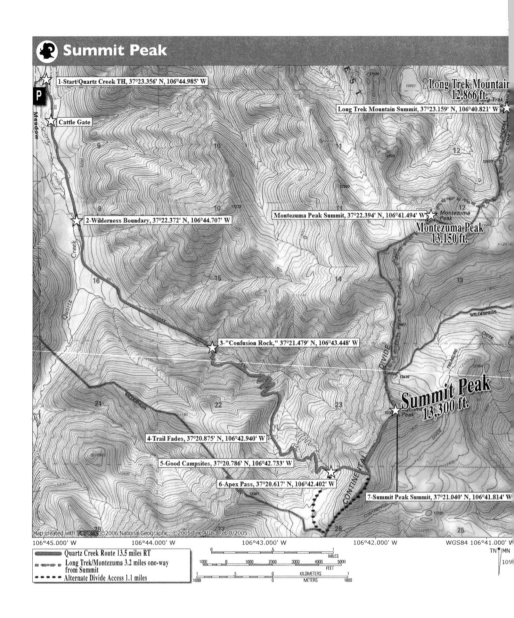

1-Start/Quartz Creek TH, 37°23.356' N, 106°44.985' W

Long Trek Mountain 12,866 ft.

Long Trek Mountain Summit, 37°23.159' N, 106°40.821' W

Cattle Gate

2-Wilderness Boundary, 37°22.372' N, 106°44.707' W

Montezuma Peak Summit, 37°22.394' N, 106°41.494' W

Montezuma Peak 13,150 ft.

3-"Confusion Rock," 37°21.479' N, 106°43.448' W

Summit Peak 13,300 ft.

4-Trail Fades, 37°20.875' N, 106°42.940' W

5-Good Campsites, 37°20.786' N, 106°42.733' W

6-Apex Pass, 37°20.617' N, 106°42.402' W

7-Summit Peak Summit, 37°21.040' N, 106°41.814' W

Map created with TOPO!® ©2006 National Geographic; ©2005 Tele Atlas, Rel. 8/2005

106°45.000' W   106°44.000' W   106°43.000' W   106°42.000' W   WGS84 106°41.000' W

Quartz Creek Route 13.5 miles RT	
Long Trek/Montezuma 3.2 miles one-way from Summit	
Alternate Divide Access 1.1 miles	

MILES
FEET
KILOMETERS
METERS

TN/MN

33 **Summit Peak** *Good Overnight!*

Isolation and peace are the themes for this seldom-visited route to Summit Peak. If you are looking for a beautiful escape and a great walk on the Continental Divide, read on.

Round Trip Distance	13.5 miles
Hiking Time	7 ½–10 hours
Difficulty	5/10
Class	2
Start Elevation	8,917 ft., at Quartz Greek Trailhead
Peak Elevation	13,300 ft.
Total Elevation Gain	4,460 ft.
Terrain	Good trail leading to pristine wilderness area
Best Time to Climb	July–September
Gear Advisor	Gaiters, trekking poles, GPS, sandals for river crossing
Crowd Level	Low

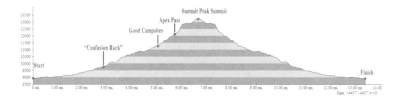

Location   San Juan Mountains in the San Juan Wilderness/San Juan National Forest outside of Pagosa Springs

Intro   Sometimes you just want to get away. Summit Peak and its attendant trail take you deep into the wilderness, where there will be no signs of civilization in sight. This hike is a catalog of natural wonders: thundering waterfalls, spacious alpine meadows, soulful forests, elaborate rock formations, dark woods, and grassy plateaus. This serene setting is ideal for a relaxing overnight journey, complemented by a good trek up to Summit Peak. Add the optional Montezuma Peak and Long Trek Mountain into the mix, and you have a trio of summits sure to rejuvenate your soul.

Why Climb It?   This is not a hike for adrenaline junkies! That's not to say there are not challenges; you'll need to navigate an overgrown basin and push up steep slopes to reach the Continental Divide. The raw natural splendor will have you reaching for your camera at every turn. Quartz Creek is especially fetching, as the cold mountain water runs clear over a bed of white and light gray rocks. Once you are on the Divide, Summit Peak opens up a wonderful world of gentle ridges and glorious vistas.

Driving   Tough passenger cars can make the trailhead, but if there has been a lot of rainfall (which is common in the San Juans), there may be trouble. When East Fork Road drops down next to the river around mile 7.0, there are several runoffs and mud puddles that bisect the road; heavy rain can make these puddles traps for two-wheel drive vehicles. On Forest Service Road 684, there is a wide river crossing where the water normally flows about a foot and a half deep. If you can clear this, you're home free to the trailhead. SUCs, SUVs, and 4x4s will be fine.

How to Get There   From the intersection of US Highway 84 and US Highway 160, east of Pagosa Springs, travel 9.7 miles north on US 160 to the East Fork Road turnoff on your right (east). If you are approaching from the north, this turn is roughly 10 miles from the top of Wolf Creek Pass. Turn onto East Fork Road (Forest Service Road 667) and follow it for 9.2 miles. Turn right onto FS 684 (Quartz Meadow Road). At mile 0.1, there is a river crossing that is often too deep for passenger cars, which will have to park here if the water is too high. One plus to this crossing is that the bottom is lined with rocks, not mud. Continue up the road, where a large cattle gate may be closed, depending on the time of the year; it's not locked, but you'll have to get out of your vehicle to open and close it. Turn left at mile 2.8 and park at the obvious trailhead near a large meadow. Make sure not to drive into the woods past the trailhead.

Fees/Camping   There are no fees to hike or camp in this area. Drive-in camping is available at East Fork Creek Campground's 25 sites at $8 per night, but there are plenty of places to pull off and car camp along the way, including at Quartz Creek Trailhead.

Route Notes   I'd highly recommend this hike as an overnight; you can set up a high camp protected by trees at several flat sections around 11,270 feet in the high basin. These spots are mentioned in the route description.

Mile/Waypoint   **0.0 mi (1)**   Start at the Quartz Creek Trailhead. Get on the Quartz Creek Trail and head south through the open meadow. Don't bother the cows that may be grazing in the area. (Seriously, these are not your normal cows. Alpine cows are a tough breed. They've come to chew cud and kick butt… and they're all out of cud.) Pass through a cattle gate and enjoy this trail. For the most part, it is easy to follow, though there are some sections that seem to be washed out, where runoff from the east intersects the trail. If there is a washout, continue south and eventually you'll regain the well-worn tail.

1.2 mi (2)   Wilderness boundary sign. From here, you begin to go away from the creek and enter a pine forest draped with hanging moss. The trail is still easy to follow and gradually gains altitude.

2.8 mi (3)   Welcome to "Confusion Rock." Confused? The trail you have been following goes down a little hill to the creek. There are faint trails on your side of the river, and they all apparently dead-end. When you are standing at this point, you'll see a giant rock that looks like a big, gray potato. You need to cross the river and get on the right side of this rock, where the

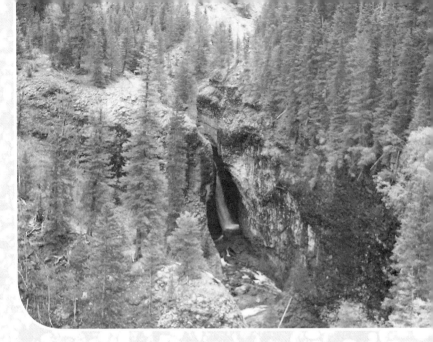

This hidden waterfall can be seen from the top of "Confusion Rock."

trail resumes in a series of steep switchbacks. This means you'll need to go downstream a little to get across to the rocky, steep hill. It's a bear to lug a backpack up that section, but once you are up, the trail magically reappears and the going is easy again. When you hike to the top of Confusion Rock, look to the east. You'll see a secret waterfall running in the notched entrance of a cave.

The next section of the trail is easy to follow, but there were a lot of trees down on it in the summer of 2006. The switchbacks are well-designed as they climb higher. With luck, you won't scare any camouflaged pheasants, who will in turn scare the tar out of you with their loud, flapping wings.

4.7 mi (4) As you enter the big, sloped basin, the trail gets overgrown. You need to start heading southeast. If the trail is visible, take it. If not (which was the case when I was last there), find a good route through the foliage. There are several ways to gain the Continental Divide here, but stay on route.

5.0 mi (5) In many of the pockets of pine trees, you can find level ground. These sites are great for camping. They are sheltered, close to water, and have great views. This is a good place to pitch a tent and call it a night. Dayhikers will want to continue up toward the grassy slopes below Apex Pass.

5.8 mi (6) This is the base of Apex Pass (12,100 feet), a smooth, loose, scree slope that grants access to the Continental Divide. Starting at the grassy slopes above timberline, march to the base of the pass and push up to the Divide—a gain of 700 feet. Those looking for an easier (but longer) way to gain the Divide can go south and get on the ridge via mild slopes (this is the way the trail should go, but it's faded out).

6.2 mi Once you are on the divide, the way to Summit is obvious. Walk northeast on the gentle grassy ramp to Summit's highest point.

6.8 mi (7) Summit's summit! You'll feel like the king of your own private empire up here. Continue on the optional route or return the way you came. A GPS is helpful for retracing your tracks. Once you're on the trail on the west side of the basin, it's easy going back down the Quartz Creek Trail.

13.5 mi Finish your hike.

Options If you overnight at the camp spot (waypoint 5), you set yourself up for a great day of peak-bagging! Gain the ridge via Apex Pass and begin a long, easy, class 2 stroll north. The Continental Divide Trail runs along the peaks here. Montezuma Peak (13,150 feet) is 1.8 miles from Summit. The hermit's haven of Long Trek Mountain (12,866 feet) is 3.2 miles from Summit. From high camp, the round-trip mileage to Long Trek and back is 10 miles—a very full day. On the divide, it's easy to hike quickly, so you can do this out-and-back in about four to six hours. Start early (at sunrise) and get back to camp to avoid summer storms. All three summits as a dayhike from Quartz Creek Trailhead? You're looking at 20 miles. Fit trail runners may be able to do it, but it would be tough. Break it up and you have two full days of great hiking.

Quick Facts At least Summit Peak's bland name is accurate: it's the highpoint of Archuleta County. This fact brings a few county highpoint peak-baggers to Summit every year.

Montezuma is named for the ancient deity who had significance to both the Aztec and Pueblo people. It is also the incorrectly cited as the name of two flesh-and-blood emperors of the Aztec empire. Their names were actually Monteczuma I and Monteczuma II: Esta Vez Esto Es Personal. (Every sequel needs a tagline: "This Time It's Personal" seems to work for most!)

Contact Info San Juan National Forest
Pagosa Ranger District
180 Second Street
P.O. Box 310
Pagosa Springs, CO 81147
(970) 264-2268

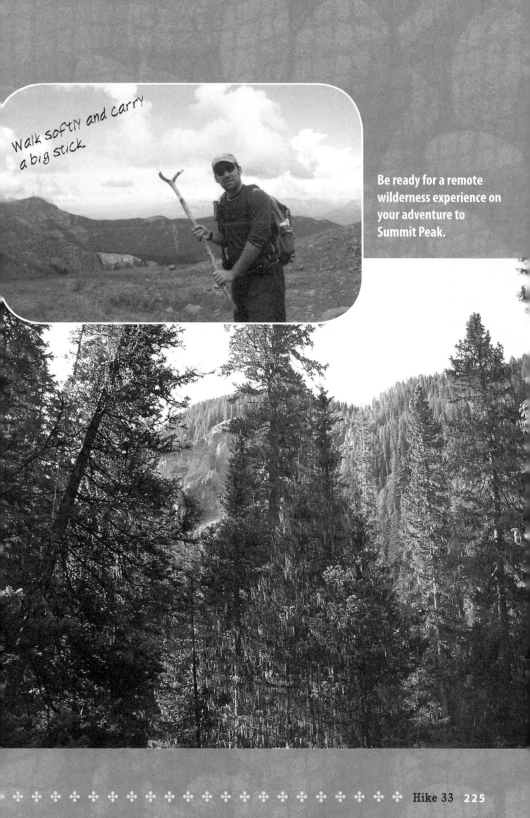

Walk softly and carry a big stick.

Be ready for a remote wilderness experience on your adventure to Summit Peak.

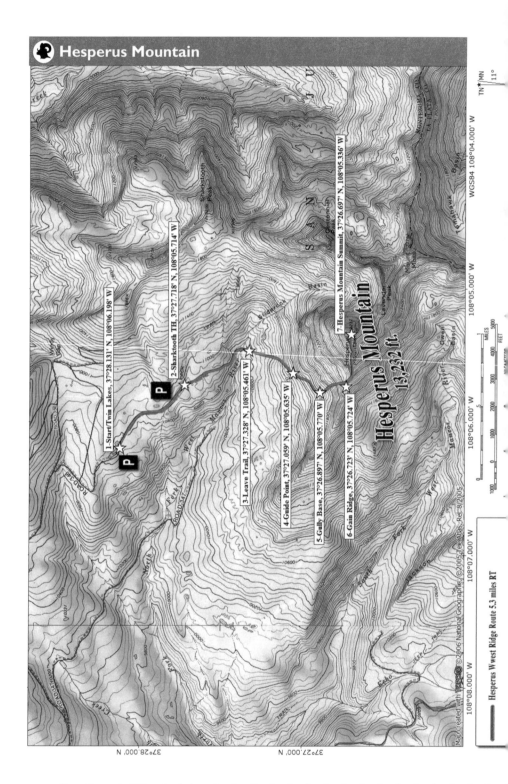

Hesperus Mountain

Hesperus Mountain
13,232 ft.

1-Start/Twin Lakes, 37°28.131' N, 108°06.198' W

2-Sharktooth TH, 37°27.718' N, 108°05.714' W

3-Leave Trail, 37°27.328' N, 108°05.461' W

4-Guide Point, 37°27.059' N, 108°05.635' W

5-Gully Base, 37°26.897' N, 108°05.770' W

6-Gain Ridge, 37°26.723' N, 108°05.724' W

7-Hesperus Mountain Summit, 37°26.697" N, 108°05.336' W

WGS84 108°04.000' W

108°05.000' W

108°06.000' W

108°07.000' W

108°08.000' W

37°28.000' N

37°27.000' N

TN MN
11°

Map created with TOPO! ©2006 National Geographic; ©2005 Tele Atlas, Rel. 8/2005

Hesperus West Ridge Route 5.3 miles RT

34 Hesperus Mountain

Red and white stripes decorate the face of Hesperus; it's a truly unique Colorado color scheme. Go off-trail and make your way to the top of this most sacred mountain.

Round Trip Distance	5.3 miles
Hiking Time	5–7 hours
Difficulty	7/10
Class	2+
Start Elevation	10,780 ft., at Sharkstooth Trailhead
Peak Elevation	13,232 ft.
Total Elevation Gain	2,840 ft.
Terrain	Short but good trail leads to rocky, rugged gullies and ridge walk
Best Time to Climb	June–September
Gear Advisor	GPS, trekking poles
Crowd Level	Low

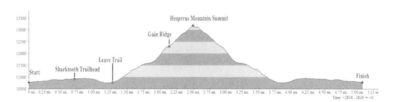

Location La Plata Mountains in the San Juan National Forest outside the town of Mancos.

Intro It's easy to see why the Navajo people consider this sacred mountain a special place on earth. They call it *Dibé Nitsaa*, which translates to "Big Mountain Sheep." Each of the four sacred mountains was assigned a color that related to its spiritual significance; Hesperus was noted not for the red and white stripes, but for the black, powdery obsidian found on its ridges. Obsidian was an important rock to the Navajo because it could be shaped into tools and arrowheads. Dibé Nitsaa is the sacred mountain of the north (more about the other peaks in the "Quick Facts" section on page 231).

   The Navajo believe these mountains are vital to their existence; not only do they designate the boundaries of the land given to the Navajo by the Great Spirit, but they are places where the people can connect with all living things, renew the spirit, and gaze with wonder upon the same lands as their ancestors.

Why Climb It? I would be lying if I said I didn't feel a spiritual pull to Dibé Nitsaa. The striking profile and coloration of the peak stands out from miles away. Views from the top are incredible, mimicking an eagle's persective of the land below. Sharkstooth Peak rises from an ocean of talus to the north, and the craggy, broken face of Lavender Mountain shares a busted ridge to the west. The hiking is tough at times, but once you have gained the west ridge, you're in business. What begins as a steep ridge on broken plates of rock gives way to better scrambling the higher you climb. It's short mileage-wise, but it's a challenging hike that will take some time and route-finding.

Driving Tough passenger cars can make it most of the way; the route described here starts at the car parking area at Twin Lakes. Sport utility cars, SUVs, and 4x4s can push on the final 0.7 mile to Sharkstooth Trailhead. The dirt road is rocky and washed out in places; large mud puddles are the main obstacles for two-wheel-drive vehicles.

How to Get There From the charming town of Mancos, on US Highway 160, find the intersection of US 160 and Colorado Highway 184. Turn north onto CO 184 for 0.3 mile and turn right onto County Road 42 (there will be signs for Mancos State Park/West Mancos Road/Jackson Lake). This is also known as Forest Service Road 561. It begins as a paved road and turns to dirt at 1.2 miles.

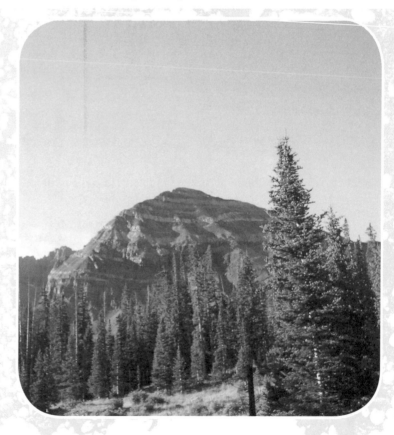

Hesperus is considered a sacred mountain by native people.

Follow this road past the Transfer Campground and Aspen Guard Station, and at mile 12.0, take a right onto Forest Service Road 350 (Spruce Mill Road). There will be signs for the Sharkstooth Trailhead (mile 7.5) here. Stay on this semirocky road 6.0 miles (there are nice camping options the last mile), and then turn right and downhill onto Forest Service Road 346. The turn isn't well marked; there are signs for the Aspen Loop ATV Trail, a Mancos 17 sign, and eventually a sign for Twin Lakes and Sharkstooth Trailhead. The road gets significantly rougher here. Cars can make it to within 1.0 mile of Twin Lakes and park on the right; the route described here starts at this point. SUCs, SUVs, and 4x4s can brave some big mud puddles and deeply rutted chunks of road to travel the remaining 0.7 mile to the Sharkstooth Trailhead at the end of the road.

Fees/Camping   There are no fees for hiking or camping in this area. The closest pay sites with facilities can be found at the Transfer Campground, where sites are $10 per night. The backcountry car camping is quite good the last 2.0 miles of FS 350.

Route Notes   This route is off-trail most of the way. A GPS will help, as will trekking poles.

Mile/Waypoint   **0.0 mi (1)**   Start the hike at Twin Lakes parking area. Hike or drive up the remaining 0.7 mile to the formal Sharktooth Trailhead.

0.7 mi (2)   This is the official trailhead, at 10,925 feet. A few trails start here. You want to go south on the West Mancos Trail #621. This trail doesn't see a ton of traffic, so it's a little faded. It's an easy start—you go downhill! Stay on trail as you drop down to the river. A sign that reads NORTH FORK OF THE WEST MANCOS is visible. Cross the river and stay on trail, due southwest.

1.3 mi (3)   From the trail, you'll see a grassy clearing to your left (south). It's time to get off-trail, but take a good look first. There is a teardrop of talus in the middle of the slope; to the right of that are some weeds and bushes, and to the right of them is a row of pine trees. Aim to climb on the left fringe of the pine trees, up a grassy slope and right, to the top of the talus pile. From there, you will begin to go right and line up a good path to gain the ridge.

1.6 mi (4)   Use this waypoint to stay on course. Under the giant north face, continue to skirt up and right (southwest) toward a grassy slope west of the rocky face. Stay above the patches of willows. I've seen some people trying to get a more direct route up these rocky ledges and they struggled mightily. The line may be more direct, but it's also on bad rock—rotten, broken, and steep. Keep going right (southwest) through a few pine trees and gullies. Stay low on the flatter parts of the slope while you traverse over.

1.9 mi (5)   At 11,646 feet, you will be at the base of a gully with a moderate grade (it's the second big gully after the rocky shoulder of the ridge). The gully is defined by a plethora of scree and a coating of obsidian powder at the top. GPS users should check the waypoint. If it still looks too steep, you can continue to traverse westward and connect with the ridge farther down.

Enjoy your moment of enlightenment on the summit of Hesperus.

2.2 mi (6) After a tough push, you've gained the west ridge. From here, all you need to do is head east and get up the ridge. Most of the terrain on the ridge is class 2+, perhaps easy class 3. Staying on the spine of the ridge makes travel easier; the frosted flakes of rocks in the beginning aren't good for your knees. There are some nice notches and gullies to scramble up, just make sure you don't go onto the north face. There is always a class 2 option to your right (south) if the terrain gets too tricky for you. Continue up, past bands of white rock and work to the highest point on the horizon (which may be blinded out by the east-rising sun). Eventually, you'll top out; hike about 60 feet north, and you'll be at the summit.

2.6 mi (7) Hesperus Mountain Summit! You are standing on the white top of the sacred mountain. There is a summit register here maintained by a very dedicated individual. The views up here rival that of any 14er. As you gaze out upon the homelands of the Navajo, consider this quote:

"We, the five-fingered beings, are related to the four-legged, the winged beings, the spiritual beings, Father Sky, Mother Earth, and nature. We are all relatives. We cannot leave our relatives behind."
—*Betty Tso, Navajo*

Give your thanks to the Great Spirit of your choice and return down the way you ascended. A GPS will help you retrace your tracks back to the trailhead.

5.3 mi Finish.

Options From Hesperus, ridges to other points are fraught with peril. The southeast ridge to Lavender Peak looks to be a tough ticket; I have not tried it, but it appears to be at least class 3+/4. If you're an enterprising scrambler, it may be a fun way to reach Lavender and Centennial peaks. Oh, and if you're the kind of freak who loves knee-twisting, ankle-wrenching talus fields, you can go up to Sharkstooth Peak from the Sharkstooth Trailhead. Your orthopedic surgeon thanks you in advance.

Quick Facts Hesperus gets its name from the Hesperus Mine that spawned a boomtown of the same name in 1882, founded by John Porter. The name transferred to the mountain; in Latin it means "the Evening Star," which referred to the planet Venus.

The four sacred mountains of the Navajo delimit the land of their ancestors. The mountains are:

Mount Blanca (*Tsisnaasjini'*—Dawn or White Shell Mountain)
Sacred Mountain of the East

Mount Taylor (*Tsoodzil*—Blue Bead or Turquoise Mountain)
Sacred Mountain of the South

San Francisco Peak (*Doko'oosliid*—Abalone Shell Mountain)
Sacred Mountain of the West

Mount Hesperus (*Dibé Nitsaa*—Big Mountain Sheep—Obsidian Mountain) Sacred Mountain of the North

Thanks to www.lapahie.com, a Navajo webpage, for this information.

Contact Info San Juan National Forest
Dolores Ranger District
100 N. Sixth Street
P.O. Box 210
Dolores, CO 81323
(970) 882-6841

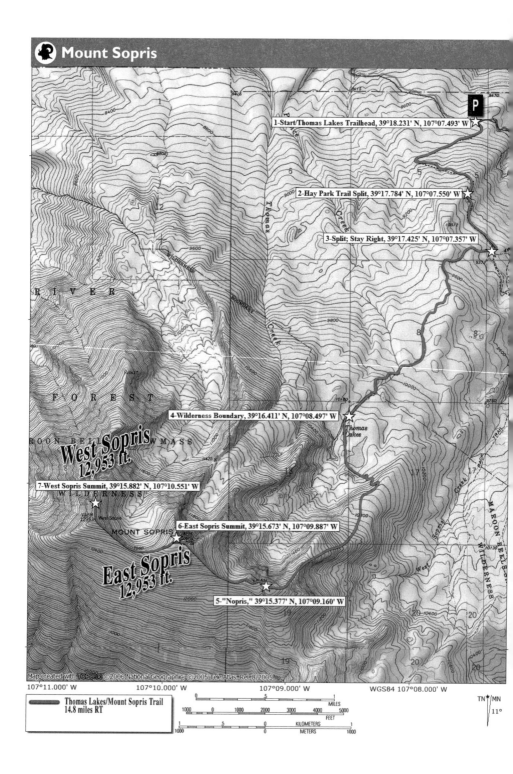

1-Start/Thomas Lakes Trailhead, 39°18.231' N, 107°07.493' W

2-Hay Park Trail Split, 39°17.784' N, 107°07.550' W

3-Split; Stay Right, 39°17.425' N, 107°07.357' W

4-Wilderness Boundary, 39°16.411' N, 107°08.497' W

West Sopris 12,953 ft.

7-West Sopris Summit, 39°15.882' N, 107°10.551' W

6-East Sopris Summit, 39°15.673' N, 107°09.887' W

East Sopris 12,953 ft.

5-"Nopris," 39°15.377' N, 107°09.160' W

Thomas Lakes/Mount Sopris Trail
14.8 miles RT

35   **Mount Sopris**

Sopris is perhaps the most impressive standalone mountain in Colorado, especially when viewed from Carbondale. Both east and west summits boast the exact same official elevation; I got the same results with my GPS!

Round Trip Distance	14.8 miles
Hiking Time	7½–10 hours
Difficulty	6.5/10
Class	2
Start Elevation	8,635 ft., at Thomas Lake/Sopris Trailhead
Peak Elevation	12,953 ft.
Total Elevation Gain	5,072 ft.
Terrain	Good trails to good ridge traverse
Best Time to Climb	June–September
Gear Advisor	Normal gear
Crowd Level	Moderate

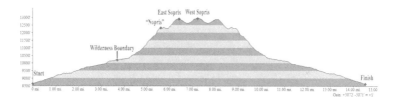

Location   Elk Range in the Maroon Bells-Snowmass Wilderness/White River National Forest outside of Carbondale

Intro   By all accounts, 12,953-foot Mount Sopris *looks* like the biggest mountain in Colorado, when viewed from the north. The twin summits rise over 6,500 feet from the nearby town of Carbondale. That would be like having a 13er smack dab in downtown Denver! In comparison, the mountains behind Boulder rise to only 8,500 feet. Not only is this a great-looking mountain, it's a great hike. What seems like an arduous task to ascend both summits turns out to be an easy, 1.0-mile saddle traverse between the two. Don't let the high mileage discourage you—this is a very viable dayhike. The approach to Thomas Lakes goes by quickly on class 1 trails.

Why Climb It?   Sopris is yet another peak that begs to be climbed. The long trail to Thomas Lakes is quite scenic and travels through open meadows and friendly forests. Once you reach Thomas Lakes you'll tour the twin summits via the east ridge. This is one of my favorite ridge walks in all of Colorado. After an initial push on rocky talus to the top of "Nopris," you are granted access to the rolling ridge to the East Summit. Views of the river of gray talus that flows down the north face are stunning; there are even ripples and contours that make it look like a molten lava flow (or a giant river of cake batter). Gaining the two summits will leave you scratching your head and wondering which is truly higher.

Driving   Passenger cars can make it to the Thomas Lakes Trailhead. The dirt road is well maintained and poses no difficult sections.

How to Get There   From Carbondale, go south on Colorado Highway 133. From the south end of town, go 0.92 mile from the intersection of CO 133 and the last major road, Snowmass Drive. Pay attention! You want to take a left onto Prince Creek Road, which is very easy to miss. It has an irregularly small blue sign, and it comes up just after passing the high school on your left. If you pass a fish hatchery on the right, you've gone too far.

Stay on the road as it passes through Bureau of Land Management lands. There will be signs for Dinkle Lake along the way. At mile 6.0, you'll come to a somewhat confusing junction. You want to bear right onto County Road 6A, which is marked with signs for Dinkle Lake; essentially this is your second right. The first right is a private road with a gate (which may or may not be open)—do not take it! Staying left on W. Sopris Road is also a mistake. Get on County Road 6A and stay the course as it climbs through aspen groves. At 1.85 miles, there is a parking area atop a hill (this comes up before Dinkle Lake). The parking area (on the left) has a large, fenced-off area for horse trailers, and a restroom. The Thomas Lakes Trail starts on the right (south) side of the road through a grassy meadow.

Fees/Camping   There are no fees to hike to camp in the area, though there may be a free permit system incorporated in the future. There are backcountry campsites at Thomas Lakes.

Route Notes   None.

Mile/Waypoint   **0.0 mi (1)**   Get on the marked Thomas Lakes Trail on the south side of the road. This trail starts as a single track through a grassy meadow and then joins a wider dirt "road" as it enters the woods. Note that the road is not used by automobiles—it's a snowmobile path. Stay on this trail as it climbs through the woods.

1.1 mi (2)   The Hay Park Trail splits to the left here; stay on the Thomas Lakes Trail.

1.7 mi (3)   There is another trail split; again stay right on the Thomas Lakes Trail as it goes up a hill to a grassy meadow. There are very good views of Carbondale from here.

3.7 mi (4)   After a pleasant walk through the forest, you arrive at the Maroon Bells-Snowmass Wilderness boundary. If the free permit system has been implemented, please take the time to fill one out. Just past this sign are the Thomas Lakes. Stay on the main trail that runs between the two of them. There is a signed trail for Mount Sopris in this area. Note that any side trails simply lead to backcountry campsites.

After passing the east lake, the trail begins to climb steadily on switchbacks to timberline.

4.9 mi At 11,060 feet, you clear treeline and have a good look at the ridge before you (as well as amazing views of the lakes and landscape to the north). The hardest section of hiking is coming up—a steep trail cut into the talus slopes en route to "Nopris." It's a lung-burner, even for veteran hikers!

5.7 mi (5) The strong push up the ridge leads to "Mount Nopris," officially, an unnamed 12,463-foot subpeak of the Sopris massif. You can skirt this summit to the left, or scramble up to the top. From here, the east summit looks huge. The little saddle between Nopris and the east summit is one of my favorites. Continue along the ridge westward to the broad East Sopris Summit.

6.5 mi (6) East Sopris Summit! This is the more spacious of the two tops, with room to stretch out and enjoy lunch. There is a register here and a wind shelter. When you are ready, continue west along the ridge to West Sopris Summit. This stretch is 0.9 mile one way on similar terrain, though the very end, near the west summit, is a bit rockier. There are some interesting homemade memorials just off the east summit on the west side: perhaps the ashes of a relative or a pet?

7.4 mi (7) West Sopris Summit! A skinny, 7-foot cairn seems to force the issue of which mountain is truly higher. Cheaters never win, West Sopris. Enjoy the views and return the way you came, bypassing the south side of East Sopris to save a little time. For a relatively long walk back, it does not get as tedious as other descents.

14.8 mi Finish.

Options There are no other routes to speak of on this hike; you're climbing on most of everything that is available. There are some alternate ridges on the north face you can try if you'd like a new way up. Good luck with the talus!

Quick Facts I once had an interesting encounter on Sopris. On my way down, I met a woman from Utah (her name slips my mind) who is a direct descendant of the man for whom the peak is named, Captain Richard Sopris. Captain Sopris surveyed the area in 1860 (he never climbed the peak), and went on to prominence as the mayor of Denver. His present-day relative had driven from Salt Lake City to see the mountain named after her great-great-great-grandfather. As afternoon storm clouds moved in, she realized she wouldn't make the summit. That's ok, since neither did her great-great-great-grandpa!

Nearby Carbondale takes its name from Carbondale, Pennsylvania. It was coincidence that coal mining later helped the economy flourish. Carbondale was originally a "feeder" town, providing potatoes and other foods to nourish the hungry miners working in the nearby silver mines of Aspen. "Potato Days" celebration in October is still a big event for the town.

Contact Info White River National Forest, Sopris Ranger District
620 Main Street
P.O. Box 309
Carbondale, CO 81623
(970) 963-2266

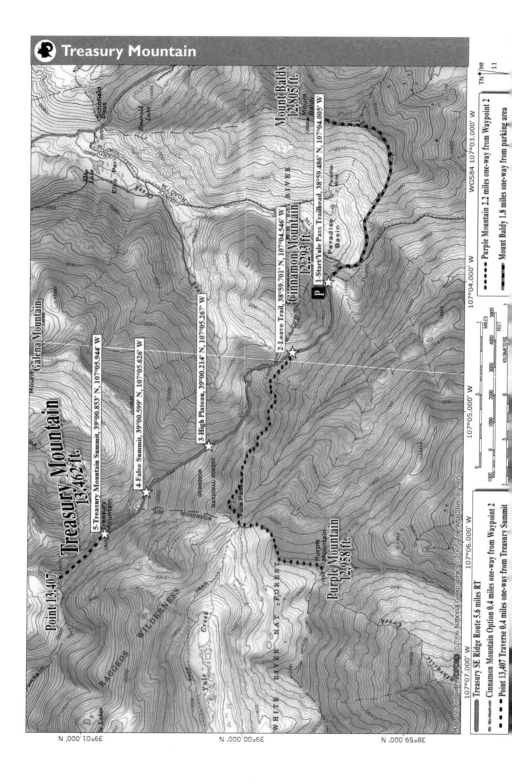

Treasury Mountain

Treasury Mountain 13,462 ft.

Point 13,407

5-Treasury Mountain Summit, 39°00.853' N, 107°05.944' W

4-False Summit, 39°00.599' N, 107°05.626' W

3-High Plateau, 39°00.214' N, 107°05.267' W

Cinnamon Mountain 12,293 ft.

2-Leave Trail 38°59.701' N, 107°04.546' W

1-Start/Yule Pass Trailhead, 38°59.486' N, 107°04.005' W

Mount Baldy 12,805 ft.

Purple Mountain 12,958 ft.

Schofield Pass

Mount Galena Mountain

Paradise Basin

Map created with TOPO!® ©2006 National Geographic (©2005 Lee's Atlas, Rel. 8/2005

Treasury SE Ridge Route 5.6 miles RT

Cinnamon Mountain Option 0.4 miles one-way from Waypoint 2

Point 13,407 Traverse 0.4 miles one-way from Treasury Summit

Purple Mountain 2.2 miles one-way from Waypoint 2

Mount Baldy 1.8 miles one-way from parking area

TN / MT 11

WGS84 107°03.000' W

MILES

FEET

KILOMETERS

107°04.000' W

107°05.000' W

107°06.000' W

107°07.000' W

RAGGEDS WILDERNESS

GUNNISON NATIONAL FOREST

WHITE RIVER NAT FOREST

PACK TRAIL

Yule Creek

36 Treasury Mountain

Often seen but seldom visited, Treasury Mountain is part of the awesome Raggeds Wilderness. The greatest treasure this mountain offers may be the dramatic views!

Round Trip Distance	5.6 miles
Hiking Time	4–6 hours
Difficulty	5.5/10
Class	2+
Start Elevation	11,350 ft., at Yule Pass Trailhead
Peak Elevation	13,462 ft.
Total Elevation Gain	2,127 ft.
Terrain	Off-trail ridge walk
Best Time to Climb	July–September
Gear Advisor	Normal gear
Crowd Level	Low

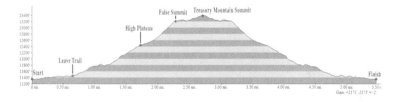

Location Elk Range in the Raggeds Wilderness/Gunnison National Forest and White River National Forest outside of Crested Butte

Intro The Elk Mountains are notorious for harsh weather, often holding onto patches of snow year-round. Treasury Mountain anchors the eastern reaches of a massif that serves as an intermediary between the Elks and the gradual declination of the Rocky Mountains to the west. Treasury is often seen from points in the Maroon Bells–Snowmass Wilderness, notably from West Maroon Pass. A great and little-known hike, Treasury is a part of Colorado that is a little more untamed than other areas!

Why Climb It? Treasury's setting brings to mind visions of the Greek underworld, with dark, stormy mountains and precipitous drop-offs into vertigo-inducing canyons. The area is wild, rugged, and teeming with elemental malice—storms that hit the area often unleash their fury with amplified force. Treasury sits on the edge of the turmoil, offering views to the benevolent Maroon Bells–Snowmass Wilderness peaks to the north, and to the more sinister-looking Raggeds Wilderness peaks to the south.

Of course, if you get a blue, sunny day, it's simply a heck of a mountain with incredible views. The ridge is a splendid experience, reaching a broad alpine plateau before the final summit push. The 300-million-year-old marine shale atop the peak is decorated with fossils of fish, plants, and shells—keep your eyes open. These may be the best treasures found on the mountain.

Driving Tough passenger cars can make it the Yule Pass Trailhead, though it may be a dramatic experience. Schofield Pass is a maintained dirt road; the last 2.5 miles on Paradise Divide Road are rougher. The road is generally passable and in good shape, but there is one particular hill that low-powered vehicles will strain to climb (my Accord barely made it up, floored and in first gear).

How to Get There From Crested Butte, follow Colorado Highway 135 north out of town to Gothic Road (Forest Service Road 317). Pass Mount Crested Butte and continue on Gothic Road, which turns to dirt. Follow this road 10.5 miles to Schofield Pass, bypassing the mysterious town of Gothic en route. At the top of Schofield Pass, 10,707 feet, turn left (west) onto Paradise Divide Road (County Road 734). The road gets a little rougher as it drops down to the flats of Elko Park. Stay left at 0.6 mile, and head up a steep hill that will challenge four-cylinder vehicles. At 1.6 miles, stay right on the main road at the junction with an old 4x4 road. At 2.3 miles, you'll reach the flats of Paradise Divide, where the road splits. The left split will go downhill, and there will be two roads uphill to the right—both lead to Yule Pass Trailhead. Take the one farther right, as the other is a gratuitous 4x4 road. The road will have signs giving the mileage to Yule Pass; note that this is the distance to the actual pass, not the parking area. Proceed 0.2 mile to the Yule Pass Trailhead (which isn't marked; the road reaches a closure gate near a small pond with spaces for about five or six vehicles).

Fees/Camping There are no fees to camp or hike in this area. There are dozens of magnificent camping areas along Schofield Pass and the Paradise Divide Road. You can pitch a tent in the area around the trailhead, but the ground is a bit lumpy.

Route Notes None.

Mile/Waypoint **0.0 mi (1)** Start at the Yule Pass Trailhead and proceed on the Yule Pass Trail. This rocky but solid trail is cut into the hillside and has amazing views of the Slate River Canyon to the left (south).

0.7 mi (2) At the low saddle between Cinnamon and Treasury mountains, leave the trail and gain the southeast ridge of Treasury Mountain. There is no trail on the ridge, but the spine is easy to follow as it curves northwest. This ridge undulates as it heads toward the mountain's highest point, now visible on the horizon.

1.8 mi (3) After climbing a few hills, you'll come to a broad plateau and slope with very good views. Push northwest up the hill, hiking just to the left (east) of the ridge for the best footing.

2.3 mi (4) Oh, man! After that big push up the long slope, the highpoint on the ridge turns out to be a false summit at 13,215 feet. Luckily, the plateau over to the summit is mild and has quite an ethereal atmosphere. Follow the plateau to a short, enjoyable scramble to the summit.

2.8 mi (5) Treasury Mountain Summit. Look at the rocks beneath your feet—fossils abound. From here, you can continue your trek northeast to the Treasure Mountain massif via the optional northwest ridge. Otherwise, return down the ridge the way you came.

5.6 mi Finish.

Options   There are lots of options from Treasury to extend your day. The most obvious side trip is a quick but steep 0.4-mile push up to Cinnamon Mountain Summit (only 0.8 mile, round trip, from waypoint 2).

From waypoint 2, stay on the Yule Pass Trail to Yule Pass, and challenge the north ridge of Purple Mountain, a class 3 scramble to Treasury's sister summit.

From the parking lot (or Paradise Divide), it's 1.8 miles one way to the eastern summit of Mount Baldy; this is a nice hike that gives you great views of Treasury.

Finally, traverse northwest from Treasury's summit to Point 13,407, one of the high peaks that grace the Treasure Mountain massif to the northwest.

One option not on the map is a trek down Treasury Mountain's east ridge (from the false summit, waypoint 4) to Galena Mountain. It is 1.5 miles one way from the false summit to Galena's top.

Quick Facts   Treasury Mountain is so named for the silver mines that were dug into its flanks. There were many mining camps set up in the area, with mixed results.

A few of the features in the area, including Yule Pass and North Pole Basin, are based on a Christmas theme.

Contact Info   White River National Forest
Aspen Ranger District
806 W. Hallam
Aspen, CO 81611
(970) 925-3445

Gunnison National Forest
Gunnison Ranger District
216 N. Colorado
Gunnison, CO 81230
(970) 641-0471

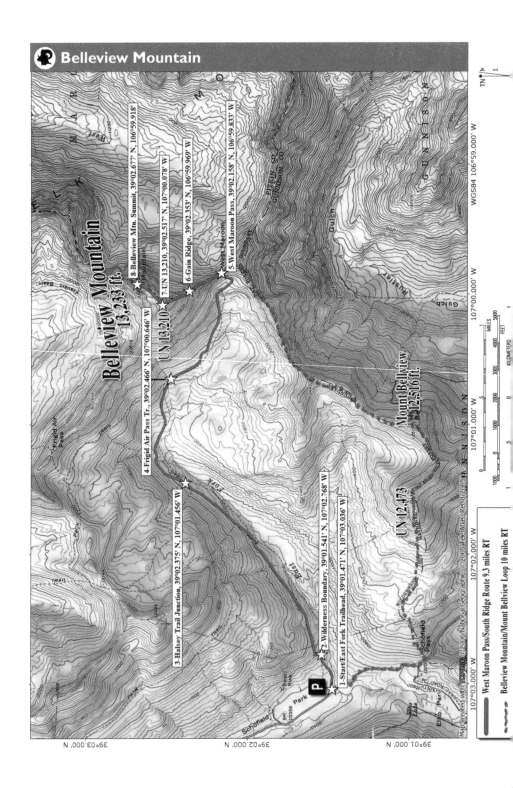

Belleview Mountain

Belleview Mountain
13,233 ft.

8-Belleview Mtn. Summit, 39°02.677' N, 106°59.918'
7-UN 13,210, 39°02.517' N, 107°00.078' W
6-Gain Ridge, 39°02.353' N, 106°59.969' W
5-West Maroon Pass, 39°02.158' N, 106°59.833' W

UN 13,210

4-Frigid Air Pass Tr., 39°02.466' N, 107°00.646' W

3-Halsey Trail Junction, 39°02.375' N, 107°01.456' W

Mount Belleview
12,516 ft.

UN 12,473

2-Wilderness Boundary, 39°01.541' N, 107°02.768' W

1-Start/East Fork Trailhead, 39°01.471' N, 107°03.036' W

P

Map created with TOPO!® ©2006 National Geographic; ©2005 Trek Atlas. Rev8/2005 R.

West Maroon Pass/South Ridge Route 9.3 miles RT

Belleview Mountain/Mount Belleview Loop 10 miles RT

37   Belleview Mountain

Belleview's name doesn't pull any punches: you'll have spectacular views of the fabled Maroon Bell peaks. A fine scramble to the summit has a few hidden surprises as well...

Round Trip Distance	9.3 miles
Hiking Time	6–8 hours
Difficulty	8/10
Class	3
Start Elevation	10,410 ft., at East Fork Trailhead
Peak Elevation	13,233 ft.
Total Elevation Gain	3,120 ft.
Terrain	Good trail leads to scrambling on crumbly, semisolid rock
Best Time to Climb	Late June–September
Gear Advisor	Boots that do well in loose scree, helmet
Crowd Level	Low on peak; moderate on trail

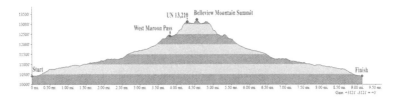

Location   Elk Mountains in the Maroon Bells–Snowmass Wilderness/White River National Forest just outside of Crested Butte or Aspen, depending on your approach

Intro   The Maroon Bells are amongst the most popular and photographed mountains in Colorado. When it comes to hiking them, it's a different story. The stratified layers of ruddy rock hide a shell of molting marine shale that makes hiking unstable and loose. Belleview offers a nice change of pace from its more photogenic neighbors to the north. Terrain on Belleview is still loose, but the ridge from West Maroon Pass has good scrambling and less exposure. Views from the summit are incredible, as this peak is centrally located between Aspen and Crested Butte. If you're thinking of challenging the big bells, why not preview this nifty 13er first? You may prefer it to its 14er kin!

Why Climb It?   Belleview's south ridge starts from the top of West Maroon Pass, a beautiful trail that runs from Aspen to Crested Butte. No matter which approach you prefer, you're already a winner—views of the Elk Mountains on both sides of the pass are exquisite. The ridge on Belleview has a tricky start, but the scrambling is fun and you always have an "out" on the west side of the mountain. Once you clear a trio of rocky obstacles, you have a clean line up to Unnamed Peak 13,210 (a nice peak in its own right). The short stroll between UN 13,210 and Belleview reveals wild rock formations and great views of Halsey Basin and the Maroon Bells. Much of the brown rock you'll see is hardened mud that once lined the bottom on an ancient sea. I have found several fossils in this area, including dozens of seashells.

Driving Tough passenger cars can make it to the East Fork Trailhead. (The dirt road to Schofield Pass was in very good shape in the summer of 2006. The only part that was tough on my car was the rutted-out parking lot.)

How to Get There From the town of Crested Butte, follow Highway 135 north, where it becomes Gothic Road (County Road 317). Pass the resort village of Mount Crested Butte and stay on Gothic Road north of town as it turns to dirt. This road is maintained and is passable by cars, though in rainy weather it can get mucky. From the start of the dirt road, it's 10.5 miles to the top of Schofield Pass. Note that you'll pass the eerie "research town" of Gothic, which I am convinced is a zombie-testing facility, 4.0 miles up the road.

Go over the pass 1.0 mile north to the large, rutted parking area; East Fork Trailhead is on your right (east) side, just after a shallow stream crossing.

Fees/Camping There are no fees to hike or camp in this area. Campsites abound along Gothic Road, though you'll be fighting with mountain bikers for spots in the summer. More good camping can be found in Elko Park, which is just west of the Schofield Pass summit on Forest Service Road 519 (Paradise Divide Road).

Route Notes None.

Mile/Waypoint **0.0 mi (1)** Start at the East Fork Trailhead. Head east on the West Maroon Pass Trail #1970 and begin your adventure.

0.3 mi (2) There's a smashed cabin just before the wilderness boundary; go up a small hill to an expansive meadow. Continue along the West Maroon Pass Trail. There are a few faint side trails along the way; just stay the course on the well-worn main trail.

Note: On some maps, this trail appears to follow the flat land directly next to East Fork Creek. Do not go down to the river! The trail is actually side-cut into the slope above the river, as shown on this map.

1.9 mi (3) A small sign in the grass denotes the split of the Halsey Trail to the left (west). Go right and remain on the West Maroon Pass Trail as it begins to arc east.

2.8 mi (4) The junction for Frigid Air Pass Trail cuts in to your left (north). Stay the course and continue on the main trail toward the pass. You won't be able to see Belleview yet, which is to the north (left), but you can see Unnamed Peak 13,210, which looks most impressive from the open alpine valley. The mountain on the ridge to your right (south) is Mount Bellview—not to be confused with Belleview Mountain.

3.9 mi (5) Hike up the mild switchbacks to the top of West Maroon Pass. You finally get your first views of Belleview Mountain from here. The ridge to the summit is on your left. Ditch any trekking poles here and get ready to scramble.

The crux of this scramble is the first 0.3 mile from the pass to waypoint 6. The terrain is easy class 3 but rather crumbly, so you'll need to be keen in your route-finding. Staying to the left (west) side offers the path of least resistance. There's a brief, grayish scree gully that avoids the steepest-looking pinnacle. Don't stray too far from the spine of the ridge, which you will rejoin at waypoint 6.

4.2 mi (6) After clearing the initial obstacles, gain the broad ridge and enjoy the easy class 2 terrain to the summit of UN 13,210.

4.4 mi (7) Go up and over this fine 13er and continue north to the obvious summit pyramid of Belleview Mtn. Views here are sublime!

As you near the base of the Belleview's final scramble, the way up may not be obvious. If you traverse to the east and northeast faces, you'll find lots of good chutes that will offer easy class 3 scrambles to the top.

4.6 mi (8) Belleview Mountain's summit! You can't beat the views from here. To the north is the enormous bulk of South Maroon Peak (also known as Maroon Peak). To the northeast, Pyramid Peak dominates a striated ridgeline. To the west is the Treasure Mountain massif, including Treasury Mountain, another fine hike (Hike 36) in this book.

Watch your step on the way down, and return the way you came.

9.3 mi Finish.

Options If ridge walks are your thing, try the optional exit that goes south from West Maroon Pass and follows a class 3 ridge over to Mount Bellview and Unnamed Peak 12,473. Follow the southwest ridge of UN 12,437 down to Schofield Pass; almost all of this route will be easy to visually follow. It's possible to intersect with the fabled 401 Trail, one of Colorado's best mountain bike rides. Continue west to Schofield Pass and walk back down to your car. This option is roughly a 10-mile loop.

Quick Facts *Belle vue* in French means "beautiful view." This is a fitting name for the mountain and a double entendre, for Belleview offers great views of the Maroon Bells. Mount Bellview and Belleview Mountain have slightly different spellings, but that doesn't make me any less forgiving of the geographers who were too lazy to come up with original names.

Schofield Pass is named for the immortal B.F. Schofield, who mined for silver in this area in 1879. He ran his camp from Schofield Park, a quarter mile north of the East Fork Trailhead parking lot.

Contact Info Maroon Bells Wilderness/White River National Forest
Aspen Ranger District
806 W. Hallam
Aspen, CO 81611
(970) 925-3445

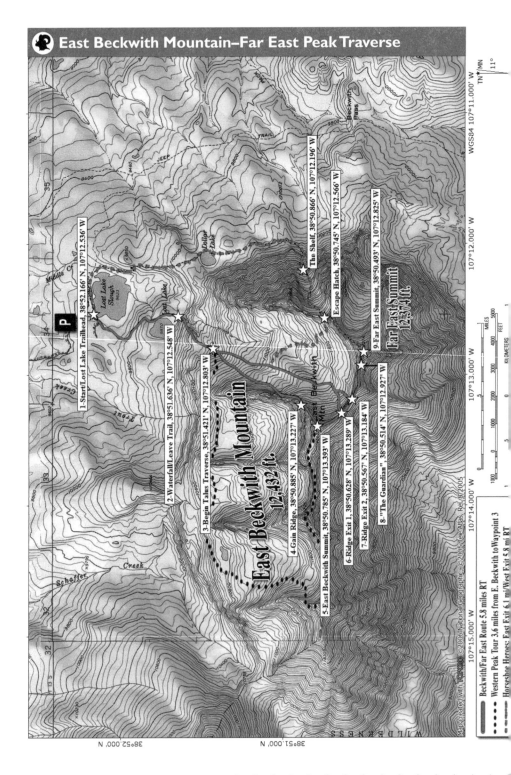

East Beckwith Mountain–Far East Peak Traverse

1-Start/Lost Lake Trailhead, 38°52.166' N, 107°12.536' W

2-Waterfall/Leave Trail, 38°51.636' N, 107°12.548' W

3-Begin Talus Traverse, 38°51.421' N, 107°12.803' W

4-Gain Ridge, 38°50.885' N, 107°13.227' W

5-East Beckwith Summit, 38°50.785' N, 107°13.393' W

6-Ridge Exit 1, 38°50.628' N, 107°13.289' W

7-Ridge Exit 2, 38°50.567' N, 107°13.184' W

8-"The Guardian", 38°50.514' N, 107°12.927' W

9-Far East Summit, 38°50.493' N, 107°12.825' W

The Shelf, 38°50.866' N, 107°12.196' W

Escape Hatch, 38°50.745' N, 107°12.566' W

East Beckwith Mountain 12,432 ft.

Far East Summit 12,374 ft.

East Beckwith Mtn

Lost Lake Slough

Dollar Lake

Beckwith Pass

Beckwith/Far East Route 5.8 miles RT
Western Peak Tour 3.6 miles from E. Beckwith to Waypoint 3
Horseshoe Heroes: East Exit 6.1 mi/West Exit 5.8 mi RT

Map created with TOPO!© ©2006 National Geographic; ©2005 Tele Atlas, Rel. 8/2005

38 East Beckwith Mountain–Far East Peak Traverse

The East Beckwith massif looks as cool in person as it does on the map. Go for the twin summits or saddle up your courage and go for the optional Horseshoe Heroes loop!

Round Trip Distance	5.8 miles
Hiking Time	5–7 hours
Difficulty	7.5/10
Class	2+/3
Start Elevation	9,625 ft., at Lost Lake Trailhead
Peak Elevations	East Beckwith Mountain: 12,432 ft.;
	Far East Peak: 12,374 ft.
Total Elevation Gain	3,000 ft.
Terrain	Trail to rocky, talus ridge and basin; mostly off-trail
Best Time to Climb	July–October
Gear Advisor	Normal gear, GPS
Best Time to Climb	July–October
Crowd Level	Low

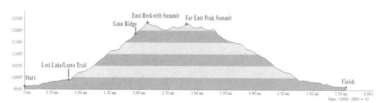

Location Elk Mountain in the Raggeds Wilderness/Gunnison National Forest outside of Paonia/Crested Butte

Intro East Beckwith is a remarkable glacially carved massif that is in the heart of aspen country. Many people consider the drive to the trailhead via Kebler Pass the most scenic in Colorado; it's a favorite of tourists, mountain bikers, campers, and runners. At Lost Lake, East Beckwith's rocky horseshoe of peaks rises to the south like an incredible, natural coliseum. The peak sees few visitors, however, due to a lack of trail and a tough talus field below the ridges. If you're up for a little work, the trip to the top is worth it. And if you're up for some *real* work, try the rough Horseshoe Heroes Loop to get most of the peaks above the basin.

Why Climb It? These peaks give hikers something lacking in most areas: an untamed mountain that is raw, rugged, and challenging—but has easy access. Most of the hike is off-trail, and while it's easy to navigate, it's on some very loose and unsettled talus fields in sections. All that is forgotten once you gain the ridged rim of the horseshoe, which bestows a good class 2+/3 scramble to Beckwith's isolated summit. A short walk over to "Far East Peak" is part of the standard route. Incredible views are everywhere, especially of the high Elk Range peaks to the north in Aspen (the Maroon Bells, Treasury Mountain, etc.). If you're a fan of truly rugged off-trail mayhem, the Horseshoe Heroes Loop is waiting.

Driving Passenger cars can make it to the trailhead. Kebler Pass is a maintained dirt road with a few rough spots; under normal conditions, all vehicles can make this beautiful drive. This applies to both sides of the pass.

How to Get There The access road to Lost Lake Trailhead is off Kebler Pass Road (County Road 12) on the west side of the pass. It's approximately 15 miles from either entrance on the pass.

To access the trailhead from Crested Butte (east side), take the Kebler Pass Road (County Road 12/Whiterock Avenue) west off Highway 135; this turn is right in town. Follow the road 16 miles up and over the pass, and turn left (south) onto Forest Service Road 706; follow the signs for LOST LAKE SLOUGH/CAMPGROUND. It's 2.2 miles on FS 706 to the Lost Lake Slough Trailhead and Campground; at 2.0 miles the road forks, and the parking area is to the left.

From the west side, locate the junction of Colorado Highway 133 and CR 12, about 14.0 miles north of Paonia. This turn is just south of Paonia Reservoir. If you're taking this route from the north, go over McClure Pass and turn east onto County Road 12 after the long reservoir. Note that this road has a lot of signs, but none that explicitly says it is CR 12 (look for Kebler Pass signs instead). Follow it 15.2 miles and turn right (south) onto FS 706—again, there will be signs for Lost Lake Campground. It is 2.2 miles to the trailhead on this road; the parking area is to the left at mile 2.0 (where the road forks).

Fees/Camping There are no fees to hike in the area or to camp at the primitive sites. The developed sites at the campground at Lost Lake Slough are $10 per night, though there are plenty of places to pull off on Kebler Pass and car camp for free.

Route Notes None.

Mile/Waypoint **0.0 mi (1)** Start at the Lost Lake Trailhead. Go south on the Three Lakes Trail #843 toward Lost Lake. This is a pleasant introduction on a good trail; note that the large body of water in front of you is Lost Lake Slough, not Lost Lake. (Slough, meaning: an area of soft, muddy ground; swamp or swamplike region.)

0.8 mi (2) After a "river crossing" on the north side of Lost Lake, continue to the east shore on trail. At a bend in the trail where a waterfall meets the lake, go off-trail. Cross the waterfall and begin a climb up to the basin. This off-trail section is not difficult, but it is steep. Gradually diverge southwest from the waterfall, where the ridge is easier to hike up. The goal is to get into the basin at this point, not onto the north ridge. The north ridge may look good from here, but just out of view it reaches a broken section that is difficult to climb.

1.2 mi (3) At the base of the talus basin, the real grunt work of the hike begins. Even though the boulders here are a good size, the footing is still bad. A lot of the rocks are unstable, so test your steps. You are better off staying left on the flatter section for the time being and making the push up to the north ridge in one effort. As you get higher, you'll be able to scan the north ridge for a good line up. I waited until I was past the broken gap

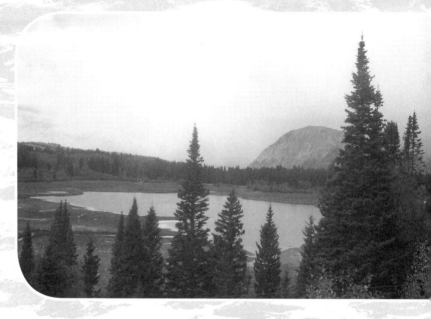

st Lake Slough is where your adventure begins.

and then made my way to the ridge via a strong push at mile 1.9. You'll need route-finding skills to find the best way up; it's steep but still class 2 talus terrain.

2.0 mi (4) At 11,880 feet, you're on the ridge proper, and the hard part is easy class 3 move will get you over small outcrops. There is some exposure, but the ridge never gets narrow enough to freak out about. Carry on south to the summit.

2.2 mi (5) East Beckwith Summit. It's a photographer's dream up here. Continue on toward Far East Summit via the southeast ridge.

2.5 mi (6 and 7) In the saddle between East Beckwith and Far East, I have marked two good exit chutes that return to the talus basin. You may want to take one or the other on the way back. These are both easy class 3 scrambles and are preferable to returning to the north ridge to descend.

2.8 mi (8) "The Guardian" is a formidable-looking rock section that is the last obstacle before Far East's summit. Once you are up close, it turns out to be a piece of cake! Easy class 2 scrambling will grant you passage to the top.

2.9 mi (9) Far East Peak's summit! There are great views of East Beckwith from here. There's no easy way down; returning to the saddle and dropping down at waypoint 6 or 7 (6 is the easiest) is the way to go. Once you are in the talus basin, return the way you came. You can use the waterfall as a guide to get you back to Lost Lake if you are without a GPS, or if you aren't handy with a compass. Once on the trail, it's an easy hike back.

5.8 mi Finish. The mileage for this hike isn't a lot, but you'll be tired. Why not enjoy the rest of the day at this lovely area? I hear the fishing in these lakes is quite good...

Options From East Beckwith's summit, you have some major options. The first is a westward traverse that goes over several unnamed peaks and drops down in the farthest cirque. From there, skirt east along the base of the massif and return to the top of the waterfall. This option tacks 3.6 miles onto your route, from the top of East Beckwith back to waypoint 3.

The Horseshoe Heroes route is for expert scramblers only, and you may want to bring a helmet along. Once you get to Far East, continue north to several unnamed peaks that are connected by a sloping, and at times narrow, ridge. This is exciting stuff! You'll pass through a neat rock gap as you descend; it's class 3 downclimbing most of the way. The rock is rotten in places, so test all your handholds. At several points, there are steep but feasible scrambles that break off west, back into the talus basin. At the "Escape

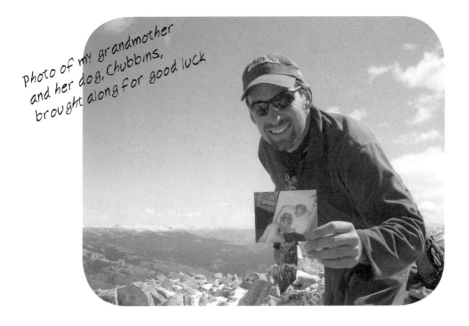

Photo of my grandmother and her dog, Chubbins, brought along for good luck

Hatch" waypoint is probably the best way back (via the western chutes). Me, I decided to make things difficult for myself and go east.

Note that a straight traverse north over the final northern peak gets into class 3+ or 4 terrain on broken rock—no fun! You'll need to exit the ridge; west is better, but I went east for a steep crawl down to a wide gully. On the map, it looks like a good way to close the loop. If you choose to take the recommended direction to exit, you're wise enough to find your own way down to Lost Lake Slough and back out. On the other hand, if you make the foolhardy choice of following in my misbegotten footsteps, the following account may be useful.

After a steep, knee-grinding descent on snowy talus, I reached the halfway point in the gully, only to find that it's almost entirely cliffed out. At "the Shelf," I traversed left (north) into the shrubs, where the terrain is passable—though a hiker needs great route-finding skills to reach the bottom of this gully. At times it was quite fun, sliding through tunnels of shrubs and grabbing their roots to prevent myself from skidding off 10- to 12-foot cliffs. Finally, I made my way down. Looking up at the cliffed-out section, I saw a prime wall for ice climbing come winter…interesting. I then skirted northwest to Dollar Lake, where a nice class 1 trail led me home. Do I recommend this route? Not really. Did I have a blast doing it? Absolutely!

Quick Facts   This mountain is named for Lieutenant E.G. Beckwith, who joined Captain John Gunnison on his surveying trip to the area in 1853. West Beckwith Mountain is not connected to the East Beckwith massif; a low saddle separates the two, but it is possible to climb them both in one long day. (While sitting in my car after the hike, I was reading a Dave Barry article about anagrams. Thus inspired, I discovered the letters in "East Beckwith" can be arranged to read "be a thick stew" and "beast chew kit.")

Kebler Pass is named for J.A. Kebler, who served as an official for the Colorado Fuel and Iron Company.

Contact Info   Gunnison National Forest
Paonia Ranger District
P.O. Box 1030
N. Rio Grande Avenue
Paonia, CO 81428
(970) 527-4131

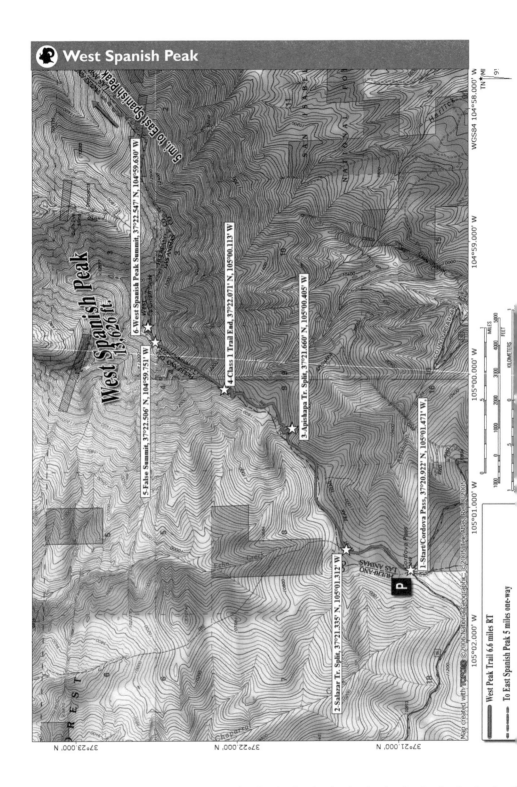

West Spanish Peak

West Spanish Peak
13,626 ft.

6-West Spanish Peak Summit, 37°22.547' N, 104°59.630' W

5-False Summit, 37°22.506' N, 104°59.751' W

4-Class 1 Trail End, 37°22.071' N, 105°00.113' W

3-Apishapa Tr. Split, 37°21.660' N, 105°00.405' W

2-Salazar Tr. Split, 37°21.335' N, 105°01.312' W

1-Start/Cordova Pass, 37°20.922' N, 105°01.471' W

5mi. to East Spanish Peak

To East Spanish Peak 5 miles one-way

West Peak Trail 6.6 miles RT

Map created with TOPO!® ©2006 National Geographic; ©2005 Tele Atlas, Rel. 8/2005

39 West Spanish Peak

The contrast between the enormous Spanish Peaks and the surrounding farmland is striking. These standalone mountains dominate the southern landscape and offer good climbs.

Round Trip Distance	6.6 miles
Hiking Time	4–6 hours
Difficulty	6/10
Class	2
Start Elevation	11,256 ft., at Cordova Pass
Peak Elevation	13,626 ft.
Total Elevation Gain	2,929 ft.
Terrain	Good trail leading to a rocky summit push
Best Time to Climb	May–September
Gear Advisor	Trekking poles
Crowd Level	Moderate

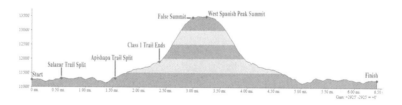

Location   Sangre De Cristo Range in the Spanish Peaks Wilderness/San Isabel National Forest south of the small town of La Veta

Intro   Gazing at the gargantuan profile of the Spanish Peaks for the first time, I got the *I can't believe I'll be standing on the top of that tomorrow* feeling. The two mountains that make up the Spanish Peaks explode from a flat valley, dominating the landscape with pure, massive, mountain goodness. Only Mount Sopris (which is very similar in design) rivals the Spanish Peaks in perceived height. The entire mountain is flanked on all sides by the Great Spanish Dykes—long walls of rock that fortify the lowlands.

Why Climb It?   West Spanish Peak is the lower of the two mountains (the other being 13,683-foot East Spanish Peak). When mountains rise straight out of the ground like West Spanish, you are guaranteed spectacular views. To the south, the views open up into New Mexico, including the distant Wheeler Peak, at 13,161 feet, the state highpoint. "Forbidden" Culebra Peak and the Culebra Range dominate the western horizon. (Culebra Peak is the only privately owned 14er; the owners charge $100 per person to hike it.) To the north, the fortress-like Mount Blanca group juts into the clouds.

The Spanish Dykes look like manmade walls, but are in fact natural formations (more on this in the "Quick Facts" section). In addition to the views, this is a good hike, with a graceful prelude trail leading to a challenging and steep summit pyramid.

Driving Passenger cars can make it to Cordova Pass without any trouble, thanks to J.J. Cordova's dream come true (read more on him in "Quick Facts"); the dirt road is well maintained.

How to Get There Find the intersection of US Highway 160 west and Colorado Highway 12, roughly 7.0 miles west of the town of Walsenburg (located in southern Colorado along Interstate 25). Turn left (south) onto CO 12 and stay on this road for 22.3 miles, heading for Cucharas Pass. You will go through the small town of La Veta (follow the signs for CO 12 through town). After passing La Veta, keep your eyes out for the walls of the Spanish Dykes on your left (east). Drive past the village of Cuchara and continue all the way to Cucharas Pass. At mile 22.3, turn left onto the dirt road to Cordova Pass (Las Animas County Road 46). Another 6.0 miles will bring you to the top of the pass, and to the trailhead for West Spanish Peak.

Fees/Camping There is a $4 day-use charge for hiking in the Spanish Peaks Wilderness. There is a self-pay box at the trailhead. There are also a few campsites, which are $6 per night; at the time I visited the area, there were only six sites available. Note that if you camp up here, there are no water sources, so bring enough for camping and the hike.

Route Notes None.

Mile/Waypoint **0.0 mi (1)** Start on the north side of Cordova Pass on the West Peak Trail. The first 2.5 miles of this class 1 trail are nearly flat, taking you through forests and open meadows. At the onset of the hike, there is a plaque on a rock (on the right) that proclaims the Spanish Peaks designation as a National Natural Landmark. Stay on the West Peak Trail.

0.3 mi (2) There is a split for the very faint Salazar Trail to the left (west); stay on the main West Peak Trail.

1.5 mi (3) Pay attention at mile 1.5. The Apishapa Trail splits from the West Peak Trail. There is a hard-to-notice brown forest marker designating the split. The mellow pace of the trail up to this point can lull you into not noticing that the Apishapa Trail goes straight (then turns southeast). You need to turn left (northeast) to remain on the West Peak Trail.

2.4 mi (4) At a clearing with good views, the formal class 1 trail ends. You will be at the base of the southwest ridge, which you will climb to reach the top. Get off-trail and prepare for a 1,500-foot push to the top.

Note that there are a few cairned trails and worn paths on the way up. It gets very rocky; the less crumbly stuff can be found just below the ridge on your left (north) side. If you stay on the southwest face, the rocks will be loose and frustrating. Staying left gives you better footing. About halfway up, there are random wind shelters built into the mountain at various points, some on trails, some not. Continue your push, aiming for the highest point you see.

3.1 mi (5) Surprise! After all that work, you're at a false summit! At 13,450 feet, it really isn't that bad. The remaining 180 vertical feet are on easy, relatively flat terrain.

3.4 mi (6) West Spanish Peak's true summit is the first major rock pile/cairn that you encounter on this summit block. There is a register here. I swore that the gleaming, large cairn to the northeast was the top when I first got here. It *looks* higher from the true summit. However, after taking the short walk over to it, my GPS reported it as being slightly lower. And, to add to the optical confusion, now the *real* summit looked higher. Just to be sure you've topped out, visit them both.

Descend the way you came up, picking your best line down the mountain to return to the trees where the class 1 West Peak Trail terminated (waypoint 4). Pick up the trail again and follow it all the way back.

6.6 mi Finish.

Options
The cheese truly stands alone here! There aren't many options off West Spanish Peak. The obvious question is: can you do both peaks in one day? From the summit of West Spanish, you can follow the east ridge to a saddle that connects the two, and then ascend the west ridge of East Spanish Peak (not shown on this map). There is an intermittent trail. This option is class 2, but it's 5.0 miles one way from the summit of West Spanish Peak. Done as an out-and-back, that's over 17 miles. (If you are creative, you can make a one-way trip using two cars; however, since these peaks are a long drive

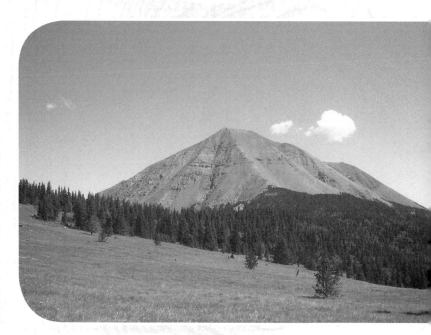

West Spanish Peak cuts an impressive profile.

from most areas, you'll probably only have one car at your disposal.) From the saddle between the two, a pack trail (#1304) heads north to Wahatoya Camp, a possible parking option for a second car if you were trying the two-car idea. It may be more fun to hike East Spanish Peak the next day. You can fill the post-hike afternoon with tours of the Great Spanish Dykes if you'd like more hiking.

Quick Facts
When explorer Zebulon Pike first saw the Spanish Peaks in 1806, he called them the Mexican Mountains. At that time, the peaks were still within the boundaries of Spanish-controlled territory, thus the name morphed into its present form.

Native people called the mountains Wahatoya, which translates to "the breasts of the earth." This proves that the lonely French fur trappers who dubbed the Grand Tetons in Wyoming weren't the only mountain men longing for the company of women.

Native tribes as widespread as the Apache and the Aztecs were familiar with the Spanish Peaks.

The striking geology, including the Spanish Dykes, was formed when continental pressures pushed the entire Sangre De Cristo Range sky high (irregularities in the uplifted plate explain the gaps between mountains in the range). Molten rock cooled in gaps under the earth, forming granite batholiths known as "stocks." (Batholith is a large body of intrusive igneous rock believed to have crystallized at a considerable depth below the earth's surface.) Some of these stocks formed in narrow veins and cracks in the earth; when the land was pushed up, these hard igneous batholiths went up as well. Both Spanish Peaks were formed this way; thus they are not true volcanic mountains. The dykes were pushed up with the peaks. When the sedimentary rock eroded, the tougher granite of the dykes remained, creating the long walls we see today.

There is an interesting sign at the top of Cordova Pass telling the story of Jose de Jesus Cordova and his dream of connecting the town of Aguilar and Cucharas Pass. Spurred on by his vision, the road was completed in 1934 and named after the man himself in 1978. It was a very practical dream, and he made it come true. Three cheers for J.J. Cordova!

Contact Info
San Isabel National Forest
Main Pueblo Office
2480 Kachina Drive
Pueblo, CO 81008
(719) 553-1400

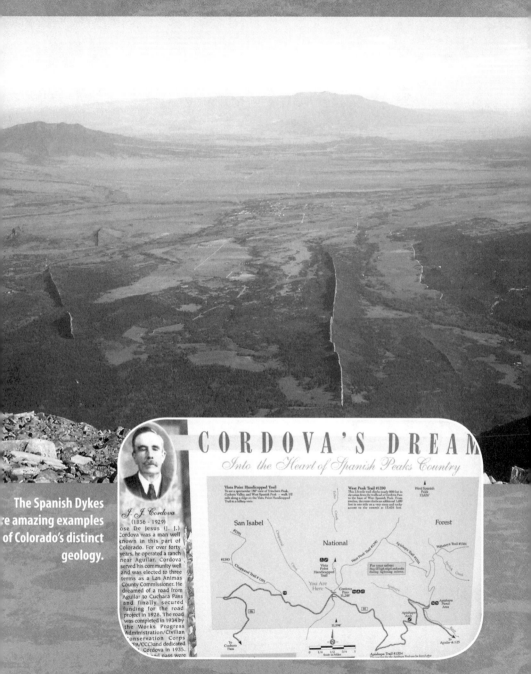

The Spanish Dykes
are amazing examples
of Colorado's distinct
geology.

J. J. Cordova
(1856 - 1929)

Jose De Jesus (J. J.)
Cordova was a man well
known in this part of
Colorado. For over forty
years, he operated a ranch
near Aguilar. Cordova
served his community well
and was elected to three
terms as a Las Animas
County Commissioner. He
dreamed of a road from
Aguilar to Cuchara Pass
and finally secured
funding for the road
project in 1928. The road
was completed in 1934 by
the Works Progress
Administration/Civilian
Conservation Corps
(WPA/CCC)and dedicated
to Cordova in 1935.
...and pass were

CORDOVA'S DREAM
Into the Heart of Spanish Peaks Country

Vista Point Handicapped Trail
To see a spectacular 180° view of Trinchera Peak,
Cuchara Valley, and West Spanish Peak — walk 1/2
mile along a ridge on the Vista Point Handicapped
Trail to a hilltop vista.

West Peak Trail #1390
This 2.6-mile trail climbs nearly 800 feet in
elevation from the trailhead at Cordova Pass
to the base of West Spanish Peak. From
treeline, the route climbs an additional 1,600
feet in one mile on a very steep and rocky
ascent to the summit at 13,626 feet.

West Spanish
Peak
13,626'

San Isabel

National

Forest

#1391

Dodson Creek

Chaparral Creek

#1390

Chaparral Trail #1391

Vista
Point
Handicapped
Trail

West Peak Trail #1390

Apishapa Trail #1324

Wahatoya Trail #1304

For your safety:
Stay off high ridges and peaks
during lightning storms.

Cordova
Pass
11,248'

You Are
Here

Apishapa Trail #1324

Southern

11,394'

Apishapa
Picnic
Area

Apishapa
Arch

To
Cuchara
Pass

0 1/4 1/2 3/4 1
Scale in Miles

To
Aguilar & I-25

Apishapa Trail #1324
The trailhead for the Apishapa Trail can be found after

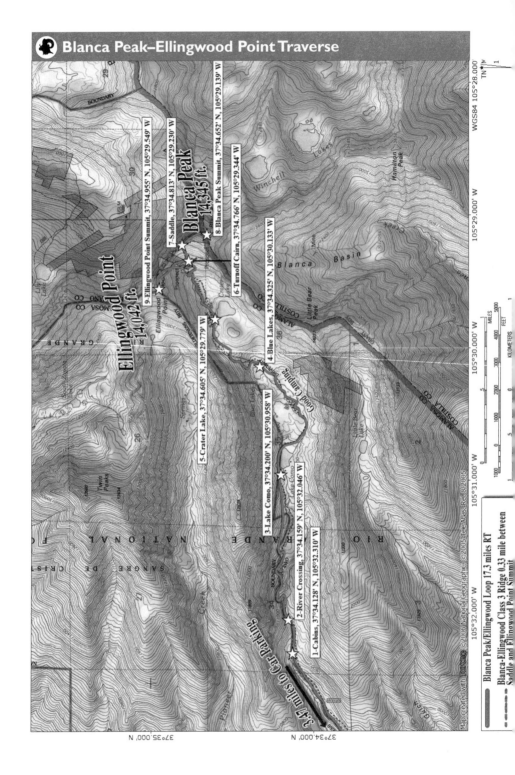

Blanca Peak–Ellingwood Point Traverse

Blanca Peak
14,345 ft.

Ellingwood Point
14,042 ft.

9-Ellingwood Point Summit, 37°34.955' N, 105°29.549' W
7-Saddle, 37°34.813' N, 105°29.230' W
8-Blanca Peak Summit, 37°34.652' N, 105°29.139' W
6-Turnoff Cairn, 37°34.766' N, 105°29.344' W
4-Blue Lakes, 37°34.325' N, 105°30.133' W
5-Crater Lake, 37°34.605' N, 105°29.779' W
3-Lake Como, 37°34.200' N, 105°30.958' W
2-River Crossing, 37°34.159' N, 105°32.046' W
1-Cabins, 37°34.128' N, 105°32.310' W

3.4 miles to Car Parking

Blanca Basin

Winchell Lakes

Hamilton Peak

Little Bear Peak

WGS84 105°28.000

TN★/N

105°29.000' W

105°30.000' W

105°31.000' W

105°32.000' W

3703 5,000' N

3703 4,000' N

Map created with TOPO! ©2000 National Geographic; ©2005 Tele Atlas, Rel. 8/2005

— Blanca Peak/Ellingwood Loop 17.3 miles RT
--- Blanca-Ellingwood Class 3 Ridge 0.33 mile between Saddle and Ellingwood Point Summit

MILES
FEET
KILOMETERS

40 Blanca Peak– Ellingwood Point Traverse

Good Overnight!

Blanca Peak is the high point of a high alpine oasis featuring a great scramble and magnificent scenery. This hard-earned peak is my favorite climb of all the 14ers.

Round Trip Distance	17.3 miles
Hiking Time	2 days (13–15 hours of hiking from car parking and trailhead)
Difficulty	7/10
Class	2+
Start Elevation	7,860 ft., at Lake Como Road (4x4s can start a few miles higher)
Peak Elevations	Blanca Peak: 14,345 ft.; Ellingwood Point: 14,042 ft.
Total Elevation Gain	7,225 ft.
Terrain	Long access road, good scramble to Blanca; loose scramble to Ellingwood
Best Time to Climb	May–September
Gear Advisor	Bug gear in mid-summer; backpacking boots; sandals for river crossing
Crowd Level	Low to moderate

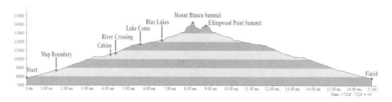

Location   Sangre De Cristo Range in the Rio Grande National Forest near the town of Alamosa

Intro   Blanca Peak is the sacred mountain of the east to the Navajo people. It's easy to see why Blanca Massif, home to three other 14ers, would inspire spiritual awe. At the base of the group, the land is dry and hot, evidenced by the nearby Great Sand Dunes National Monument. Elevated from the scorching heat, the secret alpine garden in the Blanca basin is an oasis of lakes, streams, and snow. Climb to the top of Blanca and traverse over to Ellingwood Point to grab your second 14er in one day.

This is a great overnight trip; the camping in Blanca's basin is incredible (though it may be buggy mid-summer). It is possible to climb these two peaks as an epic one-day hike, but you'll be missing out on the extraordinary experience of spending time in Blanca's covert campground.

Why Climb It?   Mount Blanca is the highest mountain in Colorado outside of the Sawatch Range. It is the king of the Sangre De Cristos and the fifth highest peak in Colorado (the eighth highest in the lower 48 states and 27th highest in the US). In the past, many people thought this was the highest Colorado mountain, and you can't blame them; Blanca cuts a much more regal profile than the state's true highpoint, the gentle giant Mount Elbert. The Lake Como Road that you'll be hiking up is a testpiece for advanced 4x4 drivers. Unlike other 4x4 roads in Colorado, this road is more like a wide class 2 trail that a few maniacs attempt to drive up. The stiff elevation gain (over 7,000 feet total) has a silver lining—you get to observe ecosystems gradually transform from parched desert land to lush meadows of alpine lakes. The hike up to Blanca's apex is a scrambler's delight, following a rocky but solid ridge to a small summit platform.

I added in Ellingwood Point for those hoping to bag another 14er. The class 2 traverse over from Blanca is a pain. (I find staying high on the ridge, which is a class 3 option, preferable.) The rock is very loose and the angle is steep, meaning you'll be spinning your wheels all the way up and slippin' and slidin' all the way down. It does have some great views, especially of Blanca, but it's a scrappier climb.

Driving   Passenger cars and TPCs should park 1.5 miles up the road, before it gets super rocky. Sport utility cars, SUVs, jeeps, and 4x4s will be able to push it another 2 to 3 miles before the obstacles get too great—look for good turnoffs to park before it gets too late (see sidebar, "Good Spots to Park SUVs and 4x4s Along the Lake Como Road" on page 259). Only true, dedicated, modified 4x4s with super-high clearance, mega-suspension, and necessary adaptations (like winches and roll cages) should attempt the drive to reach Lake Como.

How to Get There   Find the intersection of US 160 and US 150; this is roughly 26 miles east of the Alamosa. Those coming from the metro areas will probably pick up 160 in the town of Walsenburg. Turn north onto Hwy. 150, which will have a sign for the Great Sand Dunes National Monument. Follow this road for 3.2 miles and turn right (this turnoff is not well marked, so be sure to check your odometer). You'll go over a grate and find yourself in a very sandy lot. This is the start of the fabled Lake Como Road, also known as Forest Service Road 975 and hiking trail #886. All passenger cars can drive to the large lot on the left (north) side of the road at mile 1.5. If you value your car, park here. SUCs and SUVs can struggle up another 2.0 miles and park at one of the pulloffs along the way. Jeeps and 4x4s can likely get to mile 4.5; after that, the only vehicles capable of clearing the road are specialized 4x4s, driven by experienced (i.e. crazy) drivers.

Fees/Camping   There are no fees to hike and camp in this part of the Rio Grande National Forest. Be aware that if you camp on the lower part of the road, there will be no water sources.

Route Notes This hike begins 1.5 miles up Lake Como Road at the car parking area. From the paved road (CO 150), the road is 7.3 miles to Lake Como. From the car parking area, the first good campsites at Lake Como are at 5.8 miles, though the better spots are a bit higher, around mile 6.0. Please note that mile 0.0 in the hike description is 1.5 miles up Lake Como Road.

Good Spots to Park SUVs and 4x4s Along the Lake Como Road

These mileages are measured from the start of the Lake Como Road, where it intersects with 150.

1.5 mi Car parking; a good place to drop a trailer if you brought ATVs to get up the road: 37°32.147′ N, 105°34.825′ W

2.5 mi Parking/camping spot 1: 37°32.734′ N, 105°33.992′ W

3.1 mi Parking/camping spot 2: 37°33.067′ N, 105°33.6′ W

3.8 mi SUV max camp (farthest recommended point for SUVs and SUCs): 37°33.413′ N,105°33.469′ W

4.2 mi 4x4 camp 1: 37°33.591′ N, 105°33.321′W

4.8 mi High 4x4 camp: 37°33.713′ N, 105°32.99′ W

These are just my suggestions; you are welcome to bash your vehicle as you see fit. Amazingly, the highest "normal" vehicle I saw on the trail was parked at mile 5.5, which is just before the first 4x4-exclusive obstacle, known as "Jaws 1." More amazingly, this vehicle was a Suzuki XL7.

For those of you who are curious, the three "Jaws" obstacles can be found at miles 5.74, 6.31, and 6.64. You'll know them when you see them.

For those of you who are curious, the three "Jaws" obstacles can be found at miles 5.74, 6.31 and 6.64. You'll know them when you see them.

Mile/Waypoint **Note:** This description assumes a two-day trip with an overnight in the Lake Como Area.

0.0 mi (off map) Start at mile 1.5 on the Lake Como Road. Walk up the road as it starts in shrubs, passes through aspen, and eventually reaches Lake Como. The main road is easy to follow; the few side roads you see are mostly parking areas.

You have at least 5.8 miles to go before reaching comfortable campsites around Lake Como.

4.1 mi (1) At 10,510 feet, you'll pass some cabins on your right. You're getting closer!

4.4 mi (2) There is a sizeable river crossing here, even if you're on foot. After this, the big rock obstacles in the road seem impossible to pass in a vehicle, but people do it.

5.6 mi (3) Finally, you are at Lake Como. There is decent camping here, but for better sites, look between here and the Blue Lakes at mile 6.7. Just above Lake Como are good sites in the trees. If you prefer to camp above treeline, there are lots of places around the Blue Lakes to pitch a tent. I would not recommend going to Crater Lake, as it is very rocky (though if you are determined to pitch a tent there, look to the south side of Crater Lake for a few flat, grassy spots).

6.7 mi (4) The Blue Lakes region, and incredibly, the formal end of the 4x4 road—at 12,200 feet! The trail finally becomes suitable strictly for foot traffic; follow it northeast and stay on the right (east) side of the Blue Lakes. Past the Blue Lakes, head up the rocky and steep slope to Crater Lake. Stay on the left (west) side of Crater Lake and the small sublake that precedes it.

7.3 mi (5) Crater Lake. From here, you must go northeast toward the saddle between Blanca and Ellingwood Point. The trail has cairns occasionally, but the Colorado Mountain Club has blazed the "official" trail with whisker markers in the ground. Follow these for the easiest route to the saddle.

7.8 mi (6) Stay right at this cairned intersection and continue toward the saddle. (The left is the class 2 route to Ellingwood Point.)

8.0 mi (7) At 13,700 feet, gain the saddle. Turn east and begin a very enjoyable scramble on class 2+ terrain to Blanca's summit.

8.3 mi (8) Blanca's summit! Amazing, isn't it? It's obvious from this vantage that Blanca is considerably higher than Little Bear Peak and Ellingwood Point. Return down to waypoint 7. Those comfortable with class 3 scrambling can take the optional (and in my opinion, better) ridge walk to Ellingwood, though it is quite exposed and a little crumbly. Otherwise, return to waypoint 6.

8.7 mi (6) Back at the turnoff cairn, follow a faint trail north to the east ridge to Ellingwood Point. This slope is loose and the trail dissolves after a while. Slog up to the ridge, clear a minor false summit, and continue to the true summit of Ellingwood.

9.0 mi (9) Ellingwood's summit! The hike up isn't pretty, but the views sure are. Brace your knees for the descent on the loose rock and scree; find the best line down, and rejoin the main trail above Crater Lake. From Crater Lake, reverse your route back to your car.

17.3 mi Finish at the car parking lot. With luck, you were able to cut a few miles from this hike by driving to a higher starting point than I could reach in my Honda Accord.

Options This is such a long hike, you probably won't want to do much more. There is an option to climb 14,037-foot Little Bear Peak from the basin. It is a class 3+/4 route, and given its technical nature, is not covered in this book.

The option to stay high on the ridge between Blanca and Ellingwood has some good but exposed scrambling. This high traverse is only 0.33 mile one way from the "saddle" waypoint to Ellingwood's summit.

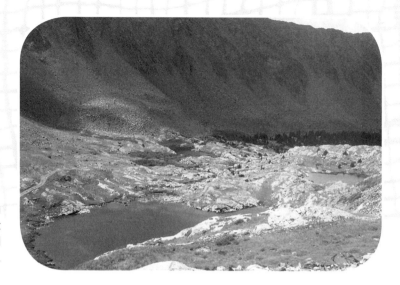

Camping in Blanca's basin is a pleasure. The best campsites can be found around Lake Como.

Blanca is one of the four sacred mountains of the Navajo. (Read more about the sacred mountains in the "Quick Facts" section for Hike 34 on page 231.) Blanca is Spanish for "white," a name that reflects the peak's often snowy summit.

Ellingwood Point was "officially" ratified as a 14er in 1990; before then, some considered it a mere subpeak of Blanca. The rule to determine if a peak is an official 14er is that the summit must be at least 0.25 mile from the "mother" peak, and there must be a saddle that drops at least 300 feet. between the two. After enough surveying, Ellingwood was welcomed into the club.

Ellingwood is fittingly named after Albert R. Ellingwood, a truly inno vative and bad-ass climber. He was one of the first three people to scale all the 14ers, including first ascents of Crestone Needle, Crestone Peak, and Kit Caron Peak—in 1916! Even more impressive was his gutsy ascent (with Barton Hoag) of the crumbling Lizard Head formation in 1920, an incredible feat at the time, as the 400-foot tower had to virtually be free-climbed. He also pioneered two major routes on 14ers: Ellingwood Ridge on La Plata Peak, and Ellingwood Arete on Crestone Needle.

When he wasn't putting up routes, this Rhodes Scholar taught political science at Colorado College. He died at the young age of 46, having lived more than most men twice his age.

Contact Info Rio Grande National Forest
1803 W. Hwy 160
Monte Vista, CO 81144
(719) 852-5941

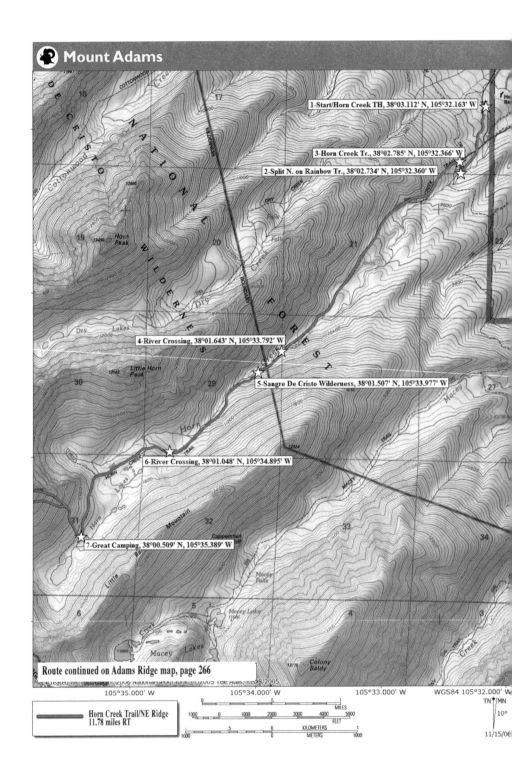

Mount Adams

1-Start/Horn Creek TH, 38°03.112' N, 105°32.163' W

3-Horn Creek Tr., 38°02.785' N, 105°32.366' W

2-Split N. on Rainbow Tr., 38°02.734' N, 105°32.360' W

4-River Crossing, 38°01.643' N, 105°33.792' W

5-Sangre De Cristo Wilderness, 38°01.507' N, 105°33.977' W

6-River Crossing, 38°01.048' N, 105°34.895' W

7-Great Camping, 38°00.509' N, 105°35.389' W

Route continued on Adams Ridge map, page 266

Horn Creek Trail/NE Ridge
11.78 miles RT

41 Mount Adams   *Good Overnight!*

Adams is located in the heart of the Sangre De Cristo Range yet remains relatively unknown. Adams is a great adventure, with one of the best ridge scrambles in Colorado!

Round Trip Distance	11.78 miles
Hiking Time	10–12 hours / 2-day option
Difficulty	9/10
Class	3; class 2 hike in
Start Elevation	9,095 ft., at Horn Creek Trailhead
Peak Elevation	13,931 ft.
Total Elevation Gain	4,898 ft.
Terrain	Rugged, steep, solid rock scramble on long ridge
Best Time to Climb	July–September
Gear Advisor	Trekking poles, gaiters, sandals: there are two or three river crossings, plus mud
Crowd Level	Low on Horn Lakes Trail, hermit on the peak

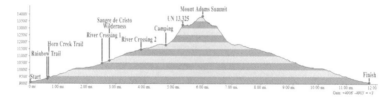

Location Sangre De Cristo Range in the Sangre De Cristo Wilderness/San Isabel National Forest outside of Westcliffe

Intro If it were a little bit taller, Adams would be one of the most talked about peaks in Colorado. Measuring in at 13,931 feet, Adams is just a 69-foot whisker short of 14er status. It also has a rather generic name: there are two Mount Adams in the state (the other is in Rocky Mountain National Park), and dozens of other "Adams" features—lakes, rivers, towns, etc. Nonetheless, this is an Adams you should get to know! Not only do you get to scramble a premier class 3 ridge to the summit, your path to the mountain takes you to the beautiful Horn Lakes Basin. Be ready for some steep hiking and amazing views.

Why Climb It? The northeast ridge of Adams is an absolute delight. The scramble is roughly 0.25 mile on classic Crestone-style conglomerate and granite rock; that means lots of knobby holds! From the base of the ridge, finding the line looks like a thoroughly daunting prospect. Once on the ridge, however, the line becomes apparent, as the mountain reveals its best route. The exposure is diminished by switching from the south side of the ridge to the north and back; there is always a safe class 3 option to negotiate obstacles.

The hike/backpack in is very scenic. Camping at Horn Lakes is awesome. The amphitheater of enormous peaks surrounds you to the southwest, while your view to the northeast shows the flat, peaceful farmland and city lights of Westcliffe. This is a perfect late-summer or early-autumn trip, best done as a two-day adventure. It is certainly possible as a hearty dayhike, but the area is so pristine and beautiful, I see no reason to rush the experience.

Driving   The Horn Creek Trailhead is off a paved road and is reachable by any vehicle.

How to Get There   From the town of Westcliffe, take Colorado Highway 69 south out of town. Drive 2.8 miles south, and turn right (west) onto Schoolfield Road (County Road 140). Go west 1.8 miles and turn left (south) onto Macey Lane (County Road 129). Go south 1.9 miles and turn right onto Horn Road (County Road 130). It is 2.97 miles west on Horn Road to the Horn Creek Trailhead; signs for the trailhead are well marked. Stay on Horn Road after you pass Horn Ranch Creek (which will have you bearing right at an intersection). As you come up the road, you may see a small parking area with a sign for the Rainbow Trail on the right; bypass this parking area and continue to the end of the road, where you will come across a large parking area with a sign kiosk, restroom, and ample space for horse-trailer parking.

Fees/Camping   There are no fees for hiking Mount Adams or for camping in this section of the San Isabel National Forest.

Route Notes   The Horn Creek Trail #1342 follows a canyon that begins in conifer trees and eventually passes through a striking aspen stand. As you near Horn Lakes, you'll pass into the Sangre De Cristo Wilderness. Upon reaching the open lakes area, you'll have a stunning view of the black wall between Fluted Peak and Unnamed Peak 13,325—Adams will still be blocked! There are three sections of lakes here; the middle and upper lakes are optimal campsites.

To reach the northeast ridge, you have to march directly up a more than 1,500-foot slope, which is grassy and steep but has excellent footing. The route described here includes the summit of UN 13,325, though it's possible to shortcut from the slope to the saddle between it and Adams (the footing is actually better if you scale UN 13,325, but the choice is yours). From the saddle, the ridge is a fine scramble to the blocky summit of Adams. Views to the south of the Crestone and Carson mountains and Humboldt Peak are breathtaking!

Mile/Waypoint   **0.0 mi (1)**   From the Horn Creek Trailhead, take the obvious marked trail into the woods. Note that this connector will bring you to the Rainbow Trail, your first goal. There are some trails that come in from the north before you intersect the Rainbow Trail; stay on the large obvious trail bearing southwest.

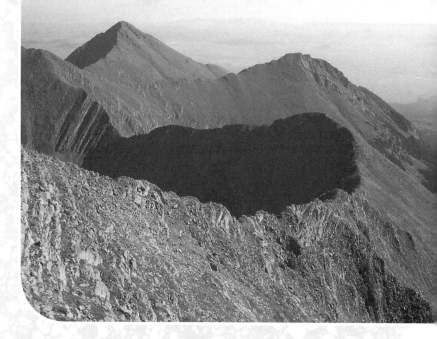

The ridgeline on Adams can be intimidating until you unlock its secrets.

0.5 mi (2) Here you intersect with the actual Rainbow Trail, which runs north and south. Head right (north), following the signs for Horn Lakes and Horn Creek Trail. Do not head toward Macey Lakes, even though you may be lured by the nearby sound of rushing water.

0.6 mi (3) Your stay on the Rainbow Trail is short lived. Turn left (west) onto Horn Creek Trail 1342; the marked sign also mentions the Horn Lakes. From here on out, the trail is class 2, with rocks, roots, and mud. Despite the obstacles, this is still a maintained trail that is good for backpacking. Elevation gain is gradual, and it's easy to set a good pace on the lower section of the trail.

2.6 mi (4) River crossing number one! In early spring, this stream can flow quite high.

2.8 mi (5) Cross into the Sangre De Cristo Wilderness. From here, the trail gets muddier and has steeper sections. In other words, it's time to get dirty and sweaty.

4.0 mi (6) As you finally begin to emerge from the trees, you'll be surrounded by Little Baldy Mountain on your left and Little Horn Peak on your right. As you reach a clearing, you'll come to your biggest river crossing (which is also at the base of the first of the Horn Lakes). Check out the incredible blackish eastern wall of Fluted Peak to your right.

4.8 mi (7) Here you reach the middle group of the Horn Lakes; this is a great place to set up camp. Camping at the largest Horn Lake is an option, too; in fact, you'll have to pass just over 5.0 miles to actually see the summit block of Adams, to the northwest.

Right around this area, you'll want to get off-trail and begin the grueling push up the giant grassy slope to Unnamed Peak 13,325. Consult the Adams Ridge map for this and the rest of the route. From camp, at around 11,800 feet, it is 1,325 feet straight up to UN 13,325's summit. I found that staying north on the slope offered much better footing, mostly grass. While the lines may look more direct to the south, the terrain is talus-filled and rocky. Set the line of your ascent north to the next waypoint, a small rock outcrop I call "the Cornerstone."

5.1 mi (8)   Reach the "Cornerstone," and head directly for the summit of UN 13,325. If you don't mind off-camber hiking (or you want to bypass UN 13,325), you can traverse diagonally to the saddle of Adams.

5.4 mi (9)   Reach the summit of Unnamed Peak 13,325. You'll have a stunning, somewhat intimidating view of the ridge to Adams. Drop down southwest to the saddle and get ready to scramble.

5.6 mi (10)   The saddle is a good place to ditch your trekking poles. From here, it's a mere 0.4 mile and 800+ vertical feet to the summit—this is where the fun begins!

Navigating the northeast ridge of Adams is not as hard as it looks. It will take some route finding, but the challenge is never overwhelming. I offer the following tips:

You can stay on the spine of the ridge for most of this climb, but there are a few sections where you may want to diverge. Pinnacle 1 **(11)** will be easy to scramble up and maintain the ridge. Get up the pinnacle notch **(12)** and stay on the ridge to Pinnacle 2 **(13)**.

Pinnacle 2 is your first real challenge. If you are feeling bold, scramble directly up (class 3+) and walk on a short, exhilarating section I call the "Adams Skyway." If you prefer a safer traverse, divert to the north (right) side of the ridge, which will likely be in shadows and has snow year-round.

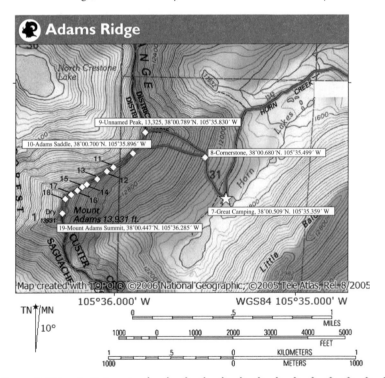

Here, you'll find a nice detour with solid terrain. Rejoin the ridge (14), where you'll exit the Skyway.

Next, you'll encounter Pinnacles 3 (15) and 4 (16). You again have the option of a direct scramble or an easier detour; this time, the detours are safer on the south (left) side of the ridge. Once you climb Pinnacle 4 or detour around it, get back up on the ridge for the best part of the hike! It may be tempting to head for the loose, rocky slopes on Adams' east face, but stay on (or close to) the ridge.

Pinnacle 4 may have seemed tough, but once you are atop it you have it free 'n' easy to the summit. Begin "Skyway 2" (17) and follow it to Adams Side Summit (18) at mile 6.0 of your hike.

From Side Summit, head south to the prized main summit. I found it easiest to divert left (southeast) of the ridge and get out a bit on the east face, where a faint path zigzags up to the summit proper block. Enjoy the awesome views, especially those to the south. You've earned it!

6.1 mi (19) Mount Adams Summit! Take your photos and return down to the saddle.

6.6 mi (10) Once at the saddle, pick up any jettisoned gear and begin your descent; there's no reason to revisit UN 13,325. The off-camber route is easier to descend than to ascend, so I recommend it for the way down. Aim for Cornerstone and regain the Horn Creek Trail at mile 7.1. Walk out the way you came.

11.8 mi Finish.

Options The Sangres rise from the plains like a giant, natural amusement park. There's always a lot to see and explore in each distinct basin. Because Adams is such a demanding route, it will probably be the focus of your trip, but if you are feeling robust, you can go for Little Horn Peak and connect it to Fluted Peak. The ridge between UN 13,325 and Fluted Peak looks possible, but you drop down quite a bit in the saddle. Little Baldy Mountain has several summits you can scale, most easily by slogging up the northeast slopes that begin at the lower section of Horn Lakes. Also note that Adams has an easier ascent route from the west side, starting at Willow Creek Trailhead— but the northeast ridge is much more fun!

Quick Facts The origin of Mount Adams's name is somewhat shrouded in mystery, as there were a few notable "Adams" to choose from. Most think the peak is named for Colorado Governor Alva Adams, who served two full terms and won the election in 1904; the third term was contested by legislature, and Adams was forced out. Oddly, there was a second Colorado politician named Alva Adams (Alva B. Adams), a senator for whom the *other* Mount Adams is named.

Sangre De Cristo, which translates as "the Blood of Christ," is rumored to have been uttered by a Spanish missionary upon his first sight of the deep red alpenglow over these impressive peaks.

Contact Info San Isabel National Forest
2480 Kachina Drive
Pueblo, CO 81008
(719) 553-1400

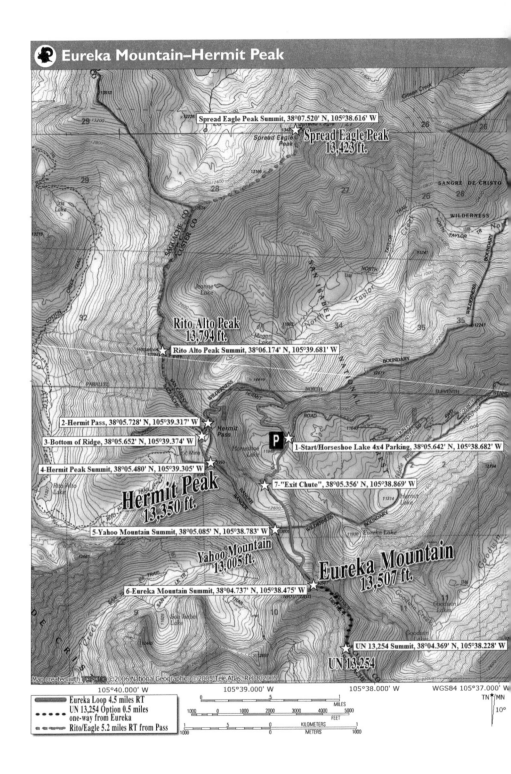

Spread Eagle Peak Summit, 38°07.520' N, 105°38.616' W

Spread Eagle Peak
13,423 ft.

SANGRE DE CRISTO

WILDERNESS

TAYLOR

Rito Alto Peak
13,794 ft.

Rito Alto Peak Summit, 38°06.174' N, 105°39.681' W

BOUNDARY

2-Hermit Pass, 38°05.728' N, 105°39.317' W

3-Bottom of Ridge, 38°05.652' N, 105°39.374' W

Hermit Pass

1-Start/Horseshoe Lake 4x4 Parking, 38°05.642' N, 105°38.682' W

4-Hermit Peak Summit, 38°05.480' N, 105°39.305' W

7-"Exit Chute", 38°05.356' N, 105°38.869' W

Hermit Peak
13,350 ft.

5-Yahoo Mountain Summit, 38°05.085' N, 105°38.783' W

Eureka Lake

Eureka Mountain
13,507 ft.

Yahoo Mountain
13,005 ft.

6-Eureka Mountain Summit, 38°04.737' N, 105°38.475' W

UN 13,254 Summit, 38°04.369' N, 105°38.228' W

UN 13,254

Map created with TOPO! © 2006 National Geographic; ©2005 Tele Atlas, Rel. 8/2005

105°40.000' W   105°39.000' W   105°38.000' W   WGS84 105°37.000' W

TN ↑ MN
10°

Eureka Loop 4.5 miles RT
UN 13,254 Option 0.5 miles
one-way from Eureka
Rito/Eagle 5.2 miles RT from Pass

MILES
FEET
KILOMETERS
METERS

42 **Eureka Mountain–Hermit Peak**

BONUS PEAK: YAHOO MOUNTAIN

Shouts of joy are commonplace on these two picturesque Sangre De Cristo Peaks. Snag a bonus summit en route from Hermit to Eureka's grand apex.

Round Trip Distance	4.5 miles from Horseshoe Lake (15 miles from car parking)*
Hiking Time	3–6 hours from Horseshoe Lake
Difficulty	6.5/10
Class	2+
Start Elevation	12,050 ft., at Horseshoe Lake
Peak Elevations	Eureka Mountain: 13,507 ft.; Hermit Peak: 13,350 ft.; Yahoo Mountain 13,005 ft.
Total Elevation Gain	2,290 ft.
Terrain	Off-trail ridge walking on good rock
Gear Advisor	Trekking poles
Best Time to Climb	June–September
Crowd Level	Hermit

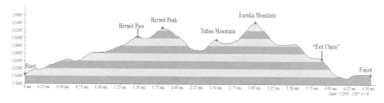

*__Note on Hiking Distance:__ The road to Horseshoe Lake is very rocky and rough. Passenger cars will be lucky to make it to the first parking area. Sport utility cars can get higher but are better off not pushing it on the higher parts of the road (the same may be said for SUVs). Those 4x4s with good clearance will be able to slowly claw their way up to Horseshoe Lake. It is 5.5 miles one way from the wilderness boundary (where the road gets bad) to Horseshoe Lake.

The road is actually a very nice hike in itself. Unlike other roads, which can be tedious, this feels more like a wide hiking trail. I did this hike from the very bottom of the road and enjoyed it. SUVs and SUCs can brave the road at their own discretion, resulting in a 7- to 9-mile round-trip hike, depending on where you park.

Location   Sangre De Cristo Range in the Sangre De Cristo Wilderness/San Isabel National Forest outside of Westcliffe

Intro   Eureka and Hermit are often overlooked in favor of more glamorous 14ers of the Sangre De Cristo Range. Isolation has its benefits, however; a pristine wilderness is yours to discover when you undertake this hike. Eureka

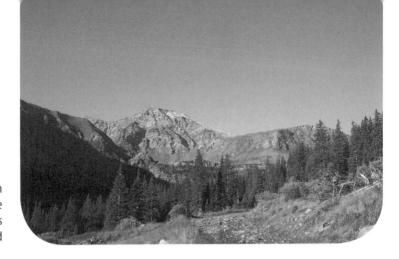

Eureka Mountain as seen from the rugged Hermit Pass Road

in an especially photogenic peak. Mountaineering fans will notice that the striated northeast face bears a strong resemblance to Mount Everest's summit pyramid. The route between these two mountains is a fun class 2+ traverse that doesn't have high exposure. Optional routes can make this a very full day from Hermit Pass.

Why Climb It? Relatively unknown peaks with fun, beautiful traverses are my favorite mountains to climb. Taken from Horseshoe Lake, this isn't a strenuous loop, but it still gives you a good workout. Views to the south from Eureka are marvelous. The Crestone group (as well as Mount Adams, Hike 41) rise like enormous tombstones. As far as Sangre hikes go, these peaks are more for hikers than technical climbers, so everyone can enjoy them. Camping in the area is a distinct pleasure and a great way to spend an autumn weekend.

Driving You're going to need a high-clearance 4x4 vehicle or a beefy SUV to make it to Horseshoe Lake. The way up is extremely rocky in places, especially on steep sections of the road. It's a bit frustrating that many of the rugged sections are followed by long stretches of perfectly smooth dirt roads. SUCs that put up a good fight can make it 2.1 miles up the road. One good thing is that there are plenty of good primitive campsites along the way. SUVs with good clearance and a strong low gear can make it up to Horseshoe Lake. As mentioned before, hiking this road isn't a miserable experience; in fact, you may enjoy the hike more by starting it a bit lower, such as at the trailhead for Hermit Lake.

How to Get There From Colorado Highway 69 in the town of Westcliffe, turn west onto County Road 160, also known as Hermit Road and Hermit Pass Road. This road begins as pavement and then turns into a well-maintained dirt road, passable for all. Old-timers (well, not that old) may recognize this as the way up to the extinct Conquistador Ski Area. Stay on CR 160 for 7.2 miles to the wilderness boundary. Once you reach the boundary, CR 160 turns into Forest Service Road 301 (Hermit Pass Road) and becomes an utter mess. Rocks galore litter this part of the road. Tough passenger cars may end up sacrificing parts struggling 0.1 mile up to the parking area on the right (when the road turns left).

SUCs, SUVs, and 4x4s can continue on for varying distances. Several side roads split off to campsites, but the main road is obvious—stay on it. One tricky section comes at mile 2.1, where the road splits into two seemingly good sections (there is also a wilderness preservation sign). Go right, up a very rocky hill. Note, however, that the smooth, sandy flat road to the left is a great place for SUCs to park/camp. Keep fighting up this road, passing the Hermit Lake Trailhead at mile 4.0, until you reach a small parking area at Horseshoe Lake, at mile 5.5 (elevation 12,050 feet). The road keeps going up, 1.5 miles to Hermit Pass, but since the loop ends at Horseshoe Lake, do not park there (unless you want to climb back up over Hermit Peak, which is another 800 feet of elevation gain). Horseshoe Lake has several parking spots and good areas to pitch a tent.

Fees/Camping   There are no fees to hike or camp in this area; please do not camp before reaching the wilderness boundary.

Route Notes   The route detailed here does not include the mileage you may incur hoofing it up Hermit Pass Road from parking areas before Horseshoe Lake.

Mile/Waypoint   **0.0 mi (1)**   Start at the parking area at Horseshoe Lake. Hike up the wide switchbacks on Hermit Pass Road up to Hermit Pass—this is a good warm-up.

1.5 mi (2)   Reach the top of Hermit Pass, at 13,050 feet. There's a sign-in register here. Fill out your information and start south toward Hermit Peak, just off to your left.

1.6 mi (3)   Here, at the bottom of the ridge, leave the road and scramble directly up to the summit of Hermit Peak. This short ascent covers about 270 vertical feet, depending on where you begin on the ridge.

1.8 mi (4)   Hermit Peak Summit. Getting here was the easy part; now you have to downclimb over to Yahoo Mountain (which looks like a real mountain from here). Stay due south and climb all the way down to the saddle (at 12,680 feet) between Hermit and Yahoo. Hike/scramble the ridge up to the top of Yahoo.

2.6 mi (5)   Yahoo Mountain Summit! Now that you are up here, you realize this isn't so much a mountain as it is a raised shoulder of Eureka Mountain. Drop down into a saddle at 12,870 feet, and get ready to ascend Eureka's northwest ridge. Staying on the spine of the ridge is the most fun! There are plenty of handholds on this class 2+ scramble and they are made of knobby Crestone conglomerate rock. If you feel a bit uneasy on the ridge, stay to the left and ascend the rocky slope. The higher you get on this ridge, the less humble Yahoo Mountain looks like a mountain.

3.1 mi (6)   Eureka's summit! Views to the south will make your jaw drop. When you descend, it's faster to storm down the north slope to the plateau between Yahoo and Eureka. Stay on this plateau and descend, slightly rising to pass a bump that is lined up with Yahoo Mountain. Continue down to the "Exit Chute," where you'll have a good view of Horseshoe Lake and your vehicle below.

4.0 mi (7) At the Exit Chute, find a good line down the scree hill and make your way back to Horseshoe Lake. The upper parts of this descent are loose, so be careful. Going a bit farther north will bring you to the exact chute listed on the map (waypoint 7), which is a relatively easy class 2+ descent.

4.5 mi Finish.

Options The short, 0.5-mile traverse (one way) to UN 13,254 from Eureka's summit gives good views of Eureka to the north and Venable Pass to the south. It's not mind-blowing, but it is a good way to extend your day if you parked at Horseshoe Lake.

A good secondary hike is the out-and-back trip north from Hermit Pass (waypoint 2) to Rito Alto and Spread Eagle peaks (5.2 miles). This is a class 2 hike on similar rock that you can do as one long day (roughly 11 miles if you do them all). On this route, you'll also summit two unnamed 13ers—meaning if you do the full loop in a day (not including UN 13,254), you'll summit seven 13ers. Wow! On the other hand, if you are spending a weekend up here, why not do this trek on your second day?

Quick Facts "Eureka" is Greek for "I found it!" This was a buzzword of the late 1800s and the peak was named in honor of this exclamation. Hey, it's better than "Consarnit Mountain."

One last interesting note concerns the short-lived Conquistador Ski Area that once operated east of the spot where County Road 160 crosses the wilderness boundary. Westcliffe residents resisted the development, knowing full well there wasn't enough snow to make the area worthwhile. Nonetheless, developers tried. From 1978 to 1988, the ski area operated four lifts. The resort last operated in 1992. A comeback in 1996 fell short, and the lifts were removed forever. The current owner plans to make the area a mountain resort not focused on skiing.

Contact Info San Isabel National Forest
Salida Ranger District
325 Rainbow
Salida, CO 81201
(719) 539-3591

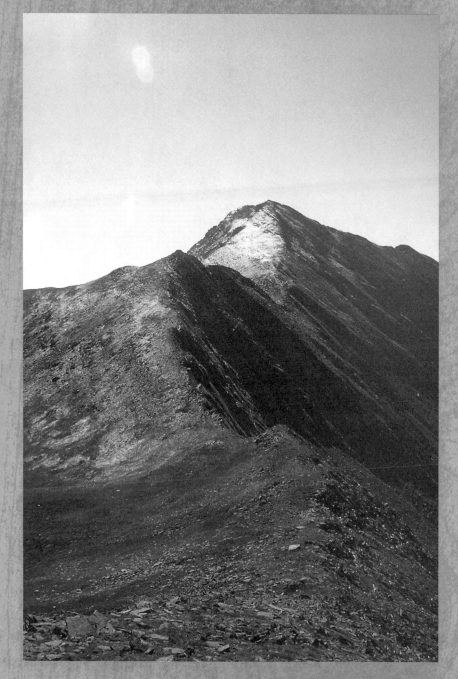

A great look at the traverse to Yahoo Mountain with Eureka Mountain in the background

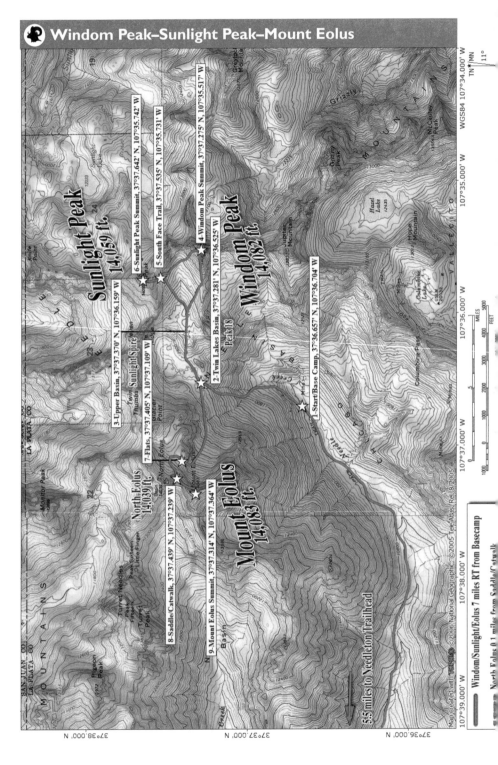

Sunlight Peak
14,059 ft.

Windom Peak
14,082 ft.

Mount Eolus
14,083 ft.

North Eolus
14,039 ft.

6-Sunlight Peak Summit, 37°37.642' N, 107°35.742' W

5-South Face Trail, 37°37.535' N, 107°35.731' W

4-Windom Peak Summit, 37°37.275' N, 107°35.517' W

3-Upper Basin, 37°37.370' N, 107°36.159' W

2-Twin Lakes Basin, 37°37.281' N, 107°36.525' W

1-Start/Base Camp, 37°36.657' N, 107°36.704' W

Peak 18

7-Flats, 37°37.405' N, 107°37.109' W

8-Saddle/Catwalk, 37°37.439' N, 107°37.239' W

9-Mount Eolus Summit, 37°37.314' N, 107°37.364' W

5.5 miles to Needleton Trailhead

WGS84 107°34.000' W

TN MN
11°

Windom/Sunlight/Eolus 7 miles RT from Basecamp

North Eolus 0.1 miles from Saddle/Catwalk

43 Chicago Basin 14er Circuit: Windom Peak–Sunlight Peak–Mount Eolus *Good Overnight!*

A trip to Chicago Basin is an unforgettable experience. Ride the Durango & Silverton train to a remote stop in the San Juans and prepare to embark on an amazing journey.

Round Trip Distance	21 miles from Needleton Trailhead; 7-mile loop when camping in Chicago Basin
Hiking Time	3–4 days; Hiking time depends on route, but expect 10–12 hours for the three 14ers in one day from camp
Difficulty	8/10
Class	2+/3
Start Elevation	8,233 ft., at Needleton Creek Trailhead
Peak Elevations	Windom Peak: 14,082 ft.; Sunlight Peak: 14,059 ft.; Mount Eolus: 14,083 ft.
Total Elevation Gain	8,220 ft.
Terrain	Train ride; long class 1 trail to Chicago Basin; class 2+/3 scrambling
Best Time to Climb	July–September
Gear Advisor	Camping gear, GPS, quad maps, trekking poles, camera, helmet
Crowd Level	Moderate

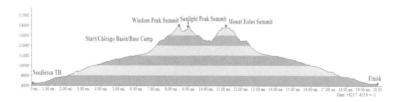

Location   San Juan Mountains in the Weminuche Wilderness/San Juan National Forest outside of Durango and Silverton

Intro   There's nothing like the feeling of taking the old steam train to Needleton Trailhead, grabbing your pack, and watching the old locomotive chug away. All grows quiet except the soothing rush of water in the Animas River. From here, you're in the backcountry! A 5- to 6-mile approach (depending on where you set up camp) lets you set up a real, honest-to-goodness base camp, from which you'll have many options regarding how to climb these mountains. Your 14ers on this hike come in three different flavors—quite a nice bit of diversity for three peaks so close to one another. Gear up and get ready to get away from it all!

Why Climb It? The train ride to Needleton is obviously a nice touch, but you're here for the hiking, not the choo-choo! The great part about hiking these three mountains is that they sample different climbing styles: Windom is class 2/2+ on big, blocky boulders. Sunlight has a good class 3 route that culminates with a fun scramble to an exposed summit. Eolus has sustained class 3 scrambling along narrow catwalks and rocky ledges. Some people do all three in one day (about 10 miles round trip from camp), but my preferred option is to hike Windom and Sunlight in one trek (about 5.3 miles round trip from camp), and on a second day to hike Eolus and optional North Eolus (about 4.2 miles round trip from camp).

Driving Needleton Trailhead is accessed by train, specifically the Durango & Silverton Narrow Gauge Railroad. Costs for tickets are $65 per person round trip (for the year 2007), and you must make reservations. You can start from either of the two train stations, though most prefer to start in Durango (parking is $5 per day, so factor that into your expenses as well). The Durango station is at the intersection of US Highway 550 and US Highway 160 in the south part of town and is very well marked. The Silverton station is off Colorado Highway 110 and is also well signed. To make your reservations, or for any other questions, contact the train service:

Durango & Silverton Narrow Gauge Railroad
Reservations and General Information: (970) 247-2733
Toll Free: (877) 872-4607

Email:
General Information: info@durangotrain.com
Reservations: reservations@durangotrain.com

Durango & Silverton Narrow Gauge Railroad
479 Main Avenue, Durango, CO 81301

For those who are wondering, there is a very long trail you can take to avoid the train, aptly named the Purgatory Trail. It is 9.0 miles one way to the Needleton Trailhead (then another 5–6 miles to camp) from this route—over 30 miles of approach hiking. Not much fun, but it's a possibility if you have lots of time and no money!

How to Get There Needleton Trailhead is almost exclusively accessed by train. Check the schedule and make sure you are on a train that stops at Needleton. The folks who work for the train service are used to backpackers and will answer any additional questions you may have.

Fees/Camping There are no fees for hiking or camping in the area. Train tickets are $65 per adult (in 2007); parking on-site at the train station is $5 per day.

Route Notes The mileage for the first waypoint is approximate, based on where you camp in Chicago Basin, which may be in any number of places. My camp was at the flat north end of the basin just before the steep hiking begins. I would advise hiking into the basin for better camp spots; the good ones start once the basin opens up, about 5.3 miles in. Be prepared, as this is truly a backcountry area. There will be other people around, but you must be self-reliant.

As mentioned, I recommend hiking Windom and Sunlight in one day, Eolus and North Eolus on another day. The route description below follows that itinerary. Spending three to four days in the area is the best plan, taking a whole day each for the hike in and hike out. The less rushed you are, the more you'll enjoy the area. Make enough time to catch the train home by not overwhelming yourself with too much on your last day.

Note: If you go for all three 14ers in a day, get a very early start.

The mountain goats in the basin are numerous and nearly domesticated. Do not feed, ride, pet, chase, tackle, groom, wrestle, snuggle, touch, or engage the goats! They are wild animals that are capable of inflicting some serious damage on hikers that get too close.

A final note: USGS quad maps are *highly* advised for this hike. You'll need the following quads: *Columbine Pass, Mountain View Crest,* and *Snowdon Peak* maps.

Mile/Waypoint

Day 1: The Hike In
Mileage from Needleton Trailhead: 5–6 miles

0.0 mi Get off the train at the Needleton Trailhead and get on the Chicago Basin pack trail that crosses over the bridge spanning the river. Follow this well-worn class 1 trail up to Chicago Basin. The way up is very well marked and easy to follow. The few intersections are well marked. As you begin to get closer to the basin, views will open up and you'll be in another world. You will slowy gain about 3,000 feet of elevation. I would suggest camping around mile 5.5, at roughly 11,150 feet.

5.5 mi (1) Find a good campsite. We'll reset the trip mileage here.

Day 2: Windom and Sunlight from Chicago Basin
Round trip mileage from camp: 5.4 miles

0.0 mi (1) From camp, get back on the main trail and follow it north up the steep slopes that lead to the high basin west of Sunlight and Windom. This trail crosses the stream/waterfall and pushes straight up to the Twin Lakes, at 12,560 feet.

0.8 mi (2) You've reached the flat Twin Lakes Basin. The trail here goes right (east) to a still higher basin. There is a cairned trail as well as a few other faint trails. As you gaze up, Windom is the big block to your upper right. That's your first goal, so keep moving east in its direction.

1.3 mi (3) The upper basin has one tiny lake and many boulders. From here, gain the saddle between Peak Eighteen and Windom at its lowest point, which will be on your right. You can get to the saddle by staying on the cairned trail or by scrambling up off trail.

Once you gain Windom's west ridge, the way up is obvious (and there's a faint trail). As you near the summit, the blocks become giant cubes! Have fun on this class 2 terrain until you reach the highest point.

2.0 mi (4) Windom Peak's summit! To traverse over to Sunlight Peak's south face, you have a few options. This route follows a steep scree gully that eliminates the need to drop back into the high basin. It begins northwest of the summit and is a bit slow-going in places, but it's quicker in the long run, if you have the knees for it. The other option is to drop back down Windom's west ridge and traverse north to the basin from the saddle of Windom and Peak Eighteen.

2.5 mi (5) If you are unsure where to start the climb on Sunlight, look for the red, rocky gully east of the slopes to Sunlight Peak. From here, a whisker-marked trail goes into the south face and works its way up a series of rocky ledges. You may lose the trail or prefer to scramble up at your own pace; in any case, it's class 3 terrain. As you get higher, start heading to the left (west) and work your way over to a saddle between Sunlight and Sunlight Spire. The climbing narrows considerably and gets harder from here. Continue west by following rocky (and somewhat exposed) ledges or by walking to the west edge of the saddle and scrambling up (north) from there. Stop when you are about 20 feet from the ridge and turn right, choosing a good class 3 route to ascend.

The best way is the famous "Keyhole," a 30-foot section that is enclosed by a boulder. Scramble east up the Keyhole and toward the summit, which will be very close. The summit register and USGS marker will be on a flat section below the final summit block. It doesn't look so bad from here, does it?

2.8 miles (6) Sunlight Peak's perilous summit! The move to reach the high-point of Sunlight is a dangerous, exposed move that you must commit to; do not climb it if you are unnerved. (And don't feel bad about it if you don't: it's a dangerous, high-risk, class 4 move.) The summit block is about 30 feet tall; go up and over to your right to reach the "launching pad," a sloped rock linking the last few boulders. The gap you need to clear drops about 12 feet in front of you and about 1,200 feet on the right side. This gap is only about 2.5 feet across and to clear it you must jump onto a sloped, polished rock. Once you clear the gap, it's a quick hop (or belly crawl) to the summit. Getting down is the hardest part; the jump to clear the gap is tough because you land on a downhill-sloped boulder. There is a rock in the gap you can hop onto, but this may be even harder to land on. Having a friend spot you is a good idea.

It isn't necessary to claim the summit. If you really want to, however, you may want to bring along a pair of rock climbing shoes for extra grip (and a mental boost). It's a tough move to protect, so if you want to belay a friend, bring a 100-foot (or longer) length of static rope and set an anchor by looping it around the summit boulder.

To return, drop down the south face again, taking your time and making your way back to the lakes area (waypoint 2). Rest up, you have another summit ahead of you tomorrow (or later today, if you're linking them).

5.3 mi Finish the Windom and Sunlight hike.

Day 3: Mount Eolus
Round trip mileage from base camp to summit and back: 4.2 miles

0.0 mi (1) Start as you did for the Windom/Sunlight hike, going back up to the top of the waterfall just before Twin Lakes.

0.8 mi (2) Below (south of) the Twin Lakes, a trail hops over the stream (before it becomes a full-fledged waterfall), and heads west toward Eolus. This trail is well worn and goes up into a sloped basin. Follow it all the way to a flat section below North Eolus.

1.7 mi (7) From the flats, you'll need to scramble up to the north ridge; it's also a good place to ditch your trekking poles. There is a cairned trail, but you can also pick your own line. (Once you are in the saddle, it's a quick class 3 optional traverse up to 14,039-foot North Eolus Summit.) If your sights are set squarely on Mount Eolus, get on the ridge and head south.

1.9 mi (8) On the ridge at 13,800 feet, you'll encounter a narrow, 15-foot-long-by-2-foot-wide section known as the "Catwalk." There's nothing hard about it, but the exposure is high; some prefer to unleash their inner felines and cross it on all fours. Once you clear it, continue on to the east face.

From here, the route is semicairned. The cubic piles of rock on this mountain seem intimidating, but you can find many safe paths up the east face, where series of ledges and traverses will bring you to the summit. This requires some route-finding, so plot out your path with care. The cairns are useful but seem to trace several different routes. A helmet is suggested for this section.

2.1 mi (9) Mount Eolus's summit! Notice that the USGS marker up here uses the Greek spelling "Aeolus." The hardest part of the climb may be returning the way you came. Take your time and pick good lines back to the ridge. Retrace your path back to camp.

4.2 mi Finish.

Now that the "work" is done, you can head out whenever you please—just make sure you catch your train on time!

Options The short scramble up to North Eolus is a mere 0.1 mile from waypoint 8. It's a nice peak, and if it were a bit farther north of Eolus, it would be distinct enough to be a ranked 14er.

Quick Facts Windom is named for politician William Windom, a senator from Minnesota who went to serve as the US secretary of the treasury from 1889–91. Sunlight Peak was named by surveyor Whitman Cross in 1902; it must have been a sunny day! Mount Eolus was named after the Greek god of wind. After initially being named "Mount Aeolus" by the Hayden survey of 1874, the Wheeler survey inexplicably changed the spelling to "Eolus" on their 1878 maps.

Contact Info Information for the Durango & Silverton train is listed on page 276.
San Juan National Forest
15 Burnett Court
Durango, CO 81301
(970) 247-4874

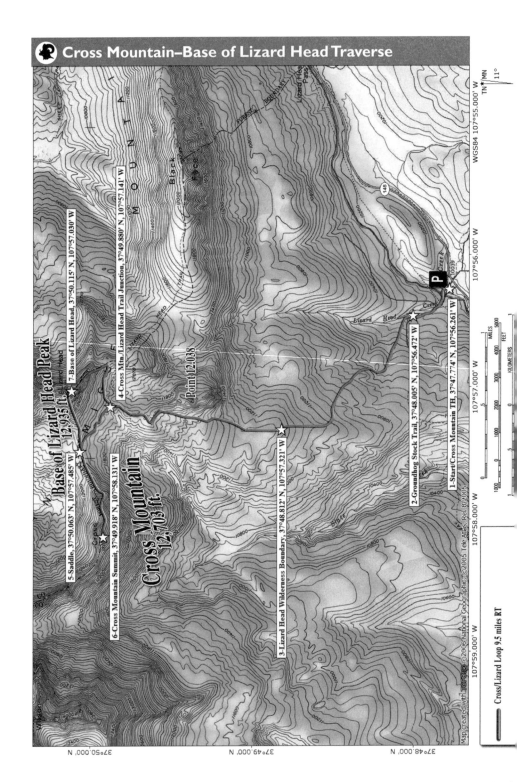

Base of Lizard Head Peak
12,935 ft.

Cross Mountain
12,703 ft.

Point 12,038

7-Base of Lizard Head, 37°50.115' N, 107°57.030' W

4-Cross Mtn./Lizard Head Trail Junction, 37°49.880' N, 107°57.141' W

5-Saddle, 37°50.063' N, 107°57.485' W

6-Cross Mountain Summit, 37°49.918' N, 107°58.131' W

3-Lizard Head Wilderness Boundary, 37°48.812' N, 107°57.321' W

2-Groundhog Stock Trail, 37°48.005' N, 107°56.472' W

1-Start/Cross Mountain TH, 37°47.774' N, 107°56.261' W

WGS84 107°55.000' W

TN ★ MN
11°

— Cross/Lizard Loop 9.5 miles RT

Map created with TOPO!® ©2006 National Geographic; ©2005 Tele Atlas, Rel. 8/2005.

44 Cross Mountain–Base of Lizard Head Traverse

Take a tour of two mystical mountains. Cross stands like an altar before a council of mountain gods while Lizard Head has dimensions that defy conventional form!

Round Trip Distance	9.5 miles
Hiking Time	5–7 hours
Difficulty	6.5/10
Class	2
Start Elevation	10,040 ft., at Cross Mountain Trailhead
Peak Elevations	Cross Mountain: 12,703 ft.; Base of Lizard Head: 12,935 ft.
Total Elevation Gain	3,565 ft.
Terrain	Class 1 trail leads to rocky scramble to Cross Summit and base of Lizard Head
Best Time to Climb	June–September
Gear Advisor	Normal gear
Crowd Level	Low/moderate

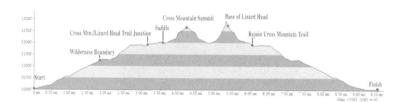

Location   San Juan Mountains in the Lizard Head Wilderness/San Juan National Forest outside of Telluride

Intro   Cross Mountain's unique position amongst a crowd of 14ers and high 13ers offers a rare perspective of the mighty San Juan Mountains. Atop its modest summit, I felt like a traveler who had come to seek the advice of a sagacious council. Cross is dwarfed by peaks from the Wilson group to the west; the effect of gazing at these enormous mountains is mesmerizing. Across the way is Lizard Head, indisputably the most difficult summit to ascend of any mountain higher than 13,000 feet in Colorado. This crumbling, 400-foot, sheer monolith is the enduring throat of an extinct volcano. This hike tours the platform beneath the cracking bust, giving you views to its upper reaches that will send chills down your spine and into your knees.

Why Climb It?   While erosion has had its way with the rock spewed forth from Lizard Head (which looks remarkably like a giant Atari joystick), the granite pipes that siphoned magma from the center of the earth have defiantly remained intact. As a result, this amazing tower is visible from many places in the San Juans (I could clearly make it out from the far-away summit of Redcloud).

Fewer people have reached its summit than have climbed Mount Everest. The technical climb to the top is only graded class 5.7–5.8, but the entire edifice is falling apart, making every handhold suspect and placements for protective gear purely ornamental. A trip to the base of Lizard Head will give you a gander at the intimidating tower from up close, and a new appreciation for Ellingwood and Hoag's first ascent—in 1920!

Cross Mountain has a different feeling than any mountain I have ever climbed. It's a fun scramble in its own right, and the views from the top are incredible. If I had a say, I would rename it "the Altar" for the way it pays homage to nearby high peaks. I wish everyone could have the experience I did when climbing the peak: a full-grown bald eagle lifted off from the summit when I was less than 20 feet away.

Driving

Any vehicle can reach the Cross Mountain Trailhead. The road is paved the entire way (though the parking lot is not).

How to Get There

Cross Mountain Trailhead is 2.0 miles south of Lizard Head Pass off Colorado Route 145; this is roughly 15 miles south of Telluride. The large parking area is on the west side of the road and is marked by signs for Cross Mountain Trail at the turnoff. If you are coming from the south, the trailhead turnoff is approximately 12 miles north on Route 145 from the town of Rico.

Fees/Camping

There are no fees to hike or camp in this area. Please note that camping in the parking area is illegal. You must pass the wilderness boundary to legally camp in the area. Just south of Lizard Head Pass are dozens of good primitive campsites on the east side of the road. These unmarked areas can be found off many of the dirt roads to the east a few miles after the pass.

Route Notes

I suggest making the loop by climbing Cross first and returning with the tour of Lizard Head's base.

Mile/Waypoint

0.0 mi (1) Start at the Cross Mountain Trailhead and head west on the Cross Mountain Trail (#637). Lizard Head stands like a granite lighthouse in the distance, serving as your beacon. When you start on this trail, make sure not to turn left or right onto the dirt road that intersects the trail very early on. The correct way is lined with a series of wooden fence posts (but no fence). A Forest Service marker at the start of the woods confirms you're on the correct trail.

0.4 mi (2) There is a split here for the bizarrely named Groundhog Stock Trail. (Are they stocking groundhogs these days?) Avoid this trail and stay the course on the Cross Mountain Trail. After this intersection, the class 1 trail is obvious. Hiking into the shadows of the pine forest is a treat and a nice way to set up the next part of the hike.

1.8 mi (3) Pass the official wilderness boundary into the Lizard Head Wilderness.

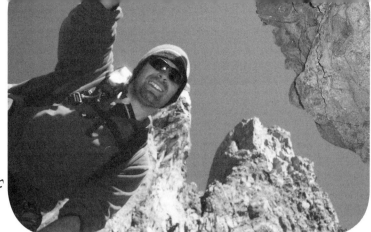

3.2 mi (4) When you clear timberline, things begin to open up. Cross Mountain is the reddish "hill" off to the west. At this point, you are at the pedestal of Lizard Head and at the junction of the Cross Mountain Trail and the Lizard Head Trail. (This is just after you hike on a short section of powdery, fine black rock.) Go left (west) on the Cross Mountain Trail to the western saddle between Lizard Head and Cross.

3.6 mi (5) At the saddle, get off the trail and head west onto the northeast ridge of Cross. Stay on the ridge spine while it is grassy. When the slope morphs to rock, hike onto the south side of the mountain, below the ridge. A faint trail leads out to a brief class 2+ scramble where the northeast and east ridges intersect. Note that staying on the spine of the ridge is a class 3 option and is perfectly acceptable. Do not attempt to climb the grayish gully; pass it and then scramble right onto steep scree to gain the ridge.

4.0 mi You're on the ridge (where you ascended determines the exact spot you've topped out). This ridge walk turns out to be quite a thrill. It has just enough exposure to keep your adrenaline glands on standby. Follow it to its western terminus.

4.3 mi (6) Cross Mountain Summit! Behold the mighty peaks to the west (from left to right): El Diente, Mount Wilson, Gladstone Peak, and Wilson Peak. From here, Lizard Head looks less saurian and more like the rotten fang of an aged predator. Return back to the saddle (waypoint 5).

5.0 mi (5) From the saddle, hike off-trail and gain Lizard Head's west ridge. This steep climb has a faint trail that switchbacks up to the base of the peak. The preview from the base may look scary, but this is a low-exposure class 2 trail, which becomes obvious when you actually get on it. Despite the fact it doesn't reach a summit, the elevation here is higher than on Cross Mountain.

5.4 mi (7) The base of Lizard Head! Be careful of falling rock; as Ellingwood put it, "pebbles rain down from the sides as readily as needles from an aging Christmas tree." The sheer profile of Lizard Head will make your knees knock. Once you've seen your fill, finish this side loop by traversing down the rocky southeast ridge and drop to your right (south) to intersect the Lizard Head Trail, which will be visible from here. Take your time on the loose terrain. Once you gain the Lizard Head Trail, follow it a short distance west to its junction with the Cross Mountain Trail.

6.2 mi (4) At the trail junction, return south the way you came on the Cross Mountain Trail.

9.5 mi Finish.

Options If you want to hike down to Bilk Basin by remaining on the Cross Mountain Trail, you'll get a good look at the 14ers as well as the couloirs on the north face of Cross. There are no other close summits, though you could scramble around on the hills south of Lizard Head (for example, Point 12,038) to get some different looks at the area.

Quick Facts Albert Ellingwood (of Ellingwood Point fame) and his inexperienced but willing partner Barton Hoag made the first ascent of Lizard Head in 1920, an incredible feat given the technology at the time. Unlike most mountains in Colorado, this first ascent probably was a first ascent by men of any skin color. Modern gear has made the climb more accessible and marginally safer. It is estimated about 10 to 20 climbers a year make their way to the summit of Lizard Head. If you'd like to try it, consult a technical climbing guidebook and wear a helmet!

Contact Info San Juan National Forest
San Juan Public Lands Center
15 Burnettt Court
Durango, CO 81301
(970) 247-4874

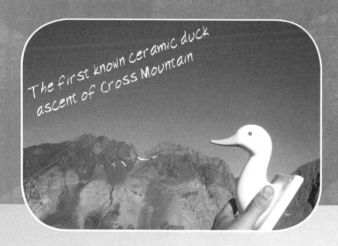
The first known ceramic duck ascent of Cross Mountain

Lizards Head stands guardian over the land.

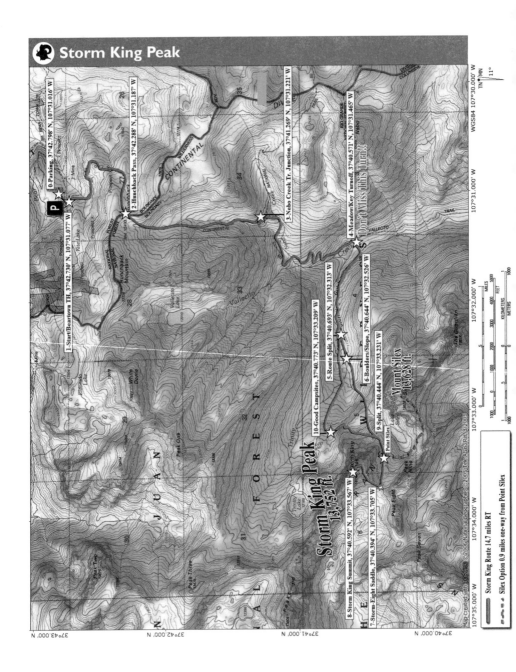

0-Parking, 37°42.798' N, 107°31.016' W

2-Hunchback Pass, 37°42.288' N, 107°31.187' W

3-Nebo Creek Tr. Junction, 37°41.269' N, 107°31.221' W

4-Meadow/Key Turnoff, 37°40.571' N, 107°31.465' W

Don't Miss This Turn!

1-Start/Beartown TH, 37°42.730' N, 107°31.077' W

5-Route Split, 37°40.693' N, 107°32.313' W

6-Boulders/Slope, 37°40.644' N, 107°32.526' W

Mount Silex
13,628 ft.

10-Good Campsites, 37°40.773' N, 107°33.209' W

9-Split, 37°40.444' N, 107°33.231' W

Storm King Peak
13,752 ft.

8-Storm King Summit, 37°40.592' N, 107°33.567' W

7-Storm-Eight Saddle, 37°40.394' N, 107°33.705' W

WGS84 107°30.000' W

TN / MN

11°

Map created with TOPO! © 2005 National Geographic © 2003 Tele Atlas, Rel. 07/2005

— Storm King Route 14.7 miles RT

--- Silex Option 0.9 miles one-way from Point Silex

45 **Storm King Peak** *Good Overnight!*

All hail the King! Storm King Peak in the Grenadier Range is as good as it gets; this is my favorite summit hike in Colorado. Get ready for a wild experience you'll never forget!

Round Trip Distance	14.7 miles
Hiking Time	2–3 days; 10–15 hours of hiking
Difficulty	10/10
Class	3
Start Elevation	11,756 ft., at Beartown Trailhead
Peak Elevation	13,752 ft.
Total Elevation Gain	5,925 ft.
Terrain	Rugged, steep off-trail and semisolid rock for extended scrambling
Best Time to Climb	July–September
Gear Advisor	GPS, camping gear, sandals for river crossing, quad maps, trekking poles, helmet, and this book.
Crowd Level	Low

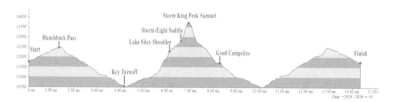

Location Grenadier Range in the Weminuche Wilderness/San Juan National Forest outside of Lake City, Creede, and Silverton

Intro This is the best summit hike I've done in Colorado. The Grenadier Range is the best-kept secret in the state; I actually feel a little guilty getting the word out. There were several other peaks in the Grenadiers that could have easily made this book; Storm King and the optional trek to Mount Silex are the best of the bunch. The difficulty rating on this hike pertains to the overall experience; just getting to the trailhead is an epic journey! Once you are there, you'll need solid backcountry navigation skills, strong legs, and good scrambling ability. This is a fantastic overnight, though it is possible as a dayhike—as a very long dayhike (that's how I did it while researching for this book). The Grenadiers feel like nothing else in Colorado—possibly like no where else in the world. Come see the secrets waiting for you in the wild, wonderful Weminuche Wilderness.

Why Climb It? Besides the pleasure of seeing an area known to only a few, Storm King's scramble has the perfect balance of challenge, exposure, and scenery. It is similar in "feel" to the Keyhole Route on Longs Peak, except that Storm

King is unmarked, so you'll need decent route-finding skills. The ridge up is airy but never exceeds class 3 (not even 3+) and the summit is a truly divine experience. Camping is great and the optional climb over to Mount Silex is just as fun. I hope this adventure will intrigue you to visit other great Grenadier climbs: Arrow, Vestal, the Guradian, the Numbers Peaks, Greystone, etc. You'll have to work hard on this hike: the elevation gain is over 5,000 feet, and that is from a trailhead start of 11,700 feet.

I have not had the time to do this (yet), but the ultimate Colorado backpacking/summit-bagging trip may start here and conclude in nearby Chicago Basin—the two areas are linkable via the Vallecito Creek Trail to Columbine Pass and then out to Needleton Trailhead.

Driving

Passenger cars and sport utility cars: forget about it. Don't even try! The access road to the Beartown Trailhead requires a high-clearance 4x4 with a powerful low gear. There is also a true river crossing, which may be high in the spring. You'll be on rocky, rutted, and steep single-lane 4x4 roads. SUVs that are geared toward actual 4x4 use (for example: Xterras, Durangos, and 4Runners) will be able to get up just fine. Hikers with good 4x4 trucks or jeeps—you're going to thoroughly enjoy the eastern approach. It's what your truck was made for! At the trailhead (which I reached in a Toyota Tacoma) I saw several Tacomas, a few Dodge Rams, an Xterra, and a Ford Explorer.

If you don't have access to a car, there is a service available out of Silverton that serves to drop off and pick up hikers at the Beartown Trailhead. Rates vary, but if you don't have access to a 4x4, give them a call:

San Juan Backcountry
P.O. Box 707
Silverton, CO 81433
(800) 494-8687
backcountry@frontier.net
www.sanjuanbackcountry.com

How to Get There

There are two ways to get to Beartown Trailhead/Kite Lake. Both require 4x4 vehicles with good clearance. SUVs are better off when approaching from Silverton. All these roads are rough, so make sure your tires and brakes are up to the task. Call the ranger station (numbers follow in the "Contact Info" section) to ensure the roads are open and passable.

From Silverton: Drive northeast out of town on Colorado Highway 110 toward Howardsville. Turn right (southeast) about 5.0 miles out of town onto County Road 4; this is the road to Stony Pass. From here it is 11.84 miles to the intersection of Forest Service Road 506. Follow the signs to Stony Pass. Turn left onto County Road 3/Forest Service Road 520 and climb up to Stony Pass. Drive down the other side and reach FS 506, the road to Beartown/Kite Lake. Directions from Beartown continue after the following paragraph.

From Lake City/Creede: Take Colorado Highway 149 to FS 520 and turn west (toward Rio Grande Reservoir). This is an easy, car-friendly dirt road for about 17 miles. At mile 18.5, you get into real 4x4 terrain. There are several river crossings, deeply rutted sections, and the rock-filled fiasco of Timberhill, a very steep hill strewn with rocks of all sizes. Stay the course for an additional 6.5 miles (making it 25 miles total from the start of FS 520), to the junction of FS 520 and FS 506.

Once you've reached FS 506, the road to Beartown goes west 6.5 miles and terminates at Kite Lake. The Beartown Trailhead is at mile 6.0. Immediately, you are forced to cross Bear Creek. In the early spring, this waterway can run high enough to prevent passage. Clear Bear Creek and the road becomes milder, passing through grazing lands.

Eventually, the road goes up some rough and rocky hills; claw your way up and reach the Beartown Trailhead (without ever seeing Beartown!) on your left at mile 6.1 There is a sign/kiosk and a trail sign for Trail #787. If you reach Kite Lake (which is worth checking out), you've gone a half mile too far. Kite Lake is the end of the road.

Important Note: Don't expect to actually see Beartown. The few ruins that remain are not visible from the road and there is little more left than old foundations and rusty nails. For all the signs, you'd think there'd be something to see!

Fees/Camping   There are no fees to hike or camp in the area. There are plenty of places to camp along FS 506 and at the trailhead. Backcountry campers can stay at dozens of places. On Trail #787, once you clear Hunchback Pass and re-enter the woods, there are lots of very nice sites next to the creek. The best camping is above Stormy Gulch, which requires a good effort to reach (it's marked on the map). Camping there gives you an easier shot at climbing both Storm King and Silex.

Route Notes   The trail maps on the sign and on topographical maps are pure confusion. In the following route description, I use the trail signs that are given along the way to avoid mixing up the routes. Even rangers were confused about the "actual" trail designations.

Mile/Waypoint   **0.0 mi (1)**   At the Beartown Trailhead, Trail #787 begins from the lot behind the sign and proceeds south and uphill to Hunchback Pass. The trail is well worn and easy to follow up to the pass.

1.3 mi (2)   The top of Hunchback Pass (12,496 feet) gives you amazing overviews of the area. The Guardian stands out from the peaks in the area; if your jaw drops, kindly close it and continue downhill.

Note: Once you are on the south side of the pass, consider this the Vallecito Trail (it will be referred to as such below).

2.6 mi (3)   The Nebo Creek Trail intersects on the left. Stay on the Vallecito Trail. Between here and the next waypoint, at 4.1 miles, there are lots of campsites. Yes, you're going to have to make up all this elevation you're losing later.

4.1 mi (4)   This is the key to your hike. Once you bottom out at about 10,500 feet, you will need to get off the Vallecito Trail. There will be an open meadow on your right with a faint hiker's trail that goes to the river and the forest beyond. Get off-trail, cross the meadow and make a river crossing at

Vallecito Creek. In the spring, this creek can really get moving, so be careful. Use your sandals here.

4.2 mi Once you have crossed the river, you should see a trail leading up to Stormy Gulch. There is a comically small hand-carved sign, but don't expect the trail to be easy to follow. There *is* a trail, but it is faint. Consider this off-trail terrain. Still, do your best to pick up the trail where you can.

5.1 mi (5) At 10,940 feet (approximately) you will have a choice. If you've followed the trail, it goes down to a river crossing that looks like it leads into weeds. If you are camping or want a longer, less direct ascent of the peak, cross the river here and snoop around for the trail on the other side. At about 11,200 feet, the weeds clear out and there are lots of good camp possibilities about 200 feet southwest of the creek (see waypoint 10). The higher you head up, the more level ground there is. You can follow the trail up to a less direct route to reach Storm King; check out the descent on the main route and take the same directions—but in reverse. Also, though camping at Lake Silex looks good on a map, in reality it's not: the entire place is a huge boulderfield. Camp lower, in the shelter of trees.

The direct ascent (which is what this route details) stays on the left (south) side of the creek, where there is no real trail.

5.4 mi (6) As you clear treeline, you'll see a very steep grassy slope heading up toward Lake Silex. It's a big push, but you can do it! Work southwest up the slopes. The creek listed on the map may or may not be running when you hike (it wasn't in August 2006). Note that your goal is not Lake Silex, but the boulder field higher and north of the lake. Keep heading southwest (right). Note: Storm King is the peak on the right of this slope; Silex is the one directly above and to the left.

6.2 mi Keep going southwest and you'll reach a boulder field below Storm King's southeast ridge. Your goal is to climb the southwest ridge, so skirt the peak and head west to Storm-Eight Saddle. When you are closing in on the saddle, it is easier to stay low and reach the low point in the saddle instead of trying to intercept the southwest ridge higher up. The footing below Storm King's south face is off-camber, loose, and cruddy. The choice is yours, but I found it quicker to stay lower and reach the saddle on better footing.

6.7 mi (7) Finally, you're at Storm-Eight Saddle (between Storm King and Peak Eight). You are within striking distance of the summit. The southwest ridge is pure, unfettered scrambling on good rock. It's all class 3, and you can stay fairly close to the spine most of the way up; staying on the left (west) side offers safer options if the ridge gets too airy. Those with good route-finding skills will blaze up this rock like a jungle gym, linking together fun scrambling sections and indulging in the thrill of the climb! Once up high, a fitting catwalk goes northwest like a red carpet to the summit of this awesome mountain.

7.07 mi (8) You are amongst royalty: Storm King's summit! Enjoy!

On the descent, you will return to the saddle (waypoint 7) and to the shoulder of boulder (Point Silex) above Lake Silex and take a slightly different route back.

8.0 mi (9)   At the trail split, go northwest on a trail that stays below the east side of Storm King's northeast ridge. There is an actual path that goes near the lower Trinity Lakes and then follows a trail to waypoint 5 at the top of Stormy Gulch. If it's faded, just work down to Trinity Creek, and follow it to the top of the gulch.

8.3 mi   The trail cuts through a big notch—more like a gash—and goes into treeline.

8.5 mi (10)   This is the camping waypoint. To get back to your vehicle, follow the creek (or the faint trail) back to the top of Stormy Gulch. Again, if you have GPS, retracing your tracks is a lot easier.

10.3 mi (4)   It's a bittersweet moment when you cross over the creek and return to the Vallecito Trail; not just because the fun is over, but also because you now have to hike uphill another 2,000 feet to Hunchback Pass (waypoint 2). Oy! Hey, if you're lucky, you'll be on Hunchback Pass just in time to see a beautiful sunset. Continue on over the pass to your car.

14.7 mi   Finish.

Options   There is so much to do here! Mount Silex (13,628 feet) is just one option. From above Lake Silex, go to the saddle between Silex and northeast shoulder of Peak 9. Once on the southwest ridge, stay about 200 feet below the top for a class 3 scramble to Mount Silex Summit, similar to the one on Storm King. Bolder scramblers can stay on the ridge proper, which is a class 4 route. This route is 0.9 mile one way from Point Silex (between waypoints 7 and 9 on the mapped route).

The other peaks in the area are similar scrambles waiting to be discovered. Get out there, have fun, and be safe. One route that looks fun on the map (though I haven't done it personally) is the traverse from Mount Silex's south side to the Guardian. Rock climbers take note: the quartzite rock here has several classic multipitch routes, some up to 1,500 feet.

Quick Facts   Storm King is one of four peaks in the state with this same name; this one is the highest (and the best!). Silex is the Latin word for "silicon." The Grenadiers are one of the few ranges in Colorado not explored by the Hayden or Wheeler surveys. Two climbers (William S. Cooper and John Hubbard) ventured into the area in 1908 and made many first ascents in the region.

With all the signs and its name still on the map, you'd think Beartown would be a bigger deal. It was founded in 1893 and brought more than 400 prospectors to the area. The Sylvanite Mine yielded a great deal of ore and was worked well into the 20th century. However, today, even the ruins are hard to find, making Beartown a true ghost town.

Contact Info   San Juan National Forest
Columbine West Ranger District
110 W. Eleventh Street
Durango, CO 81301
(970) 884-2512

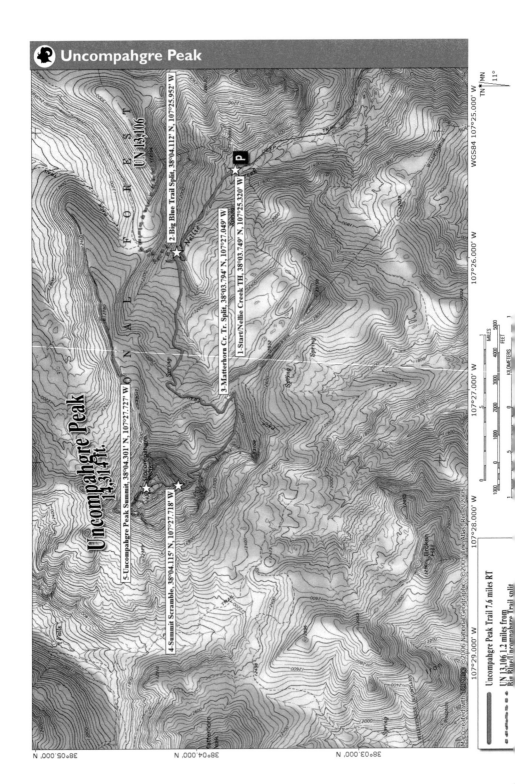

Uncompahgre Peak

UN 13,106

Uncompahgre Peak
14,314 ft.

5-Uncompahgre Peak Summit, 38°04.301' N, 107°27.727' W

4-Summit Scramble, 38°04.115' N, 107°27.718' W

2-Big Blue Trail Split, 38°04.112' N, 107°25.952' W

3-Matterhorn Cr. Tr. Split, 38°03.794' N, 107°27.049' W

1-Start/Nellie Creek TH, 38°03.749' N, 107°25.320' W

Map created with TOPO!® ©2006 National Geographic; ©2005 Tele Atlas, Rel. 8/2005

Uncompahgre Peak Trail 7.6 miles RT

UN 13,106 1.2 miles from Rio Blue/Uncompahgre Trail split

46 Uncompahgre Peak

Colorado's sixth highest mountain dominates the open plains of the San Juans, rising from the land like the bow of a sinking ship. Most of this scenic hike is above treeline.

Round Trip Distance	7.6 miles
Hiking Time	4½–6 hours
Difficulty	5/10
Class	2
Start Elevation	11,410 ft., at Nellie Creek Trailhead
Peak Elevation	14,314 ft.
Total Elevation Gain	2,911 ft.
Terrain	Good trail with some easy scrambling toward the summit
Best Time to Climb	June–September
Gear Advisor	Normal gear
Crowd Level	Low due to tough access road

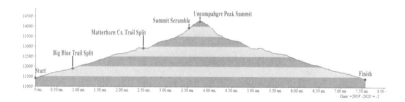

Location   San Juan Range in the Uncompahgre Wilderness/Uncompahgre National Forest near Lake City

Intro   The name alone is enough to inspire curiosity. Uncompahgre Peak is the highest mountain in the San Juan Range in southwest Colorado. The San Juans receive more precipitation than central and southern ranges, tinting the tundra with flora of green, yellow, red, and blue. There is something that draws you into Uncompahgre; perhaps it is the colorful burst of life that contradicts the apocryphal notion of mountains as barren, grim places. On clear-blue-sky days, the vivid hues and spacious views embody the refreshing rewards of being in the mountains.

Why Climb It?   The colors, the views, and Uncompahgre's distinct "wedding cake" shape will elevate your senses and psych you up to climb this peak. Most of this trek is above treeline on gentle, rolling alpine tundra. You'll be in spacious, wide-open land the entire hike. The trail is well maintained and easy to follow. After a long, gradual ascent, there are a few moderate switchbacks and a brief, easy scramble to the flat and accommodating summit. It's not a very

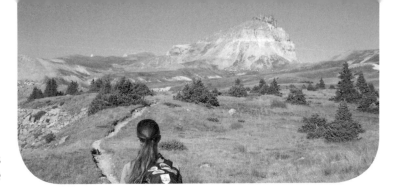

long or difficult hike, but every foot of the trail will enliven your senses
with incredible views and fresh mountain air.

Driving   You'll need a high-clearance SUV or 4x4 to get up the tough Nellie Creek
Road. Sport utility cars with good clearance and a strong low gear have a
shot at making the whole road (I saw a Honda CRV at the trailhead when I
was there). The road is steep with very sharp turns; it has some rocky sections and some major ruts. There are two stream crossings as well. If you
have a car, you'll have to park at the base of the Nellie Creek Road and hoof
it—making this a 16-mile hike with over 5,000 feet of elevation. The road
and trail are easy to hike, so if you have the time and endurance (especially
during a monotonous walk up/down the 4x4 road), give it a shot.

How to Get There   From County Road 149 in Lake City, follow the signs for Engineer Pass.
Turn west off CR 149 onto Second Street. Drive a short 0.1 mile, and you'll
begin the road up Engineer Pass (also known as Alpine Loop Scenic Byway/
Henson Road/20 Road). Drive 5.0 miles up this well-maintained dirt road
to Nellie Creek Road, passable by all vehicles. Keep an eye out on the left
(south) side of the road for an old, amazing abandoned mine operation
built into the canyon (there are a few informative plaques to learn about
the area). This is a good place to stop on your way home.

At mile 5.0, you'll reach the intersection for the Nellie Creek Road
(#877) on your right. Cars and low-clearance sport utility cars will have
to stop here and walk up. Nellie Creek Road is 4.0 miles and ends at the
Nellie Creek Trailhead and wilderness boundary. This road is rugged,
steep, rocky, rutted, and tight! At mile 2.3, there is a junction on a turn.
Stay left on the main road here. Cross two streams, muscle your vehicle up
the road, and at mile 3.7, you'll come to a flat section ideal for camping.
The trailhead is just beyond at mile 4.0; it has ample parking, a restroom,
and a small sign kiosk.

Fees/Camping   There are no fees to hike Uncompahgre Peak. There are no fees to camp at
the unimproved sites along the access road or in this area of the San Juan
Mountains.

Route Notes   None.

Mile/Waypoint   **0.0 mi (1)**   Start at Nellie Creek Trailhead. Get on the well-marked, well-
worn Uncompahgre Peak Trail. Note that the large, impressive mountain
to your right (north) is Unnamed Peak 13,106, an optional summit.

0.8 mi (2) As you come up a small hill, a field of green opens up with Uncompahgre's imperial shape finally coming into view. There is an intersection for the Big Blue Trail here; stay left on the Uncompahgre Trail. Continue over the tundra on trail.

2.5 mi (3) After climbing another short hill, you'll intersect with the Matterhorn Creek Trail at 12,920 feet. Stay right on the Uncompahgre Trail. This semiflat ridge has great views of rock formations to the left and San Juan vistas to the right.

3.2 mi At 13,460 feet, begin a brief, steep section of dusty switchbacks.

3.6 mi (4) Atop the switchbacks, at 13,930 feet, the trail splits into several worn paths (all of them with cairns!). My preferred route is to bear right (which is more straight than right) and make the class 2+ scramble up. If you go left, you'll be fine—it's a similar trail that goes onto the west face of the mountain and scrambles up.

3.8 mi (5) Uncompahgre's broad summit. As of September 2006, there were several summit markers, but no register (that will change I'm sure). The highest points are on the boulders on the flat section near the drop-off to the north, not on the western shoulder. Return the way you came.

7.6 mi Finish.

Options The wide-open, rolling terrain makes hiking and scrambling to the unnamed hills around Uncompahgre a fun diversion. There are a few 14ers and high 13ers in the area, notably 14,017-foot Wetterhorn Peak to the northwest, not on the map. For those looking for a burly challenge, try linking Uncompahgre and Wetterhorn by splitting off the Matterhorn Creek Trail at waypoint 3 after climbing Uncompahgre. (Or camp down in the basin northeast of the Wetterhorn/Matterhorn ridge, and bag the peak the next day.)

A more modest peak to grab is Unnamed Peak 13,106 (which is looming to the northwest from the Nellie Creek Trailhead parking area). Turn right (at waypoint 2) onto the Big Blue Trail for 0.5 mile, and then get off-trail and scramble up the class 2 ridge to the top. This is 1.2 miles one way from the intersection of the Big Blue and the Uncompahgre trails.

Quick Facts Unlike many other names in the San Juans, Uncompahgre is not Spanish in origin. Rather, the word comes from the native Ute Indians, who used the term *Ancapagari* (translated: "red lake" or "red water") to describe a reddish hot spring near the mountain. The name was first applied to the Uncompahgre River; the mountain was named shortly thereafter. Despite some resistance, the native title stuck, albeit with a European phonetic twist.

Contact Info Uncompahgre National Forest
Gunnison Ranger District
P.O. Box 89
Lake City, CO 81230
(970) 641-0471

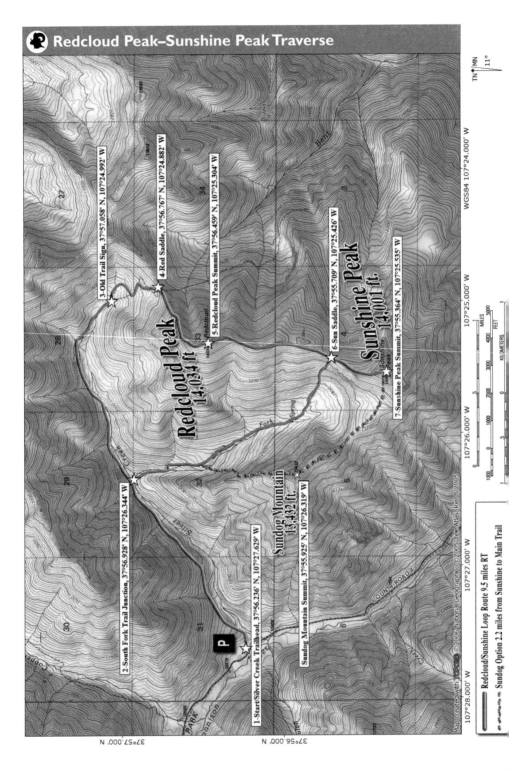

Redcloud Peak–Sunshine Peak Traverse

Redcloud Peak
14,034 ft

Sunshine Peak
14,001 ft.

Sundog Mountain
13,432 ft.

1-Start/Silver Creek Trailhead, 37°56.236' N, 107°27.629' W

2-South Fork Trail Junction, 37°56.928' N, 107°26.344' W

3-Old Trail Sign, 37°57.058' N, 107°24.992' W

4-Red Saddle, 37°56.767' N, 107°24.882' W

5-Redcloud Peak Summit, 37°56.459' N, 107°25.304' W

6-Sun Saddle, 37°55.709' N, 107°25.426' W

7-Sunshine Peak Summit, 37°55.364' N, 107°25.535' W

Sundog Mountain Summit, 37°55.925' N, 107°26.319' W

WGS84 107°24.000' W

TN MN 11°

Redcloud/Sunshine Loop Route 9.5 miles RT

Sundog Option 2.2 miles from Sunshine to Main Trail

47 Redcloud Peak–Sunshine Peak Traverse

How can you go wrong with mountains that are red and sunny? Green San Juan meadows and rusty crimson rocks give a burst of color to this beautiful landscape.

Round Trip Distance	9.5 miles
Hiking Time	5–7 hours
Difficulty	5/10
Class	2
Start Elevation	10,438 ft., at Silver Creek/Grizzly Gulch Trailhead
Peak Elevations	Redcloud Peak: 14,034 ft.; Sunshine Peak: 14,001 ft.
Total Elevation Gain	4,100 ft.
Terrain	Good trail to summits; rocky descent on medium talus
Best Time to Climb	June–September
Gear Advisor	Normal Gear; trekking poles if doing the loop descent
Crowd Level	Low

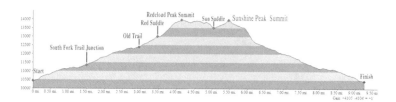

Location   San Juan Range in the Uncompahgre Wilderness/Bureau of Land Management lands west of Lake City

Intro   The San Juan Mountains owe most of their color to the precipitation that targets southwest Colorado. The increased flora is especially scenic when paired with natural red rocks that compose the upper reaches of these two peaks. Taken as a pair, they are very welcoming summits, reached by a well-maintained, nontechnical trail. Sunshine Peak is the lowest of the 14ers, clearing the height requirement with just a foot to spare!

Why Climb It?   The colorful palette of the San Juans is on display, so bring your camera. Even the clear waters of Silver Creek contribute, illuminating the gray and white rocks of the stream bed with flashes of silver when the sun shines. All the natural beauty is easy on the eyes (and the knees, thanks to a well-made trail). The loop described includes a shortcut down rocky talus that eliminates the need to reverse your route. If you are hesitant to plod down a loose, rocky slope, it's easy enough to go back the way you came. No matter how you visit these two 14ers, it's a trip well worth taking.

Driving Tough passenger cars can make it to the trailhead in normal conditions. The road is rough in places, and the shelf-road section is exciting! I was able to make it to this trailhead with my Honda Accord, but I had a few minor scrapes on the way up.

How to Get There From Lake City (which is roughly 50 miles south of Gunnison), find the intersection of Colorado Highway 149 and Hinsdale County Road 30. There will be a large sign for the Alpine Loop and Cinnamon Pass. Turn onto CR 30, which is a paved road at this point. It is 16.6 miles from here to the trailhead. Pass the beautiful Lake San Cristobel, staying on CR 30. Stay right at the southern terminus of the lake (or else you'll just loop around the east shore). CR 30 is paved for 4.2 miles and then becomes a well-maintained dirt road that passes Williams Creek and Mill Creek campgrounds. At mile 12.4, you'll come to a fork in the road; go right to start the more rugged part of your drive up to Cinnamon Pass Road (County Road 4). (Note that going left here takes you to the ghost town of Sherman.)

You'll climb on a shelf road that is washed out in places but passable by a carefully driven car. Continue along this road for 4.0 miles to the trailhead (look for mile marker 16; the trailhead is 0.6 mile after it). There are some campsites and a toilet on the left-hand side; your trailhead starts from the right-hand (northeast) lot.

Fees/Camping There are no fees for hiking or camping in this area; many parties camp at or just outside of the trailhead. Please minimize your impact.

Closing in on the summit of Red Cloud

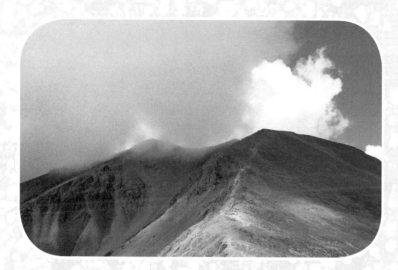

Red Cloud Mountain surrounded by white clouds

Route Notes   None.

Mile/Waypoint   **0.0 mi (1)**   Start at the Silver Gulch Trailhead. Go east on the two-lane trail that heads uphill into the woods. You'll soon parallel Silver Creek; for the ascent, stay on the left (north) side of the creek on the obvious trail.

1.5 mi (2)   You'll now be hiking next to Silver Creek. This is where you will exit South Fork Basin on your descent. There is a hard-to-see cairn designating the faint trail to the right (south-southeast) that you will be following on the way back. Note, however, that this is a poor ascent route and should be avoided for the time being. Stay on the main trail as it cuts northeast. When you get into the high part of the basin, doesn't it seem like something is missing? Unlike most mountain basins, this one has no lakes or ponds.

3.0 mi (3)   As you begin to climb to Red Saddle, you'll see a sign politely asking you to use the switchbacked trail instead of the older, more direct trail. Help lessen erosion by going on the switchbacks.

3.5 mi (4)   On top of Red Saddle (13,000 feet) you have a 1,000-foot climb to reach the top of Redcloud. The mountain looks every bit a 14er, looming to the southeast in all its crimson glory. You have two options here: attack the ridge directly by staying on the steep, rocky spine trail, or go out onto the northeast face and take the switchbacks up. Both trails go to the top and merge at a level section just before the final summit push.

4.2 mi (5)   Redcloud Peak's very red summit is beneath your boots! The trail that traverses to Sunshine is easy to follow. Head south to the Sun Saddle en route to Sunshine Peak.

5.2 mi (6)   The low point of the traverse is Sun Saddle, at 13,500 feet. The switchbacks that climb to the summit are easier than they look. The trail is still evident and easy to follow.

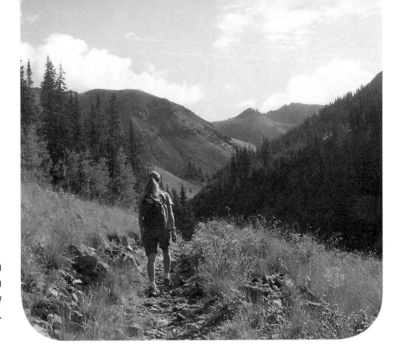

The San Juan mountains are known for their lovely approach trails.

5.6 mi (7) Sunshine Peak's flat summit has a nice wind shelter and great views. Don't rest too long if you want to try the Sundog Mountain option to the northwest. If you are following the standard route, return to Sun Saddle.

6.0 mi (6) There is a trail to the left (northwest) that descends the scree into South Fork Basin. A sign warns that this trail is dangerous. The terrain is not difficult (though it is a little annoying)—the danger is more from rocks that may get kicked down on you by other hikers. If you are in a group, stay close together so rocks don't have time to gain momentum. If others are on the trail below you, wait until they are out of the fall line before you continue down.

Once you get down the steepest section, a cairned trail through the talus leads you to the South Fork Creek. A spring supplies much of the creek's water, which seems to magically flow from the earth; it's a curious sight. Stay close to the creek as you hike out to the north. The trail fades in and out; you'll know you are out of the basin when you cross Silver Creek and the well-worn access trail reappears. (This is the trail that you avoided on the way up.)

8.0 mi (2) Return to the main trail (Silver Gulch Trail) and follow it out to the trailhead.

9.5 mi Finish.

Options The Sundog Loop is a popular alternative for those who don't want to fumble down scree nor return via Redcloud. Follow the northwest ridge of Sunshine (class 2) for 1.0 mile to the 13,432-foot summit of Sundog Mountain. This is the 299th highest peak in the state. To descend, take the northeast ridge down. Before you get into treeline, go north toward South Fork Creek. Cross the stream (possibly gaining the South Fork Trail, if it's visible), and rejoin the main trail at waypoint 2. It is 2.2 miles from Sunshine's summit to the main trail if you take this option.

Quick Facts Sunshine Peak's elevation has been accurately measured several times, and with each survey, it remains in the elite 14ers club. It's had a few iffy moments, but as of 2006 its place seems secure. Sunshine Peak was named by the USGS in 1904; before then it was known variously as Niagara Peak or Sherman Peak. Redcloud was named in 1874 by the Hayden survey, whose members thought that the red rocks resembled scarlet clouds from a distance.

There are two "Sunshine" mountains in Colorado. The other is located just outside of Telluride; despite standing only 12,930 feet, it is a very visually impressive peak that is often mistaken for a 14er.

Contact Info Bureau of Land Management
Gunnison Office
216 N. Colorado
Gunnison, CO 81230
(970) 641-0471

Bureau of Land Management
Lake City Office
(970) 944-2344

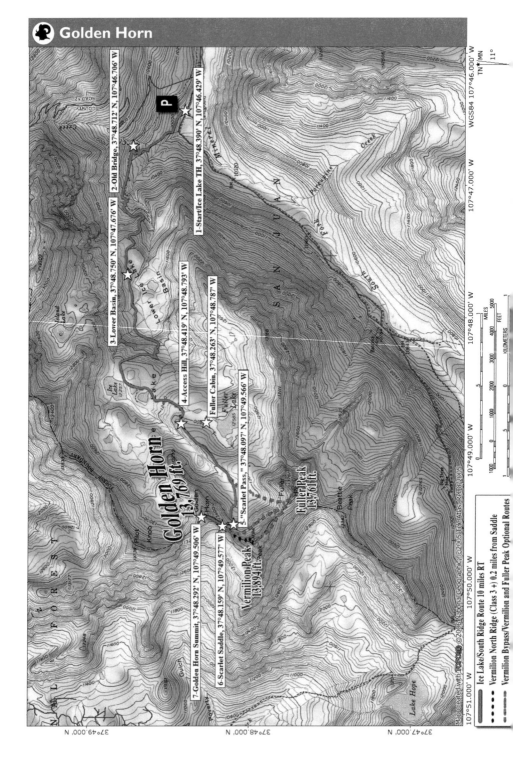

Golden Horn

2-Old Bridge, 37°48.712' N, 107°46.706' W

1-Start/Ice Lake TH, 37°48.390' N, 107°46.429' W

3-Lower Basin, 37°48.750' N, 107°47.676' W

4-Access Hill, 37°48.419' N, 107°48.793' W

Fuller Cabin, 37°48.263', 107°48.787' W

5-"Scarlet Pass," 37°48.097' N, 107°49.566' W

Golden Horn 13,769 ft.

Fuller Peak 13,761 ft.

Vermilion Peak 13,894 ft.

7-Golden Horn Summit, 37°48.292' N, 107°49.506' W

6-Scarlet Saddle, 37°48.159' N, 107°49.577' W

Ice Lake/South Ridge Route 10 miles RT

Vermilion North Ridge (Class 3 +) 0.2 miles from Saddle

Vermilion Bypass/Vermilion and Fuller Peak Optional Routes

Map created with TOPO!® ©2006 National Geographic; ©2005 Tele Atlas Rel. 8/2005

48   Golden Horn

Answer the call for adventure by scaling the best horn in Colorado! Ice Lake Basin is your gateway to this finely crafted mountain, whose profile dominates the western skyline.

Round Trip Distance	10 miles
Hiking Time	6–8 hours
Difficulty	8/10
Class	2+/Optional class 3 moves on summit
Start Elevation	9,840 ft., at Ice Lake Trailhead
Peak Elevation	13,769 ft.
Total Elevation Gain	3,890 ft.
Terrain	Good trail to rocky basin; loose but fun scramble to summit
Best Time to Climb	July–September
Gear Advisor	Normal gear
Crowd Level	Low

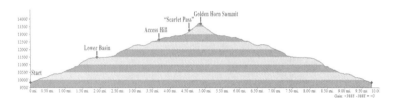

Location   San Juan Mountains in the Weminuche Wilderness/San Juan National Forest outside of Silverton

Intro   Ice Lake Basin (and the approach to reach it) is a feast for your senses. Dazzling waterfalls thunder down sheer cliffs, and colossal mountains partition the beauty into distinct compartments. At the center of it all is Golden Horn, rising like a rusty gothic castle. Your camera will be working overtime as you make your way up to the summit. Views from the top look out into the Lizard Head Wilderness and the Grenadier Range, and at several other San Juan beauties.

Why Climb It?   Golden Horn looks like a miniature version of Uncompahgre Peak, but the climbing is much different. As you can tell by its crumbly appearance, rock in this area is constantly being shed from the shattered peaks. Despite the ruinous appearance, the route to Golden Horn is on mostly solid rock. The only loose slope is found on a short scree section just below the summit. Once you get to the top, there are several places where fun scrambling offers new vantage points of the area. Bring a friend along and take photos of one another on opposing summit blocks!

<table>
<tr><td>Driving</td><td>Mineral Creek Road (Forest Service Road 585) is a very well-maintained dirt road and is passable by all vehicles under normal conditions.</td></tr>
</table>

Driving Mineral Creek Road (Forest Service Road 585) is a very well-maintained dirt road and is passable by all vehicles under normal conditions.

How to Get There From Silverton at the junction of Colorado Highway 110 and US Highway 550, drive 2.0 miles south on US 550 and turn right onto Mineral Creek Road (FS 585). If you are approaching from the south, this turn is 7.8 miles from the summit of Red Mountain Pass. There is a sign for Mineral Creek. Once on this dirt road, follow it 4.0 miles west to the South Mineral Campground. Do not take any side roads that disappear into the woods. The Ice Lake Trailhead has lots of parking and is directly across the road from the campground on the right (north) side of FS 585.

Fees/Camping There are no fees to hike or camp in the wilderness area. Camping at South Mineral Creek Campground is $14 per night; the 26 sites fill up quickly on weekends. There are several pulloffs that offer free camping on FS 585, but good luck beating the hoards of RVs to a good spot. Lower Ice Lakes Basin is the best place to set up camp if you prefer a backcountry alternative.

Route Notes None.

Mile/Waypoint **0.0 mi (1)**   Start at the Ice Lake Trailhead and get on the Ice Lake Trail. This is a well-traveled path that is easy to follow. Enjoy the experience as the secrets of the Ice Lake basins unfold before you. Stay on the path that switchbacks near the waterfall. Don't take any of the faint shortcuts. There is an easy river crossing along the way. At the top of the switchbacks, you'll see a dilapidated bridge spanning the waterfall. It looks like something out of *Indiana Jones!* Luckily, you don't have to cross it.

0.7 mi (2) At the old bridge, go left (west) and continue on-trail to the lower basin.

2.0 mi (3) The spacious Lower Ice Lake Basin is amazing. If you want to camp in the area, this is the place to do it (though in mid-summer, the bugs are fierce). Higher up, things are very exposed. Stay on-trail as you gaze at several waterfalls—many cut into notches in the cliffs that section off this area from the upper basin. Carry on toward Ice Lake and the upper basin.

3.1 mi Ice Lake is before you when you get to the top level of the upper basin. The trail fades out in this area. Continue south to the hill west of Fuller Lake (at a large boulder, there is a faint, cairned trail to the right— this is the path of least resistance).

3.7 mi (4) You're on the hill, and you can now see "Scarlet Pass." If you want to align yourself a little better, continue to hike south until Fuller Lake and the Fuller Cabin are in sight. Go right (west) from these landmarks to gain the little ridge at 12,900 feet. Once you are on the ridge, drop down into a flat "talus lake" that borders Scarlet Pass. There is a tiny lake and some old wood planks down to your right—go past these to the flat part of the talus field. Traverse this patch of rocks, checking out some of the unique boulders and old mining debris. Scarlet Pass between Vermillion Peak and Golden Horn looks tricky, but it reveals its lines when you actually get there.

4.6 mi (5) "Scarlet Pass." This hill to the saddle is much shorter than it looks from a distance. The base is at 13,250 feet. As you look at it, there are a lot of runout routes on the right (north) side. Ignore these and head to the left (south), where a series of ledges makes travel to the saddle a class 2+ walk. Close to where the gray rocks of Vermillion merge with the reddish stone of Scarlet Pass is a good place to find your starting point. There are a few old cairns along the way, but you shouldn't need them.

4.7 mi (6) Scarlet Saddle, the high saddle at 13,560 feet, opens up western views. Your remaining scramble follows this south ridge to the summit. You may want to ditch your trekking poles here. The scramble up is loose in places; a little more solid and exposed as you stay toward the left side. If the climbing is getting too difficult, stay right on the sandy slopes, and angle up. Eventually you'll reach a notch that splits the two tops of Golden Horn. Go left to make the easier scramble to an airy summit block for the true apex.

5.0 mi (7) Golden Horn's summit! What views! This, the "west summit," has a register tube, but as of August 2006 no register. (I put the only piece of paper I had on me—a picture of Blanka from *Street Fighter 2*—as a temporary log.) You can scramble around up here as you see fit. However, if you want to visit the "east summit" as well, there is a "wiggle notch" that you'll have to jam yourself into and then squirm up and through (a class 3 move) to get there. These two summits are the two photograph points I mention in the "Why Climb It?" section.

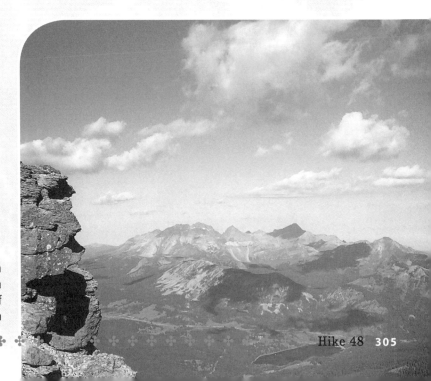

The impressive "Wilson Group" of 14ers as seen from the summit of Golden Horn

Return the way you came. The descent back to the talus field is fast. On the way down, you may want to detour over to Fuller Lake and the old Fuller Cabin. This is a good place to take shelter if storms move in before you can make it to timberline.

10.0 mi Finish.

Options From Scarlet Pass (waypoint 5), it's a mere 0.23 mile to Vermillion Peak, but the ridge is a class 3+/4 adventure with some very exposed moves on rotten rock. A lower route on sandy slopes leading to a steep, loose gully is less exposed but still difficult. Either way, the easiest way to get atop this 13,894-foot peak is to follow the sandy notch on the east face to the summit. This traverse is tougher than it may seem, and I only include it for more experienced scramblers. From Vermilion, it's a class 2+ trek of 0.5 mile over to the shapely cone of Fuller Peak (13,761 feet). Descend via the slope between Vermillion and Fuller for a 1.6-mile loop from Scarlet Pass to the small ridge and waypoint 4.

If you'd rather not go for the scramble on the north ridge of Vermillion but want to bag these two peaks, you can traverse a shelf on the east face of Vermillion Peak, at 13,400 feet, to the saddle between Fuller and Vermillion. Taking the southeast ridge up to Vermillion is much easier than the higher north ridge traverse.

Quick Facts Vermilion Peak is the highest point in San Juan County. The Ice Lake basins hold their snow into the summer, which is why I'd suggest waiting until July to try the peaks. The slopes are prime avalanche terrain. Even in July, bringing an ice axe may not be a bad idea. The cabin by Fuller Lake used to host winter trips, but it has fallen into disrepair in recent years.

Pilot Knob and other peaks in this area are technical ascents that require ropes and belays.

Contact Info San Juan National Forest
San Juan Public Lands Center
15 Burnettt Court
Durango, CO 81301
(970) 247-4874

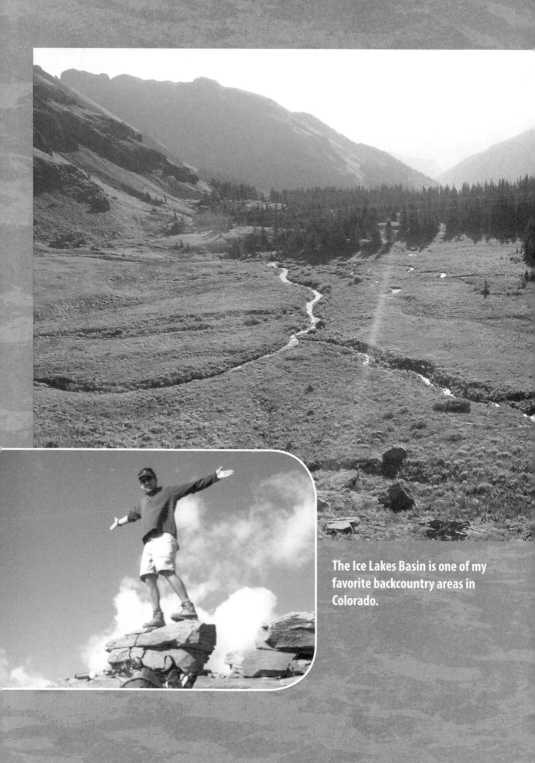

The Ice Lakes Basin is one of my favorite backcountry areas in Colorado.

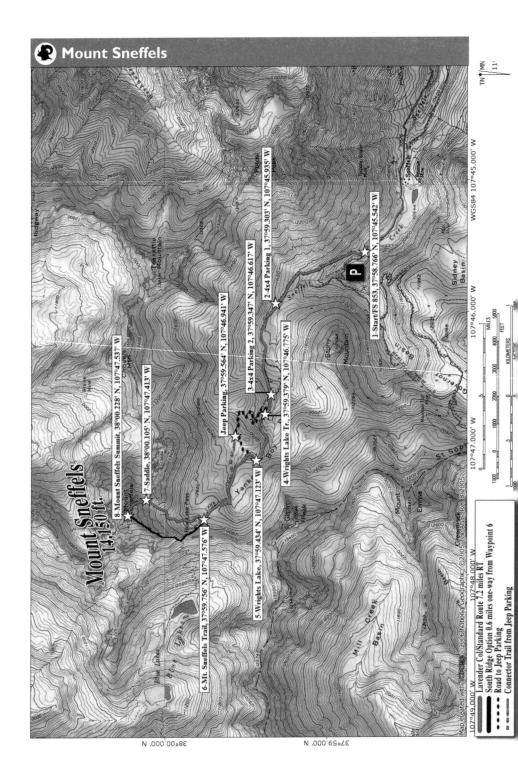

Mount Sneffels

Mount Sneffels
14,150 ft.

8-Mount Sneffels Summit, 38°00.228' N, 107°47.537' W

7-Saddle, 38°00.105' N, 107°47.413' W

Jeep Parking, 37°59.564' N, 107°46.941' W

3-4x4 Parking 2, 37°59.347' N, 107°46.617' W

2-4x4 Parking 1, 37°59.303' N, 107°45.935' W

4-Wrights Lake Tr., 37°59.379' N, 107°46.775' W

5-Wrights Lake, 37°59.434' N, 107°47.123' W

6-Mt. Sneffels Trail, 37°59.756' N, 107°47.576' W

1-Start/FS 853, 37°58.766' N, 107°45.542' W

TN/MN 11'

WGS84 107°45.000' W

107°46.000' W

107°47.000' W

107°48.000' W

107°49.000' W

38°00.000' N

37°59.000' N

Map created with TOPO! ©2006 National Geographic; ©2005 TELE ATLAS, Rel. 8/2005.

Lavender Col/Standard Route 7.2 miles RT
South Ridge Option 0.6 miles one-way from Waypoint 6
Road to Jeep Parking
Connector Trail from Jeep Parking

49 Mount Sneffels

Mount Sneffels is a photographer's favorite, but it's not just another pretty face. With great scrambling and fantastic views, you'll be salivating for Sneffels!

Round Trip Distance	7.2 miles
Hiking Time	4–6 hours
Difficulty	6.5/10
Class	2+
Start Elevation	10,784 ft., at Yankee Boy Basin Road
Peak Elevation	14,150 ft.
Total Elevation Gain	3,250 ft.
Terrain	Good trail leads to scree slope and solid, scrambly gully to summit
Best Time to Climb	June–September
Gear Advisor	Ice axe in early spring, trekking poles, boots for scree
Crowd Level	Moderate

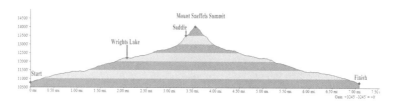

Location

San Juan Range in the Mount Sneffels Wilderness/Uncompahgre National Forest outside of Ouray

Intro

When you hike Mount Sneffels, you'll literally be climbing on a mountain of gold. Mines from its ore-rich flanks have produced more valuable gold than any other peak in the nation—and the deposits have yet to give out. Who knows, maybe you'll find a nugget or two on your hike! As is the norm in the San Juans, mountain views are tinged with green and orange, making for some of the best hiking pictures in Colorado. The scramble up Lavender Col is a solid and fun way to top out.

Why Climb It?

Yankee Boy Basin is a beautiful place to spend an afternoon. The colors of the San Juans and the views of surrounding mountains are spectacular. Many peaks in the region are over 13,000 feet; they sprawl out like a legion of stoic giants. Many wild animals call the area home. A black bear, a coyote, and several elk said hello to me the last time I was in the basin. The gully that exits just below the top is a great finishing touch. Sneffels is a good hike for people who want to try their first rugged 14er.

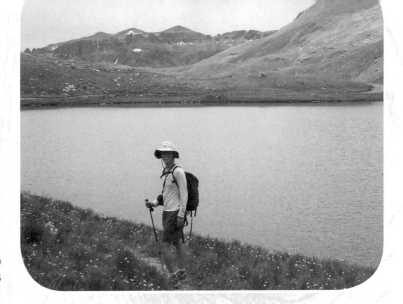

On the way to
Sneffels

Driving　Driving to the parking areas on Sneffels can be a fun and scenic ride or a sphincter-clenching thrill-ride, depending on what kind of vehicle you have. For the record, tough passenger cars can make it to the lower part of Yankee Boy Basin—my Accord made it to the junction of Sneffels Road (Forest Service Road 853) and County Road 26. For those with low-clearance vehicles, there is a section on the shelf road that is cut into solid rock and is just wide enough for one car. It's like driving through a tunnel with one open side. Cars will have to take the rock steps in the road head-on— you will have nowhere else to go. Expect to scrape—hard—a few times. When it's been raining, you may get to exit this cave by driving under a waterfall. The rest of the road is rough but passable to the aforementioned junction.

Of course, if you're driving an SUC, SUV, or 4x4, the road is fun. These vehicles can continue up the road, past the CR 26/FS 853 junction to two different parking areas. 4x4s with a short wheel base (i.e., Jeeps) can drive up to a high parking area at 12,314 feet.

How to Get There　From Ouray, drive 0.5 mile out of the southern end of town on US Highway 550 and turn right onto Ouray County Road 361; the turn is after a sharp left curve and has signs for Yankee Boy Basin. Follow this road as it gets progressivly rougher, and make sure to stay right when the road intersects with mining roads down to Camp Bird. Cars that have the guts to brave the "Sneffels Cave" (see above) can drive 6.8 miles and park at the junction of County Road 26 and FS 853 (or just below, in parking areas past the ghost town of Sneffels). SUCs, SUVs, and 4x4 vehicles can stay right on FS 853 and work up the road. There are several parking pulloffs along the way. Some of the rocky stream crossings will challenge sport utility cars. You will come to a sign warning vehicles with long wheel bases against proceeding. Jeeps and smaller 4x4s have the option of taking the road shown on the map to a high parking area, where a connector trail joins the main route. This takes a mile or two off the route.

Fees/Camping	There is no fee to hike here, but camping is restricted to designated areas. Most of the land is privately owned (mostly by mining interests) and must be respected. Call for more information, as regulations regarding camping are subject to change.
Route Notes	The route described here starts from the junction of County Road 26 and FS 853. If you drive to the jeep parking area, there is an easy-to-follow, signed connector trail.
Mile/Waypoint	**0.0 mi (1)** Start at the CR 26/FS 853 junction. Stay right (on FS 853) and hike up the road, which is quite scenic. Drivers of tougher vehicles can pull off in any number of small parking areas along the way. I've marked two on the map: at mile 0.78 **(2)**, and at mile 1.47 **(3)**.
	1.6 mi (4) When the road curves to the right, go straight on the footpath to the Wrights Lake Spur/Wrights Lake Trail. It is 0.5 mile to tiny Wrights Lake.
	2.1 mi (5) The trail forks as you near the lake. Go right, and avoid the trail on the rocks to the left (it goes to a mine). Go along the east side of the lake and stay on the footpath by turning left at the sign (west), passing the "north shore" of the lake. A jeep road goes north from the lake; do not take it (though if you do, it simply leads to the jeep parking area).
	2.9 mi (6) It's a sign! At this junction, go right (north) on the MOUNT SNEFFLES TRAIL NO. 204. There is a semivisible trail through the boulder field. Following the intended trail may not be feasible, but it lines you up for the steep scree gully you must climb to reach a saddle at 13,530 feet. This is where trekking poles are a big help.
	3.4 mi (7) From the scenic saddle, there's an impressive gully to the top on your left (northwest). Thankfully, this gully is more solid than the scree slope you just came up. A trail reappears and zigzags up. At the top, you have two options to exit. Both are class 2+ or easy class 3 moves. The first option: you can simply top out and scramble left on semi-exposed rock to the summit. The second option is a slightly easier variation: take a small chute left, just below the top—a single tricky move that leads to an easy and fun scramble on ledges to the summit.
	3.6 mi (8) Mount Sneffels's sumptuous summit! What views! You can return the way you came or, if you're up for scrambling, take the class 3 south ridge down to Blue Lake Pass. Either way, the descent is a little rough on the knees.
	7.3 mi Finish at the CR 26/FS 853 junction.
Options	If you continue to Blue Lake Pass instead of turning right at waypoint 6, you can attempt Sneffels's south ridge. This class 3 route has some exposure on solid rock and is cairned all the way to the top. Descend the standard route for a great loop.
Quick Facts	Sneffels's name has been a source of contention for years. The story that has the most artistic merit alludes to novelist Jules Verne's book *Journey to the*

Centre of the Earth. In that book, Verne refers to a real-life volcanic mountain in Iceland, known as "Snæfellsjökull," as the gateway to the center of our planet. I have no idea how to say that name, and neither did the geographers of old, since they condensed it to "Sneffels." Other rumors persist that a "Mr. Sneffels" existed, though if that entity was a man, a hamster, or a stuffed animal is unknown. A third explanation is that miners who worked on the mountain called it "Mount Sniffles," due to the cold-inducing conditions of the chilly tunnels. It's just as well, since many people call it "Sniffles" anyway.

Speaking of mines, Sneffels sits atop some of the most prolific veins of gold and silver ever mined. Even before the turn of *last* century (1900), the mines had already produced over $35 million dollars worth of ore. The Camp Bird Mine is still plugging away at the remaining ore. Thomas Walsh made his fortune from the bounty of the earth here; his daughter Evalyn Walsh McLean gained fame by being the last private owner of the supposedly hexed Hope Diamond. She was famous enough to be mentioned in the famous Cole Porter tune "Anything Goes." The reference to her goes as follows:

When Missus Ned McLean (God bless her)
Can get Russian reds to "yes" her,
Then I suppose
Anything goes.

These lines probably made a lot more sense in 1934; the best I can come up with is that "yes" in this context means something very naughty.

Contact Info   Uncompahgre National Forest
Ouray Ranger District
2505 S. Townsend
Montrose, CO 81401
(970) 240-5300

Additionally, The Yankee Boy Conservation Alliance works with private land owners to manage and maintain access to this beautiful spot. Read about them online at www.yankeeboy.org or contact them at:

YBCA
P.O. Box 1448
Ouray, CO 81427
(970) 325-4116

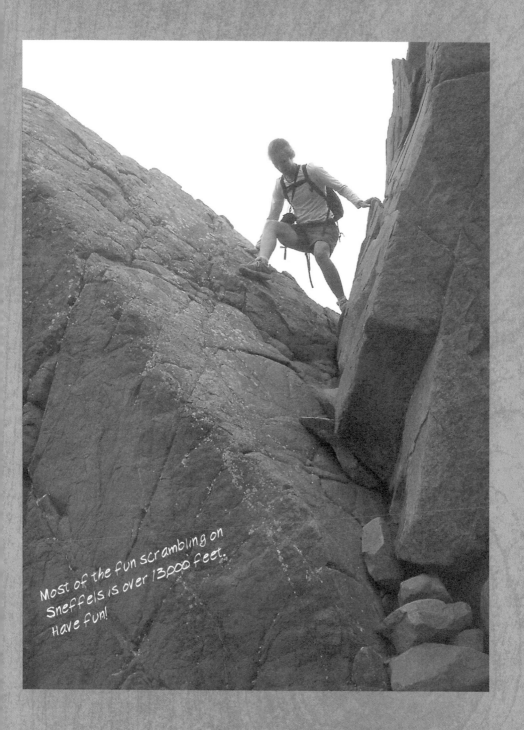

Most of the fun scrambling on Sneffels is over 13,000 feet. Have fun!

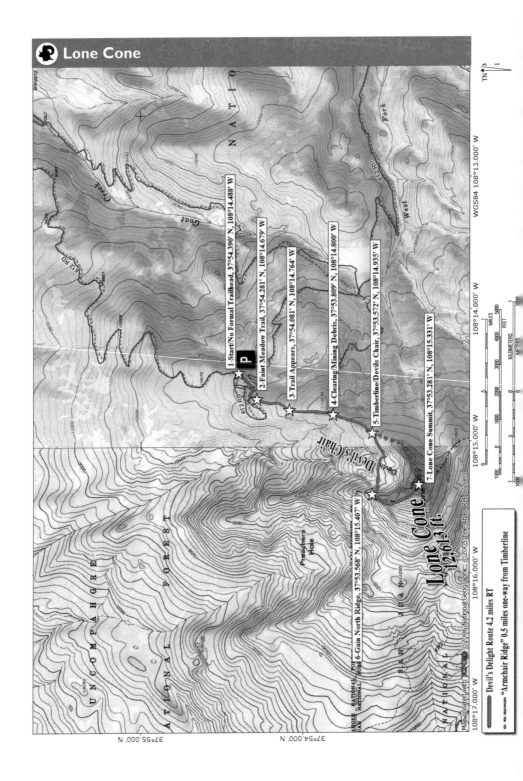

Lone Cone

1-Start/No Formal Trailhead, 37°54.390' N, 108°14.488' W
2-Faint Meadow Trail, 37°54.281' N, 108°14.679' W
3-Trail Appears, 37°54.081' N, 108°14.764' W
4-Clearing/Mining Debris, 37°53.809' N, 108°14.800' W
5-Timberline/Devils Chair, 37°53.572' N, 108°14.935' W
6-Gain North Ridge, 37°53.568' N, 108°15.407" W
7-Lone Cone Summit, 37°53.281' N, 108°15.331' W

Lone Cone
12,613 ft.

Devil's Chair

Preachers Hole

Goat Creek

West Fork

UNCOMPAHGRE NATIONAL FOREST

SAN JUAN NATIONAL FOREST

WGS84 108°13.000' W

Mapcreated with TOPO! ©2006 National Geographic; ©2005 Tele Atlas Rel. 8/2005

Devil's Delight Route 4.2 miles RT

"Armchair Ridge" 0.5 miles one-way from Timberline

50   Lone Cone

Lone Cone beckons like an oracle. This remote, standalone mountain is the last high peak in western Colorado, signaling an end of the mountains and the start of the desert.

Round Trip Distance	4.2 miles
Hiking Time	3½–5 hours
Difficulty	6.5/10
Class	2+
Start Elevation	10,790 ft. No formal trailhead
Peak Elevation	12,613 ft.
Total Elevation Gain	1,963 ft.
Terrain	Off-trail ridge leads to talus field and a climb up rocky ridge
Best Time to Climb	June–September
Gear Advisor	GPS, trekking poles, sturdy boots
Crowd Level	Hermit

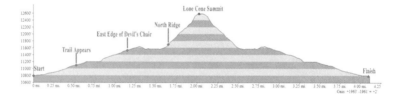

Location   Uncompahgre National Forest in the San Miguel Mountains outside the town of Norwood

Intro   There is something mystical about Lone Cone. Perhaps I've been in Boulder too long, but I sense that this mountain exudes a strange energy, a kind of surreal force whose effect is amplified by its remote and isolated nature. Crossing the Devil's Chair and gaining the north ridge reminded me of the knights of old journeying to reach a wise hermit in forbidden lands. And yet, the mountain is not far from Telluride and the Lizard Head Wilderness. Summiting Lone Cone puts you in an exclusive club of enlightened trekkers who have gained wisdom from this lonely peak.

Why Climb It?   Never mind all my metaphysical mumbo-jumbo, Lone Cone is a great climb! Mileage-wise it's short, but you'll be navigating off-trail in pine forests and rocky boulder fields, and focusing on navigation takes time. On the map, the Cone rises from the flat land and stands as the final, western vestige of the Colorado Rockies. If you like to get away from it all, this is your hike. The class 2+ scrambling is actually quite enjoyable (comparable to the summit scramble on the standard route on Mount of the Holy Cross). The Devil's Chair is an impressive sight—the entire northwest face is carved out, resembling the perfect recliner for ol' Beelzebub. Those who would deny the devil a chair anywhere but in Hell (even if the chair is metaphorical) may prefer to say it's simply a stunning natural feature. The climb seems to be inspirational, as many hikers have expressed some very personal and touching emotions in the register at the top.

Driving Tough passenger cars have a shot at making it to the start of the hike. The roads are fine up until Forest Service Road 612, which is especially troublesome if there has been a lot of rain. The road is rutted and washed out in spots, rocky and steep in others. A carefully driven car in good conditions could make it to the top. Don't be discouraged if you only have a passenger car—you can park 1.6 to 2.4 miles up the road and just hike or bike up the hill. It's a short distance, so it's not a huge deal.

Sport utility cars, SUVs, and 4x4 should have no trouble making it up to the parking area. The only real obstacle may be the huge mud puddles that form on the road. Taken too slowly, they will mire your vehicle in their slimy grasp. (Note to passenger cars: if you're gonna try 'em, get some speed!)

How to Get There Near the town of Norwood, at the junction of Colorado Highway 145 and County Road 44.Z, turn south on CR 44.Z (there will be a sign as you start down the road for the reservoirs and forest access). Stay south on this scenic, paved road. At mile 10.0, the road enters Uncompahgre National

Devil's Chair
on Lone Cone

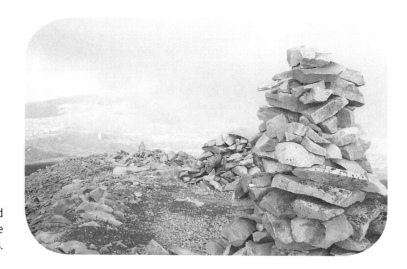

Despite being an isolated peak, the summit of Lone Cone has some nice cairns.

Forest; turns to dirt, and becomes known as CR 44.Z/Forest Service Road 610. Follow this road 2.0 more miles south (as it exits the national forest, it becomes CR 44.Z again—it's still the same road). Just past mile marker 12, turn left onto my favorite road in this whole book, Beef Trail Road (also known as County Road M44). As you start up this road, at mile 0.2, look to your right (south) at the beautiful metalwork on the sign for the Halsey Ranch. Ride the Beef Trail Road 2.5 miles to the intersection with CR 46M/ Forest Service Road 611 and turn right. This is an easy road to miss, so slow down when you near it. The road starts at a gap in a fence with NO TRESPASS-ING signs; there is also an old wood sign on the left (north) side announcing the mileage to Norwood and Beef Trail Road. You'll know you've gone too far if you start driving downhill.

Go south on FS 611 for 2.2 miles to FS 612 on your right (the turn is 0.1 miles after the WELCOME sign for Uncompahgre National Forest). FS 612 is a fairly uninviting road and will jostle the plucky passenger cars that attempt to climb it. Follow this road 4.4 miles; cars may be forced to park around mile 1.6. At mile 2.5 there is another parking area at a gate, which may serve as a good campsite. Just after this, the road starts a series of switchbacks. There are parking spots at the top of the hill at 10,780 feet. Note the GPS point if you have one with you. There is no trailhead.

Fees/Camping

There are no fees to hike or camp in the area. If you do overnight here, make sure you are within the boundaries of Uncompahgre National Forest and not on private land. The best places are along FS 612 and on the brief section of 44.Z/FS 610 before the turn onto the Beef Trail Road.

Route Notes

The entire route is technically off-trail, but there are old roads and a faint path through the woods to guide you, to a small degree. Don't rely on them, but note that they are there. Once you clear treeline at the base of the Devil's Chair, the navigation is much easier.

Mile/Waypoint   **0.0 mi (1)**   From the parking area, head west. This is the route I call "Devil's Delight." There is no formal trail, but there are a bunch of old logging roads. Head uphill to gain the highpoint of the forested ridge—you can follow the faint roads if the footing is easier, but don't rely on them.

0.3 mi (2)   This open meadow is quite scenic. From here, there is an old logging road that is overgrown but fairly easy to follow. You can use it as a guide to get to the spine of the ridge. Aim high on the ridge and continue south, leaving the meadow and heading into the dark forest.

0.5 mi (3)   As if by divine intervention, a trail materializes on the top of the ridge. It has some survey tags here and there. Again, remain on the highpoint of the ridge and don't be tempted to take any of the faint animal

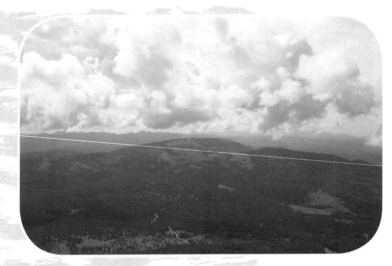

Lone Cone is Colorado's western-most 11,000-foot summit.

trails that go off into the woods. If the trail is not visible, don't be discouraged—continue along the highpoint of the ridge, heading south.

0.9 mi (4)   In a flat saddle clearing, there are the remnants of some old mining or survey equipment. There are also good views of Lone Cone. Continue south and uphill on the ridge.

1.2 miles (5)   Exit the trees at timberline, at 11,530 feet. Depending on your navigation savvy, that first section was either very easy or very difficult. From here you have a clear visual of Lone Cone, with the north ridge to the west, across the "seat" of the Devil's Chair.

Boulder-hop west across the semistable rocks of the seat, taking in wicked views of the chair to your left. Find a spot on the north ridge that suits you and climb to it (the easiest way to gain the ridge is by staying slightly to the north side).

1.7 mi (6)   Gain the north ridge and follow its rocky spine south/southeast to the high summit of Lone Cone.

2.1 mi (7) Lone Cone's secluded summit! There's a big cairn on top, as well as a summit register. Views to the east look out at the Lone Cone's partner, Little Cone, and at the high Wilson Peaks in the distance. Return the way you came. Navigation will be a little easier on the way down.

4.2 mi Finish.

Options

The east ridge of Lone Cone, also known as "Armchair Ridge," is a decent scramble that is 0.5 mile southwest one way from waypoint 5 to the summit. It is a class 3+ route with some exposed moves, but if you're up for some scrambling, it's the way to go.

It took me a few tries to realize "Devil's Delight" is the best route up Lone Cone; previously I had entered at the gate 2.5 miles up FS 612 and taken a convoluted and difficult bushwack through some ugly terrain. Forest sections were dark and eerie, and the landscape was littered with fallen trees and animal skulls. Other fearsome experiences along that route included a fast-moving lightning storm and a mad dash to escape a furious herd of angry, rogue, alpine cows. (This was the second time I was almost mauled by these supposedly peaceful ungulates. I also had to hop a cattle gate while running full speed to escape an ornery cow gang near Summit Peak. In retrospect, it may have been a couple of bulls leading the charge.) In other words, don't go this way! On the way down this bad route, I found the trail and an easier exit to the road, though I logged over 8.0 miles figuring this out. Live and learn, right? Better yet, read and beware!

Quick Facts

Lone Cone is the most fitting name for any mountain in Colorado. It's a forlorn peak, cast off from the social giants of the Sawatch or the conjoined legions of the San Juans. Technically, the San Miguel Mountains are part of the San Juans, but Lone Cone is a volcanic relic that is not attached to any other mountain.

Contact Info

Uncompahgre National Forest
Norwood Ranger District
P.O. Box 388-1150 Forest
Norwood, CO 81423
(970) 327-4261

Hike Your Heart Out

I've made the error of thinking the mountains serve to soothe the sting of my very human blunders. When seeking solace from the troubling architecture of manmade existence, I've run like a child into mother mountain's arms. I've wanted to close my eyes and feel nothing but the pure, sweet singular embrace.

And there I am greeted with dark clouds. My quest for grace is intercepted by something wicked.

I've endured withering heat and marrow-chilling cold. I've run from lightning until my lungs turned to ice on the verge of shattering. I've been lost in the fearful night. I've purpled my skin with bruises, and swollen my wrists and ankles countless times. I have felt the still malice of lurking forces intent on inflicting injury and dread. I have failed to reach summits. I've fantasized about warm meals, women, and soft beds. When I have sought comfort from the mountains, I have often made the mistake of not bringing anything to share but my self-pity. I have seen my troubles brought to life in fast-building storms, high-running rivers, and sheer cliffs.

And yet, even in my most selfish hour, even when I threaten to abandon this life of adventure for a plush couch and plasma screen TV, the mountains have imparted their wisdom. Even when my eyes have welled with tears of frustration, I have returned home again to find the food tastes sweeter, sleep comes easier, the body feels lighter. I have faced hardship with meaning, struggled in an honest kingdom, been humbled by a much wiser teacher. I have endured the tough love of the mountains and I am made better for it.

I grow. I return to the mountain wiser. I bring a gift of joy. Perhaps this solemn body of rock is curious of the ways of those who seek its heights. Instead of demanding spiritual enlightenment from the mountain, I converse with the details. I appreciate a good storm as much as the clear blue sky. And as I learn to love those details, funny things happen. The brain reprioritizes all the clutter banging around in my head, preferring to focus on faces in the rock and the symmetry of flowers. My heart pounds and my legs burn, with every vessel a throbbing affirmation of life. My legs feel the cold mud and the warm sun. When finally willing to yield my senses to the alpine world, I have received that long-sought embrace.

I admit, I'm not all that savvy in the frontcountry. Material wealth has yet to impress me enough for me to master the means by which many keep score. My ability to relate to this system has been just adequate enough to get by. Ask me what my favorite movie is and I'll struggle and stumble; to me, watching a movie is a last resort. I've found equal inspiration and despair in Eastern and Western beliefs, and I've built a totem pole from the best values extracted from each. I'm at best, a clumsy citizen of the world.

But talk with me of mountains and my eyes light up. Suddenly, I can relate and I am connected. I do not care if your journey was a quarter-mile walk to examine an alpine lake or a harrowing climb of a Himalayan peak; it is a language I understand. And while my fluency may not be as elegant as more enlightened climbers, I can finally listen and speak of an authentic world of triumph and tragedy.

I am made better by mountains. Each visit replenishes me just enough to get by until the next great adventure. Somehow, even the real world becomes more enjoyable and manageable when infused with the afterglow of a good summit hike. I hope this book gives you a chance to harvest from the mountains the goodness of life and the lessons of Mother Nature. For my own case, I will remain eager to learn from the mountains and revel in the joy of their trails and trials. When given a choice of investments during my short stint on this beautiful planet, the wealth I've received from my time in the hills has proven to be a far superior currency than any I've yet to uncover.

Appendix A

"Best" Hikes and Others of Note

Only have a half-day to hike? Got friends from out of town looking to snag a summit or two? Trying to get away from the mind numbing pace of everyday life? Here's a few suggestions for these and other situations.

Best dayhikes for out-of-town friends who aren't hardcore hikers but still want a good summit Mount Sniktau, Mount Elbert, Guardians of the Flatirons, Mount Thomas, Mount Sherman, Geissler Mountain, Treasury Mountain, Cross Mountain–Lizard Head Traverse

Best overnight adventures Fools Peak, Mount Zirkel, Storm King Peak, Chicago Basin 14er Circuit, Mount of the Holy Cross, Mount Adams, Mount Alice, Summit Peak

Best from the Denver/Boulder/Golden metro area when you have plans later that night The Citadel, Peak 1/Tenmile Peak, Mount Sniktau, Pacific Peak, James Peak, Mount Chapin group, Mount Ida group

Best hikes that get away from the crowds Lone Cone, Storm King Peak, Fools Peak, Summit Peak, East Beckwith Mountain, Golden Horn, Hesperus Mountain, Mount Powell, Mount Alice

Best hikes with excellent scrambling Navajo Peak, Lead Mountain, Mount Richthofen, Longs Peak, Mount Alice, Fools Peak, Belleview Mountain, Mount Blanca, Mount Eolus, Storm King Peak, Mount Sneffels

Best hikes for wildflowers (in season, of course) Stanley Mountain and Vasquez Peak, Treasury Mountain, Belleview Mountain, Mount Sherman, Mount Thomas, Mount Adams, Deming Mountain, Mount Hope, Mount Zirkel

Best hikes to do with your dog Huron Peak, James Peak, Clark Peak, Mount Sherman, Mount Zirkel, Mount Sopris, Uncompahgre Peak, Guardians of the Flatirons, Mount Thomas, Hahns Peak

Best hikes that stay above treeline most of the time Mount Sniktau, Stanley Mountain and Vaquez Peak, Mount Ouray, West Spanish Peak, Eureka Mountain–Hermit Peak, Uncompahgre Peak

Best off-trail adventures Jasper Peak, Lone Cone, Navajo Peak, Fools Peak, Mount Ouray, Golden Horn, Storm King Peak, Mount Adams, Treasury Mountain, Hesperus Mountain, Mount Powell, Mount Richthofen, Clark Peak

Best lungbusters Mount Powell, Lead Mountain, Peak 1, "Stanley's Wall," Mount Sneffels, Storm King Peak, Mount Adams, Mount Sniktau, Navajo Peak, Pacific Peak, Fools Peak, West Spanish Peak, Mount Richthofen

Best hikes to do when there is still spring snow Navajo Peak, Jasper Peak, Clark Peak, James Peak, Bison Peak, Hahns Peak, Mount Sniktau, Mount Sherman

Best hikes for autumn leaves and colors Mount Hope, East Beckwith Mountain, Belleview Mountain, Huron Peak, Uncompahgre Peak, Mount Powell, Mount Sopris, Fools Peak

Best social hikes (lots of people to chat with, observe, etc.) Longs Peak, Mount Elbert, Mount Shavano–Tabeguache Peak, James Peak, Huron Peak, Mount of the Holy Cross, Chicago Basin 14er Circuit, Redcloud Peak–Sunshine Peak

Best hikes with crazy and cool natural rock formations Bison Peak, Summit Peak, Belleview Mountain, Mount Zirkel, Uncompahgre Peak, Golden Horn, the Citadel, Guardians of the Flatirons, Hesperus Mountain, Mount Adams, Storm King Peak, Lone Cone

Best hikes to see wildlife Mount Sneffels, Mount Ida group, Mount Chapin group, Mount Thomas, Clark Peak, Chicago Basin 14er Circuit, Storm King Peak, Summit Peak

Best hikes to see mining ruins and ghost towns Mount Sherman, Huron Peak, Pacific Peak, Peak 1, James Peak, Golden Horn, Hahns Peak

Hikes with airplane wreckage Navajo Peak, Mount Yale, Jasper Peak, Lead Mountain

Best on-trail summit hikes Mount Elbert, Huron Peak, Guardians of the Flatirons, Longs Peak, Peak 1, Mount Sopris, Uncompahgre Peak, Redcloud Peak–Sunshine Peak, Mount Thomas, Mount Ida group

Best hikes that are named after characters in *Street Fighter 2* Mount Blanca, Bison Peak

Best hikes you can't pronounce properly Mount Shavano–Tabeguache Peak, Mount Ouray

Best hikes with names that best suit a muppet Sneffels, Zirkel, Elbert, Stanley, Sniktau, Jasper, Hahns, Eureka, Chiquita

And finally: Best hikes with the author's name or the author's cat's name in the title James Peak and "Mount Bruplex"

James Dziezynski's Top 10 Hikes

It's a question that is best asked spontaneously—what are your favorite hikes in the book? When given too much time to ponder the question, I could make a diplomatic argument for any of the 50. However, if budget cuts had reduced this book to the "10 Best Summit Hikes in Colorado," I'd have a list ready to go without second thought. Obviously it's a partisan list; the mountains included have just the right amount of all the things I like to experience on a good summit hike.

If you're like me, and I know I am, there's nothing better than a long day in the mountains. Give me steep hills, good scrambling, and great views, and I'm in heaven. Combine that with a scenic approach and good weather, and you have the perfect hike. These 10 hikes have all that plus a "special something" that makes them linger in my memory.

1. Storm King Peak A trip to Storm King is part heart-pounding climbing, part exhilarating scrambling, and part mystical spirit quest. The remote setting is an all-natural Shangri-la, a place where the trappings of mankind are left far behind. There's no place like the Grenadier Range, and Storm King reigns supreme as the monarch of these wonderful mountains.

2. Golden Horn The Ice Lakes Basin is gorgeous and the Horn serves as the centerpiece. A fine approach followed by good scrambling leads to a nifty summit.

3. Chicago Basin 14er Circuit: Windom, Sunlight, and Eolus Amplify the exotic nature of this adventure by taking the old narrow-gauge train to the trailhead. You'll feel like you're in a new frontier when you disembark for these three 14ers. The best part: all three are great climbs with distinct personalities.

4. Fools Peak Even though the rule in Colorado is "everything that can be climbed has been," you'll feel like the first person to ever stand on Fools summit. I hope no one ever puts a register on top—it would ruin the wild feeling of this marvelous mountain.

5. Mount Adams What a ridge walk! Adams always feels like it's on the verge of being unclimbable, only to reveal its secrets upon closer inspection. You never get hung out to dry, and the views are spectacular.

6. Lead Mountain Another thrilling ridge walk, this time with more exposure and less obvious route-finding. You'll have to stay on your toes, but there are always bailout points if you need them. Linking up to neighboring peaks adds to the fun.

7. Longs Peak It's the classic Colorado climb, with prolonged scrambling and a flat, spacious summit. I'm just one of its countless fans, but it really is a "must-do" hike.

8. Blanca Peak	The approach alone is worth the adventure. Watching the land change from smoldering desert to a lush basin is incredible! As if that weren't enough, the scramble up to Blanca's summit is solid, with breathtaking views along the way. A tried and true winner.
9. Bison Peak	Sometimes you have to sit back and wonder how Mother Nature was able to build such impressive monuments. Bison's rock garden is unique and inviting—and you can visit it year-round. It must be seen in person for one to appreciate its fabulous formations.
10. Peak 1 and Tenmile Peak	Even though I've already hiked these two, every time I drive by on I-70, I want to stop what I'm doing and climb 'em again. Too often, mountains with good profiles lack the quality climbing to match—not the case with these classics. Easy to access and a blast to climb, this summit hike certainly merits a spot in my top 10.

Good Weekend Getaways

Alright! You have a long weekend to go out hiking. Try pairing up the suggested hikes or go for a nice overnight in the following areas:

Good hike pairings for a long weekend:
Hope and Huron
Richthofen and Clark
Yale and Shavano/Tabeguache
Fools and Thomas
The Citadel and Peak 1/Tenmile
The Citadel and James
Yale and Geissler
Treasury and Belleview
Uncompahgre and Redcloud/Sunshine
Stanley/Vasquez and Deming
East Beckwith and Treasury or Belleview

Great two-night trips; leave Friday, return Sunday:
Deming Mountain
Lead Mountain
Clark Peak
Mount Alice
Mount of the Holy Cross
Blanca Peak
Uncompahgre Peak
Mount Adams
Fools Peak

Summit Peak
Mount Zirkel
Eureka Mountain/Hermit Peak

Additional hikes with very good backcountry camping or extended camping:
Storm King Peak
Chicago Basin 14er Circuit
Golden Horn
Mount Sopris
Mount Blanca

Honorable Mention Hikes

Following are some outstanding hikes that could have made the book but didn't quite fit the criteria for the top 50 Colorado summit hikes for one reason or another. However, each of them is definitely worth checking out—once you've finished all the hikes in this book!

Mount Audubon A nice walk up in Indian Peaks but a bit too "normal" for this book.

Twilight Peak Access is too rough on unmaintained roads for this otherwise great San Juan hike.

Vestal and Arrow Peaks Two awesome scrambles in the Grenadiers; route-finding pushes them a little into class 4 territory (though both have established class 3 routes—if you can find them).

Ice Mountain A very visible peak with a good hike, but lacks that certain zing of other Sawatch hikes.

Mount Massive Same as Ice Mountain; a good hike but it can feel very long and a bit tedious.

Pikes Peak Famous but a rather straightforward hike without a lot of bells and whistles—except for those on the cog railroad to the top!

Maroon Bells Class 4 and crumbly. The Bells are dangerous for inexperienced hikers and the terrain is unstable and exposed.

Crestone Peak Excellent class 3 route but a lot of rock-fall present.

Sheep Mountain A good mountain to hike in Telluride, but the Cross-Lizard Head loop is better!

Wilson Group These 14ers, also outside Telluride, include Mount Wilson, Wilson Peak, and El Diente Peak. They are good hikes, but the talus sections are quite long, placing them just a notch below the best hikes.

Three Over the Border

King's Peak in Utah's Uintas Mountains   Check this one out; it's just over Colorado's northwest border. The Uintas Mountains are the only major range in the Lower 48 US states that run east-west rather than north-south.

Wheeler Peak in New Mexico It's in the Sangre De Cristo Range and is the high point of New Mexico; check it out if you visit Taos.

Medicine Bow Peak in Wyoming   Just north of the border, near the town of Saratoga Springs. It's a fun climb and a shorter drive from Fort Collins than many peaks in Colorado.

Rounding Out Colorado's Next Best

Hallets Peak This Rocky Mountain National Park favorite has a very long approach via its standard route—a bit too long.

Bills and Byers Peaks Two mountains in the Vasquez Mountains. Nice hikes, but they have very long approaches and aren't as scenic as Stanley Mountain and Vasquez Peak.

Milwaukee Peak Another awesome Sangre hike, but the scrambling is class 4 in brief sections.

South Arapahoe Peak An Indian Peaks classic, it's got a great snow route but a standard hiking route. Good views all around from this big boy.

Chair Mountain A very fun Elk Range hike. Unfortunately, the peak is surrounded by private land and rangers have warned me that landowners have been less than inviting to hikers who stumble onto their property. It was a major bummer to have to omit it from the book.

North Mamm Peak Sometimes they just look better on the map then they do in person.

South Rawah Peak You'll have great views of this mountain from the top of Clarks Peak. It lacks the fun skywalk of Clark, so it only gets an honorable mention.

Appendix B

Mountain Miscellany

Colorado Mountain Trivia

Stuck in your tent? Up for 20 questions? Give these trivia questions a shot, and see how much you know about Colorado's mountains and surrounding areas:

1. What fabled 14er was originally known as James Peak in honor of the first person to climb it? *Answer: Pikes Peak, first climbed by Edwin James in 1820.*

2. Can you name all the 14ers of the Collegiate Peaks named after institutes of higher learning? *Answer: Columbia, Yale, Harvard, Princeton, and Oxford. Belford was named after James B. Belford, a territorial judge who earned the nickname "the Red-Headed Rooster of the Rockies."*

3. You may know Mount Elbert is the highest peak in Colorado. Can you name the 10 highest peaks in the lower 48 US states? *Answer (mountains are in Colorado if not specified otherwise): 1-Mount Whitney, California (14,494 ft.) 2-Mount Elbert (14,433 ft.) 3-Mount Massive (14,421 ft.) 4-Mount Harvard (14,420 ft.) 5-Mount Rainier, Washington (14,411 ft.) 6-Mount Williamson, California (14,375 ft.) 7-Blanca Peak (14,345 ft.) 8-La Plata Peak (14,336 ft.) 9-Uncompahgre Peak (14,309 ft.) 10-Crestone Peak (14,294 ft.)*

4. Which mountain in Colorado has yielded more valuable ore than any other single mountain in the US? *Answer: Mount Sneffels*

5. What is the name of the mountain in Golden that is the burial site of "Buffalo Bill" Cody? Bonus points for naming the state William Cody was born in. *Answer: Lookout Mountain. Buffalo Bill was born in Iowa.*

6. What four Colorado Mountains are within 20 feet of 14er status? *Answer: Sunlight Spire (13,995 ft.), Grizzly Peak (13,988 ft.—not the one in this book; this one is farther south in the Sawatch Range), Stewart Peak (13,983 ft.), and Columbia Point (13,980 ft.)*

7. One would think that Summit County would have the highest peak in the state, but it doesn't; that honor goes to Lake County and Mount Elbert. Can you name the summit that tops the charts for Summit County? *Answer: Grays Peak (14,270 ft.)*

8. Culebra Peak is the "forbidden 14er." The mountain is on private land and the owners demand $100 per hiker to attempt the summit. What does the word "culebra" mean in Spanish? *Answer: Snake.*

9.   Which is the only 14er that does not have "Mount," "Mountain," "Point," or "Peak" in its official name? *Answer: Crestone Needle*

10.   What mountain range in Colorado has flora that is unique to it and an Arctic island where NASA tested the Mars rover equipment before launch? (This island is the second largest in the world.) Points for the range and the island. *Answer: Indian Peaks and Devon Island in the Canadian Arctic*

11.   In 1893, what mining boomtown attempted to have the capital of Colorado moved from Denver to its city limits? *Answer: Georgetown. The 2006 population of Georgetown is roughly 1,100 people.*

12.   The Silverton & Durango Narrow Gauge Railroad is a great way to visit the 14ers in the Chicago Basin. The railroad has run every year since its inception. In what year did the trains first puff up the tracks? *Answer: 1881. The train has also been featured in several movies and TV shows.*

13.   What is the name of Colorado's oldest military fort, which was commanded by Kit Carson in 1858? Hint: you likely drive through it on your way to Blanca Peak. *Answer: Fort Garland*

14.   Who was the first person to officially climb all of Colorado's 14ers? *Answer: Who else but Albert Ellingwood?*

15.   What Colorado 14er is rumored to harbor a hidden cache of gold, jewels, and other gems buried by the Spanish in the 1700s, which has yet to be discovered? *Answer: Mount Princeton*

16.   I already mentioned in the Eureka Mountain hike that redundancy is sometimes lost in translation, such as Rito Alto Creek, which translates to "High Creek Creek" (though in today's Spanish, the word "creek" is *cara*). What Colorado town name means "hot springs springs" when translated back into the Ute Indian language? *Answer: Pagosa Springs*

17.   Colorado's mountain birds are amongst the most regal and beautiful on earth. Can you name Colorado's state bird? Bonus points if you know Colorado's state flower and animal. *Answer: The rather plain prairie lark, also known as lark bunting, is the state bird. Columbine is the state flower and Rocky Mountain bighorn sheep is our state animal.*

18.   In the winter of 1956–57, pilots were shocked to see a horse trapped in the saddle between Mount Harvard and Mount Yale at 12,500 feet. A massive effort was made to save the animal; he was finally rescued before he froze to death. What was the named of the program to save the horse, and for bonus points, what was the horse's name? *Answer: This bizarre but true story had a happy ending for the animal, who turned out to be a local Buena Vista bay horse named "Bugs." The program instituted to save Bugs was called Operation Haylift, and involved planes*

actually dropping tons of hay from their craft to the animal. The horse was fed by the "haylift" until ranchers on foot were able to rescue it when conditions improved.

19. What climber joined John W. Powell on his historic first ascent of Longs Peak? (Hint: the route they took was later named in his honor.) *Answer: L.W. Keplinger was the first of Powell's group to reach the summit; he almost summited solo the previous day while scouting a route to the top. Keplinger's Couloir is a class 3 alternative to the famous Keyhole Route.*

20. In the Geissler Mountain Rimwalk chapter, I mention that UN 13,001 (visible from the route) is the lowest ranked 13er in Colorado. What is lowest officially named 13er? *Answer: Ruffner Mountain in the San Juans, 13,003 feet above sea level*

Appendix C

Colorado's 100 Highest Peaks

Thanks to Summitpost.org for this chart. Peaks not listed with a rank are considered "unofficial," meaning they are too close to a neighboring summit to be considered a ranked mountain. Highlighted mountains are featured in this book as standard or optional hikes.

Peak Name	Rank	Elevation	Range
Mount Elbert	1	14,433	Sawatch
Mount Massive	2	14,421	Sawatch
Mount Harvard	3	14,420	Sawatch
Blanca Peak	4	14,345	Sangre De Cristo
North Massive		14,340	Sawatch
La Plata Peak	5	14,336	Sawatch
Uncompahgre Peak	6	14,309	San Juan
Crestone Peak	7	14,294	Sangre De Cristo
Mount Lincoln	8	14,286	Mosquito
Grays Peak	9	14,270	Front
Mount Antero	10	14,269	Sawatch
Torreys Peak	11	14,267	Front
Castle Peak	12	14,265	Elk
Quandary Peak	13	14,265	Tenmile
Mount Evans	14	14,264	Front
Longs Peak	15	14,255	Front
Mount Wilson	16	14,246	San Juan
Mount Cameron		14,238	Mosquito
Mount Shavano	17	14,229	Sawatch
Mount Belford	18	14,197	Sawatch
Crestone Needle	19	14,197	Sangre De Cristo
Mount Princeton	20	14,197	Sawatch
Mount Yale	21	14,196	Sawatch
Mount Bross	22	14,172	Mosquito
Kit Carson Peak	23	14,165	Sangre De Cristo
El Diente		14,159	San Juan

Peak Name	Rank	Elevation	Range
Maroon Peak	24	14,156	Elk
Tabeguache Peak	25	14,155	Sawatch
Mount Oxford	26	14,153	Sawatch
Mount Sneffels	27	14,150	San Juan
Mount Democrat	28	14,148	Mosquito
Capitol Peak	29	14,130	Elk
Pikes Peak	30	14,110	Front
Snowmass Mountain	31	14,092	Elk
Mount Eolus	32	14,083	San Juan
Windom Peak	33	14,082	San Juan
Challenger Point	34	14,081	Sangre De Cristo
Mount Columbia	35	14,073	Sawatch
Missouri Mountain	36	14,067	Sawatch
Humboldt Peak	37	14,064	Sangre De Cristo
Mount Bierstadt	38	14,060	Front
Conundrum Peak		14,060	Elk
Sunlight Peak	39	14,059	San Juan
Handies Peak	40	14,048	San Juan
Culebra Peak	41	14,047	Sangre De Cristo
Ellingwood Point	42	14,042	Sangre De Cristo
Mount Lindsey	43	14,042	Sangre De Cristo
North Eolus		14,039	San Juan
Little Bear Peak	44	14,037	Sangre De Cristo
Mount Sherman	45	14,036	Mosquito
Redcloud Peak	46	14,034	San Juan
North Maroon Peak		14,019	Elk
Pyramid Peak	47	14,018	Elk
Wilson Peak	48	14,017	San Juan
Wetterhorn Peak	49	14,015	San Juan
San Luis Peak	50	14,014	San Juan
Mount of the Holy Cross	51	14,005	Sawatch
Huron Peak	52	14,003	Sawatch

Peak Name	Rank	Elevation	Range
Sunshine Peak	53	14,001	San Juan
"Sunlight Spire"		13,995	San Juan
Grizzly Peak A	54	13,988	Sawatch
Stewart Peak	55	13,983	San Juan
Columbia Point	56	13,980	Sangre De Cristo
Pigeon Peak	57	13,972	San Juan
Mount Ouray	58	13,971	Sawatch
Fletcher Mountain	59	13,951	Tenmile
Ice Mountain	60	13,951	Sawatch
Gemini Peak		13,951	Mosquito
Pacific Peak	61	13,950	Tenmile
Cathedral Peak	62	13943	Elk
French Mountain	63	13,940	Sawatch
Mount Hope	64	13,933	Sawatch
"Thunder Pyramid"	65	13,932	Elk
Mount Adams	66	13,931	Sangre De Cristo
Gladstone Peak	67	13,913	San Juan
Mount Meeker	68	13,911	Front
Casco Peak	69	13,908	Sawatch
Red Mountain A	70	13,908	Sangre De Cristo
Emerald Peak	71	13,904	Sawatch
Drift Peak		13,900	Tenmile
Horseshoe Mountain	72	13,898	Mosquito
"Phoenix Peak"	73	13,895	San Juan
Vermilion Peak	74	13,894	San Juan
Frasco Benchmark		13,876	Sawatch
Cronin Peak	75	13,870	Sawatch
Mount Buckskin	76	13,865	Mosquito
Vestal Peak	77	13,864	San Juan
Jones Mountain A	78	13,860	San Juan
North Apostle	79	13,860	Sawatch
Meeker Ridge		13,860	Front
Clinton Peak	80	13,857	Mosquito

Peak Name	Rank	Elevation	Range
Dyer Mountain	81	13,855	Mosquito
Crystal Peak	82	13,852	Tenmile
Traver Peak		13,852	Mosquito
Mount Edwards	83	13,850	Front
California Peak	84	13,849	Sangre De Cristo
Mount Oklahoma	85	13,845	Sawatch
Mount Spalding		13,842	Front
Atlantic Peak	86	13,841	Tenmile
Hagerman Peak	87	13,841	Elk
Half Peak	88	13,841	San Juan
Turret Peak	89	13,835	San Juan
UN 13,832	90	13,832	San Juan
Holy Cross Ridge	91	13,831	Sawatch
Iowa Peak		13,831	Sawatch
Jupiter Mountain	92	13,830	San Juan
"Huerfano Peak"	93	13,828	Sangre De Cristo
Jagged Mountain	94	13,824	San Juan
"Lackawanna Peak"	95	13,823	Sawatch
Mount Silverheels	96	13,822	Front
Rio Grande Pyramid	97	13,821	San Juan
Teakettle Mountain	98	13,819	San Juan
UN 13,811	99	13,811	San Juan
Dallas Peak	100	13,809	San Juan

Works Consulted/Recommended Reading

Arps, Louisa Ward and Elinor Eppich Kingery, *Rocky Mountain National Park High Country Names*. Boulder, Colorado: Johnson Publishing Company, 1972.

Benson, Maxine, *1001 Colorado Place Names*. Kansas City: University of Kansas Press, 1994.

Bright, Wiliam, *Colorado Place Names*. Boulder, Colorado: Johnson Publishing Company, 2004.

Eberhart, Perry and Philip Schmuck, *The Fourteeners: Colorado's Great Mountains*. Chicago: The Swallow Press Inc, 1970.

Gebhardt, Dennis, *A Backpacking Guide to the Weminuche Wilderness*. Durango: Basin Printing Company, 1976.

Graydon, Don and Kurt Hanson, editors, *Mountaineering: The Freedom of the Hills*. Seattle: The Mountaineers Books, 1998.

Houston, Charles, *Going Higher: Oxygen, Man and Mountains*. Seattle: The Mountaineers Books, 2005.

Johnson, Kirk R. and Robert G. Raynolds, *Ancient Denvers: Scenes from the Past 300 Million Years of the Colorado Front Range*. Denver: Denver Museum of Nature and Science, 2006.

Schimelpfenig, Todd and Linda Lindsey, *NOLS Wilderness First Aid*. Lander, Wyoming: Stackpole Books, 2000.

Wilkerson, James A., *Medicine for Mountaineering and Other Wilderness Activities*. Seattle: The Mountaineers Books, 2001.

Online Sites Consulted

Summitpost
www.summitpost.org
This website is made up of user-contributed information about mountains, hikes, routes, and trailheads. Most of it is very reliable, though there are occasional inaccuracies and misinformation.

Wikipedia
www.wikipedia.org
Another user-contributed site, I found it useful as a starting point for a lot of information on the natural world, such as wildlife, the Laramide Orogeny, plant life, the Colorado Mineral Belt, and mining history. It's not perfect, but it's a great place to begin your research.

National Park Service
www.nps.gov
This is the official (if rather dry) source for websites for America's national parks.

Index

About the Author

James Dziezynski's love of adventure started in New England's mountains and oceans. Following a NOLS mountaineering course in Wyoming's Wind River Mountains, he was eventually drawn to Colorado. His adventures have taken him into the Arctic, Greenland, the jungles of several Caribbean islands, Mexico, the American and Canadian Rockies, and just about every US state. His work has appeared in *Outside, Backpacker, Hooked on the Outdoors, Women's Adventure, Boulder Weekly, Electronic Gaming Monthly, Gamefaqs.com,* and *Mountain Biking,* among other publications. Besides the outdoors, he is a huge fan of classic video games and has written the definitive guide for the NES classic *Ghosts N' Goblins.* James lives with his cat, Xanadu, in Boulder, Colorado, where he works as an editor and freelance writer.

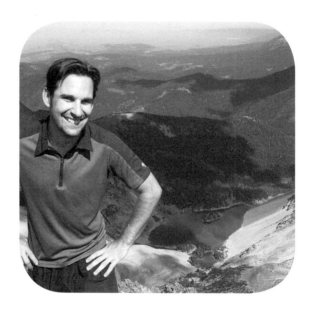